Principles and Practice of Public Health Surveillance

Principles and Practice of Public Health Surveillance

SECOND EDITION

Edited by

STEVEN M. TEUTSCH
Outcomes Research and Management
Merck & Co., Inc.

R. ELLIOTT CHURCHILL
Epidemiology Program Office
Centers for Disease Control and Prevention

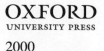

OXFORD
UNIVERSITY PRESS

2000

OXFORD
UNIVERSITY PRESS

Oxford   New York
Athens   Auckland   Bangkok   Bogotá   Buenos Aires   Calcutta
Cape Town   Chennai   Dar es Salaam   Delhi   Florence   Hong Kong   Istanbul
Karachi   Kuala Lumpur   Madrid   Melbourne   Mexico City   Mumbai
Nairobi   Paris   São Paulo   Singapore   Taipei   Tokyo   Toronto   Warsaw

and associated companies in
Berlin   Ibadan

Copyright © 2000 by Oxford University Press, Inc.

Published by Oxford University Press, Inc.,
198 Madison Avenue, New York, New York, 10016
http://www.oup-usa.org
1-800-334-4249

Library of Congress Cataloging-in-Publication Data
Principles and practice of public health surveillance /
edited by Steven M. Teutsch, R. Elliott Churchill.—2nd ed.
p. ; cm.   Includes bibliographical references and index.
ISBN 0-19-513827-9
1. Public health surveillance.
I. Teutsch, Steven M. II. Churchill, R. Elliott.
[DNLM: 1. Population Surveillance. 2. Public Health—methods.
WA 105 P957 2000]   RA652.2.P82 P75 2000   614.4—dc21   99-088755

9 8 7 6 5 4 3 2 1
Printed in the United States of America
on acid-free paper

Foreword

With the first edition of this book, it seemed necessary to emphasize that the history of surveillance went back to the origins of human history. The case was made that the adaptation of people to their environment required that they collect information, make interpretations of that information, and on that basis plan actions.

For the new reader it bears repeating that while the story is long, it is worth knowing about the individuals who pioneered this full arc of collection, analysis, and response. Edward Jenner observed the effects of cowpox on the later attenuation of smallpox, and after a decade of observations he finally used the information gathered by transferring cowpox virus from the hand of Sara Nelmes to the arm of James Phipps. A subsequent attempt to give the boy smallpox was unsuccessful, thereby simultaneously ushering in the eras of immunization, public health, and public health surveillance. Oliver Wendell Holmes, Ignaz Philipp Semmelweis, and John Snow all made bold predictions based on careful collection, analysis, and interpretation of public health facts.

New readers will miss the thrill of this book if they are unaware of the Rockefeller Foundation funding that led to the first American school of public health at Johns Hopkins University over 80 years ago. This was followed by the secondment of Wade Hampton Frost, from the United States Public Health Service, to start the first department of epidemiology. This move institutionalized epidemiology and surveillance in the academic setting. Every modern program of public health builds on this foundation of epidemiology.

The next major step in the saga was the daily use of public health surveillance, brought to fruition by Alexander Langmuir, who, following his training at Johns Hopkins University, moved to the Communicable Disease Center (CDC) in Atlanta, Georgia, to organize the Epidemic Intelligence Service. The practical aspects of surveillance were taught to officers sent to work in states and cities around the country and to other parts of the world. National systems were established to collect and interpret information on public health problems, first for malaria in 1950, and then for poliomyelitis in 1955, influenza in 1957, and finally a host of infectious diseases, chronic conditions, intentional and unintentional injuries, and environmental health problems. The principles learned were applied worldwide in the 1960s when smallpox surveillance was instituted throughout the world.

The second edition of this book not only demonstrates the value of the first but it also provides an opportunity to focus on five other aspects of surveillance.

First, for thousands of years, writers have emphasized that everything is interconnected, everything affects everything else, and as noted by Polybius, the world must be seen as an organic whole. This is true, but it is equally true that time moves in only one direction; therefore the interconnections go from causes to effects. Our epidemiology and analysis cannot be superior to the surveillance system used for collecting the facts analyzed. The analysis of those facts, the interpretation of their health implications, the interventions designed, and the programs launched are all based on the quality of the surveillance system used. Surveillance systems are therefore basic to everything that follows in public health.

Second, where once surveillance concentrated on morbidity and mortality it is now possible to anticipate health conditions by means of risk factor surveillance. Smoking rates, seat-belt use, condom use, body weight—all can be used to forecast disease states. Surveillance of market prices and patterns can anticipate food shortages. Recent studies have shown that surveillance of child abuse can predict rates of smoking, drug use, suicide attempts, and depression among those children when they reach adulthood. Everything affects everything else, and our challenge is to detect the patterns, understand what is best measured, and learn how best to obtain those measurements.

Third, since the first edition of this book, scientific inquiry has suggested that language development itself is based on every infant's developing a surveillance system that eventually separates the denominator of sound patterns into the numerator of words that are meaningful for communication. It is not a bad analogy to the public health approach of observing all of life in order to separate out the patterns that lead to pathology and those that lead to wholeness.

Fourth, no development since the first edition has been as far-reaching as the digital revolution. It is increasingly possible to collect information directly from laboratories, clinics, and hospitals, patients, and even from electronic monitors in toilets or automobiles. It is possible to automate some analysis with built-in alarm systems. Analysis of health concerns on a global basis can be received as instantaneously as we have come to expect with information about the stock market. To use these tools well has become a huge challenge.

Finally, the trends of globalization provide compelling reasons for developing useful and workable surveillance networks. Increasing travel, drug resistance, and new infections, as well as the risk of biological terrorism provide a clear message: we are all in this together. Teutsch and Churchill once again provide an excellent framework for all of us to strengthen public health by collectively improving the surveillance foundation. Our thanks for that effort.

William H. Foege, M.D., M.P.H.
Distinguished Professor
Rollins School of Public Health
Emory University (Atlanta)

Preface

Because public health surveillance undergirds public health practice, it is unfortunate that no single resource has been available to provide a guide to the underlying principles and practice of surveillance. In recent years, a small number of courses on surveillance at schools of public health have been developed in recognition of the importance of surveillance, but few definitive reference books have appeared. We published the first edition of *Principles and Practice of Public Health Surveillance* in 1994 in an effort to fill that gap, i.e., to serve as a desk reference for persons actively engaged in public health practice and as a text for students of public health. Now, moving into the 21st century, we offer Edition 2 of *Principles and Practice of Public Health Surveillance* as an update and expansion of its predecessor.

The book is organized around the science of surveillance, i.e., the basic approaches to planning, organizing, analyzing, interpreting, and communicating surveillance information in the context of contemporary society and public health practice. Surveillance provides the information base for public health decision making. It must continually respond to the need for new information, such as about chronic diseases, occupational and environmental health, injuries, risk factors, and emerging health problems. It must also accommodate to changing priorities. Issues such as long latency, migration, low frequencies, and the need for local data must be addressed. New analytic methods and rapidly evolving technologies present new opportunities and create new demands. This book addresses many of these issues. Although a number of examples of surveillance systems are included, it is not intended to be a manual for establishing surveillance of any particular condition. We believe that this generalist's approach to surveillance will provide the reader with concepts and methods that can be adapted to her or his particular needs.

The first edition grew out of a recognition by the Surveillance Coordination Group at the then Centers for Disease Control of the need to capture the art as well as the science of surveillance. Most of the authors of the second edition are current or former staff in the Epidemiology Program Office at the Centers for Disease Control and Prevention (still designated "CDC"). In their chapters these friends and colleagues have drawn on their own experience in states, diverse federal programs, and international health settings, and have interwoven the experience of others. We felt that the risks of being parochial were outweighed by the desirability of producing a consistent and systematic coverage of the subject. Although most examples are drawn from the United States, the chapters illustrate basic principles and approaches that can be applied in a wide variety of settings around the world.

In the years since its original publication, *Principles and Practice of Public Health Surveillance* has come to be viewed as the standard textbook on this topic for practitioners and students of public health in both domestic and international settings. Because we have tried to pay close attention to the feedback we continue to receive from users of the first edition, we have added to the second a number of new topics and have broadened the scope of some of the topics that appear in both editions. Among the chapters with broadened scope are Chapter 3 (Sources of Health-Related Information), Chapter 5 (Management of the Surveillance System and Quality Control of Data), Chapter 6 (Analyzing and Interpreting Surveillance Data), Chapter 8 (Evaluating Public Health Surveillance), Chapter 9 (Ethical Issues), and Chapter 12 (State and Local Issues in Surveillance). Appearing for the first time in this edition are Chapter 4 (The Changing Health-Care Information Infrastructure in the United States), Chapter 14 (Surveillance of Quality in Health Care), Chapter 15 (Surveillance of Pharmaceuticals), and Chapter 16 (Using Surveillance Information in Communications, Marketing, and Advocacy).

Our colleagues within and beyond CDC continue to be our most important resources. We thank them all—those who are listed in this book as chapter or section authors and those who are too numerous to list but whose contributions nevertheless measure large. We acknowledge, with gratitude, the valuable advice and assistance we received from Donna Stroup and Denise Koo during the planning stages for the second edition. We also owe special thanks to Sandy Ford, Beverly Holland, Carol Knowles, Brenda Lawver, Fran Moore, Maureen O'Neill, and Marlon Wolcott for their assistance and expertise in creating visual aids and in processing the manuscript for the second edition.

In addition to the authors of the second edition whose names are listed as contributors, we would like to recognize the efforts of colleagues who were authors of chapters in the first edition but did not participate in the second. Their work still represents an essential base upon which the second edition has been constructed. They include Robert F. Fagan, Robert A. Hahn, Mac W. Otten, Barbara J. Panter-Connah, Nancy E. Stroup, Richard L. Vogt, Melinda Wharton, and Matthew M. Zack.

Finally, many persons assisted in developing the contents of specific chapters. Among those whom we would like to thank for their valuable input are John Horan, James Seligman, Claire Broome, Diane Dwyer, Suzanne Sutcliff, Henry Anderson, Elizabeth Marshall, Michael Medvesky, Michael Seserman, and Peter M. Carucci.

West Point, Pennsylvania   S.M.T.
Atlanta, Georgia   R.E.C.
June 2000

Contents

Contributors

At the Centers for Disease Control and Prevention

R. Elliott Churchill, M.S., M.A.
Senior Communications Officer
Division of International Health
Epidemiology Program Office

Andrew G. Dean, M.D., M.P.H.
Chief, *Epi Info* Development Team
Public
Division of Health Surveillance and
Informatics
Epidemiology Program Office

Robert R. German, M.P.H.
Epidemiologist
Division of Public Health Surveillance
and Informatics
Epidemiology Program Office

Norma P. Gibbs, B.S. (Retired)
Chief, Systems Operation and Information Branch
Division of Surveillance and Epidemiology
Epidemiology Program Office

Richard A. Goodman, M.D., M.P.H.
Senior Advisor for Science and Policy
Financial Management Office

Samuel L. Groseclose, D.V.M., M.P.H.
Chief, Surveillance Systems Branch
Division of Public Health Surveillance
and Informatics
Epidemiology Program Office

Robert J. Howard, B.A.
Public Affairs Officer
National Center for Infectious Diseases

Lori Hutwagner, M.S.
Mathematical Statistician
Division of Public Health Surveillance
and Informatics
Epidemiology Program Office

Gail R. Janes, Ph.D., M.S.
Epidemiologist
Division of Public Health Surveillance
and Informatics
Epidemiology Program Office

Douglas N. Klaucke, M.D., M.P.H.
Director, Global Health Leadership
Officers Program (WHO Detail)

Carol M. Knowles, B.S.
Programmer Analyst
Division of Public Health Surveillance
and Informatics
Epidemiology Program Office

Denise Koo, M.D., M.P.H.
Director
Division of Public Health Surveillance
and Informatics
Epidemiology Program Office

Gene W. Matthews, J.D.
Legal Advisor to CDC
Office of the Director

Sharon M. McDonnell, M.D., M.P.H.
Chief, Training Branch
Division of International Health
Epidemiology Program Office

Verla S. Neslund, J.D.
Deputy Legal Advisor to CDC
Office of the Director

R. Gibson Parrish II, M.D., M.P.H.
Senior Public Health Scientist
Division of Public Health Surveillance
and Informatics
Epidemiology Program Office

Dixie E. Snider, M.D., M.P.H.
Associate Director for Science
Office of the Director

Donna F. Stroup, Ph.D.
Associate Director for Science
Epidemiology Program Office

Stephen B. Thacker, M.D., M.Sc.
Director
Epidemiology Program Office

Mark E. White, M.D.
Director
Division of International Health
Epidemiology Program Office

G. David Williamson, Ph.D.
Associate Director for Science
Division of Prevention Research and
Analytic Methods
Epidemiology Program Office

At Other Organizations

Janet B. Arrowsmith-Lowe, M.D.
Arrowsmith-Lowe Consulting
Ruidoso, New Mexico

Guthrie S. Birkhead, M.D., M.P.H.
Director, AIDS Institute
New York State Department of Health

Willard Cates, Jr., M.D., M.P.H.
Corporate Director for Medical Affairs
Family Health International
Research Triangle Park, North Carolina

William H. Foege, M.D., M.P.H.
Distinguished Professor
Rollins School of Public Health
Emory University (Atlanta)

Christopher M. Maylahn, M.P.H.
Director, Bureau of Health Risk
Reduction
New York State Department of Health

James F. Murray, Ph.D.
Director
Merck & Company, Inc.
West Point, Pennsylvania

Patrick L. Remington, M.D., M.P.H.
Chronic Disease Epidemiologist
Wisconsin Department of Health and
Social Services
Madison, Wisconsin

Raul A. Romaguera, D.M.D., M.P.H.
Senior Epidemiologist
Southeast Field Office
Health Resources and Services Administration
Atlanta, Georgia

Kevin Sullivan, Ph.D., M.P.H., M.H.A.
Assistant Professor
Division of Epidemiology
Rollins School of Public Health
Emory University (Atlanta)

Steven M. Teutsch, M.D., M.P.H.
Senior Director
Outcomes Research and Management
Merck & Company, Inc.
West Point, Pennsylvania

1

Historical Development

STEPHEN B. THACKER

If you don't know where you're going, any road will get you there.
Lewis Carroll

The definition for public health surveillance most often used by the Centers for Disease Control and Prevention and the Agency for Toxic Substances and Disease Registry (CDC/ATSDR) is "the ongoing systematic collection, analysis, and interpretation of outcome-specific data for use in the planning, implementation, and evaluation of public health practice" (*1*). A surveillance system includes the functional capacity for data collection and analysis, as well as the timely dissemination of information derived from these data to persons who can undertake effective prevention and control activities. Although the core of any surveillance system includes the collection, analysis, and dissemination of data, the process can be understood only in the context of specific health outcomes.

BACKGROUND

The idea of observing, recording, and collecting facts, analyzing them, and considering reasonable courses of action stems from Hippocrates (*2*). The first real public health action that can be related to surveillance probably occurred during the period of bubonic plague, when public health authorities boarded ships in the port near the Republic of Venice to prevent persons ill with plague-like illness from disembarking (*3*). Before a large-scale organized system of surveillance could be developed, however, certain prerequisites needed to be fulfilled. First, there had to be some semblance of an organized health-care system in a stable government; in the Western world, this was not achieved until the time of the Roman Empire. Second, a classification system for disease and illness had to be established and accepted; such a system only began to be functional in the 17th century with the work of Thomas Sydenham. Finally, no adequate measurement methods were developed until that time.

Current concepts of public health surveillance evolve from public health activities developed to control and prevent disease in the community. In the late

Middle Ages, governments in Western Europe assumed responsibility for both health protection and health care of the population of their towns and cities (*4*). A rudimentary system of monitoring illness led to regulations against polluting streets and public water, construction for burial and food handling, and the provision of some types of care (*5*). In 1766, Johann Peter Frank advocated a more comprehensive form of public health surveillance with the system of police medicine in Germany. It covered school health, injury prevention, maternal and child health, and public water and sewage (*4*). In addition, Frank delineated governmental measures to protect the public's health.

The roots of analysis of surveillance data can also be traced to the 17th century. In the 1680s, Gottfried Wilhelm von Leibniz called for the establishment of a health council and the application of a numerical analysis in mortality statistics to health planning (*2*). About the same time in London, John Graunt published a book, *Natural and Political Observations Made Upon the Bills of Mortality,* in which he attempted to define the basic laws of natality and mortality. In his work, Graunt developed some fundamental principles of public health surveillance, including disease-specific death counts, death rates, and the concept of disease patterns. In the next century, Achenwall introduced the term *statistics,* and during the next several decades vital statistics became more widespread in Europe. Nearly a century later, in 1845, Thurnam published the first extensive report of mental health statistics in London.

Two prominent names in the development of the concepts of public health surveillance activities are Lemuel Shattuck and William Farr. Shattuck's 1850 report of the Massachusetts Sanitary Commission was a landmark publication that related death, infant and maternal mortality, and communicable diseases to living conditions. Shattuck recommended a decennial census, standardization of nomenclature of causes of disease and death, and a collection of health data by age, gender, occupation, socioeconomic level, and locality. He applied these concepts to program activities in the areas of immunization, school health, smoking, and alcohol abuse, and introduced related concepts into the teaching of preventive medicine.

William Farr (1807–1883) is recognized as one of the founders of modern concepts of surveillance (*6*). As superintendent of the statistical department of the Registrar General's office of England and Wales from 1839 to 1879, Farr concentrated his efforts on collecting vital statistics, on assembling and evaluating those data, and on reporting both to responsible health authorities and to the general public.

In the United States, public health surveillance has focused historically on infectious disease. Basic elements of surveillance were found in Rhode Island in 1741, when the colony passed an act requiring tavern keepers to report contagious disease among their patrons. Two years later, the colony passed a broader law requiring the reporting of smallpox, yellow fever, and cholera (*7*).

Activities associated with disease at the national level did not begin in the United States until 1850, when mortality statistics based on death registration and the decennial census were first published by the federal government for the entire United States (*8*). Systematic reporting of disease in the United States began in 1874, when the Massachusetts State Board of Health instituted a voluntary plan for physicians to provide weekly reports on prevalent diseases, using a standard postcard-reporting format (*9,10*). In 1878, Congress authorized the forerunner of the Public Health Service (PHS) to collect morbidity data for use in quarantine measures against such pestilential diseases as cholera, smallpox, plague, and yellow fever (*11*).

In Europe, compulsory reporting of infectious diseases began in Italy in 1881; in Great Britain, it began in 1890. In 1893, Michigan became the first U.S. jurisdiction to require the reporting of specific infectious diseases (*9*). Also in 1893, a law was enacted to provide for the collection of information each week from state and municipal authorities throughout the United States (*12*). By 1901, all state and municipal laws required notification (i.e., reporting) to local authorities of selected communicable diseases that included smallpox, tuberculosis, and cholera. In 1914, PHS personnel were appointed as collaborating epidemiologists to serve in state health departments and to telegraph weekly disease reports to the PHS.

But in the United States it was not until 1925, following markedly increased reporting associated with the severe poliomyelitis epidemic in 1916 and the influenza pandemic in 1918–1919, that all states began participating in national morbidity reporting (*13*). A national health survey of U.S. citizens was first conducted in 1935. After a 1948 PHS study led to the revision of morbidity reporting procedures, the National Office of Vital Statistics assumed the responsibility for reporting morbidity. In 1949, weekly statistics that had appeared for several years in *Public Health Reports* began being published by the National Office of Vital Statistics. In 1952, mortality data were added to the publication that was the forerunner of the *Morbidity and Mortality Weekly Report (MMWR)*. As of 1961, responsibility for this publication and its content was transferred to the Communicable Disease Center (now, Centers for Disease Control and Prevention [CDC]).

In the United States, the authority to require notification of cases of disease resides in the various state legislatures. In some states, authority is enumerated in statutory provisions; in others, authority to require reporting has been given to state boards of health; still other states require reports both under statutes and health department regulations. Conditions and diseases to be reported vary from state to state, as do time frames for reporting, agencies to receive reports, persons required to report, and conditions under which reports are required (*14*).

The Conference (now Council) of State and Territorial Epidemiologists (CSTE) was authorized in 1951 by its parent body, the Association of State and Territorial Health Officials (ASTHO), to determine what diseases should be reported by states to the Public Health Service and to develop reporting procedures (*15*). Officially incorporated in 1955, CSTE meets annually, and, in collaboration with CDC, recommends to its constituent members appropriate changes in morbidity reporting and surveillance, including what diseases should be reported to CDC and published in the *MMWR*.

DEVELOPMENT OF THE CONCEPT OF SURVEILLANCE

Until 1950, the term *surveillance* was restricted in public health practice to monitoring contacts of persons with serious communicable diseases such as smallpox, in order to detect early symptoms so that prompt isolation could be instituted (*16*). The critical demonstration in the United States of the importance of a broader, population-based view of surveillance was made following the Francis Field Trial of poliomyelitis vaccine in 1955 (*17,18*). Within 2 weeks of the announcement of the results of the field trial and initiation of a nationwide vaccination program, six cases of paralytic poliomyelitis were reported through the notifiable-disease reporting system to state and local health departments; this surveillance led to an epidemiologic investigation, which revealed that these children had received vaccine produced by a single manufacturer. Intensive surveillance and appropriate epidemiologic investigations by federal, state, and local health departments found 141 vaccine-associated cases of paralytic disease, 80 of which represented family contacts of vaccinees. Daily surveillance reports were distributed by CDC to all persons involved in these investigations. This national common-source epidemic was ultimately related to a particular lot of vaccine that had been contaminated with live poliovirus. The Surgeon General requested that the manufacturer recall all outstanding lots of vaccine and directed that a national poliomyelitis program be established at CDC. Had the surveillance program not been in existence, many and perhaps all vaccine manufacturers would have ceased production for vaccines against polio.

In 1963, Alexander Langmuir limited the use of the term *surveillance* to the collection, analysis, and dissemination of data (*19*). Langmuir, the chief epidemiologist at CDC for more than 20 years, made pivotal contributions to public surveillance that ultimately defined current practice throughout the world (*20*). This construct did not encompass direct responsibility for control activities. In 1965, the Director General of the World Health Organization (WHO) established the epidemiologic surveillance unit in the Division of Communicable Diseases of WHO (*21*). The Division Director, Karel Raska, defined surveillance much more broadly than Langmuir, including "the epidemiological study of disease as a dynamic process." In the case of malaria, he saw epidemiologic surveillance as encompassing control and prevention activities. Indeed, the WHO definition of malaria surveillance included not only case detection but also obtaining blood films, drug treatment, epidemiologic investigation, and follow up (*22*).

In 1968, the 21st World Health Assembly focused on national and global surveillance of communicable diseases, applying the term to the diseases themselves rather than to the monitoring of persons with communicable disease (*23*). Following an invitation from the Director General of WHO and with consultation from Raska, Langmuir developed a working paper, and in the year before the 1968 Assembly he obtained comments from throughout the world on the concepts and practices advocated in the paper. At the Assembly, with delegates from approximately 100 countries, the working paper was endorsed, and discussions on the national and global surveillance of communicable disease identified three main features of surveillance that Langmuir had described in 1963: a) the systematic collection of pertinent data, b) the orderly consolidation and evaluation of these data, and c) the prompt dissemination of results to those who need to know—particularly those in position to take action.

The 1968 World Health Assembly discussions reflected the broadened concepts of *epidemiologic surveillance* and addressed the application of the concept to public health problems other than communicable disease (*22*). In addition, epidemiologic surveillance was said to imply "...the responsibility of following up to see that effective action has been taken."

Since that time, several health events, such as lead poisoning among children, leukemia, congenital malformations, abortions, injuries, and behavioral risk factors have been placed under surveillance. In 1976, recognition of the breadth of surveillance activities throughout the world was made evident by the publication of a special issue of the *International Journal of Epidemiology* devoted to surveillance (*24*).

SURVEILLANCE IN PUBLIC HEALTH PRACTICE

The primary function of the application of the term *epidemiologic* to surveillance, which first appeared in the 1960s in association with the newly created WHO unit of that name, was to distinguish this activity from other forms of surveillance (e.g., military intelligence) and to reflect its broader applications. The use of the term *epidemiologic,* however, engenders both confusion and controversy. In 1971, Langmuir noted that some epidemiologists tended to equate surveillance with epidemiology in its broadest sense, including epidemiologic investigations and research (16). He found this "both epidemiologically and administratively unwise," favoring a description of surveillance as "epidemiological intelligence."

What are the boundaries of surveillance practice? Is *epidemiologic* an appropriate modifier of *surveillance* in the context of public health practice? To address these questions, we must first examine the structure of public health practice. One can divide public health practice into surveillance; epidemiologic, behavioral, and laboratory research; service (including program evaluation); and training. Surveillance information should be used to identify research and service needs, which, in turn, help to define training needs. Unless this information is provided to those who set policy and implement programs, its use is limited to archives and academic pursuits, and the material is therefore appropriately considered to be health information rather than surveillance information. However, surveillance does not encompass epidemiologic research or service, which are related but independent public health activities that may or may not be based on surveillance. Thus, the boundary of surveillance practice excludes actual research and implementation of delivery programs.

Because of this separation, *epidemiologic* cannot accurately be used to modify *surveillance* (*1*). The term *public health surveillance* describes the scope (surveillance) and indicates the context in which it occurs (public health). It also obviates the need to accompany any use of the term *epidemiologic surveillance* with a list of all the examples this term does *not* cover. Surveillance is correctly—and necessarily—a component of public health practice and should continue to be recognized as such.

PURPOSES AND USES OF PUBLIC HEALTH SURVEILLANCE DATA

Purposes

Public health surveillance information is used to assess public health status, define public health priorities, evaluate programs, and conduct research. Surveillance information tells the health officer where the problems are, whom they affect, and where programmatic and prevention activities should be directed. Such information can also be used to help define public health priorities in a quantitative manner and also in evaluations of the effectiveness of programmatic activities. Analysis of public health surveillance data also enables researchers to identify areas of interest for further investigation (25).

The analysis of surveillance data is, in principle, quite simple. Data are examined by measures of time, place, and person. The routine collection of data about reported cases of congenital syphilis in the United States, for example, reflects not only numbers of cases (Figure 1–1), geographic distribution, and populations affected, but also indicates the effects of crack cocaine use and changing sexual practices during the past 10 years. The examination of routinely collected data show rates of salmonellosis by county in New Hampshire and in

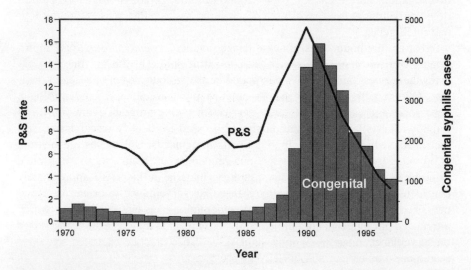

Figure 1–1 Reported cases of congenital syphilis among infants <1 year of age and rates of primary and secondary (P&S) syphilis among women—United States, 1970–1997. Note: Cases per 100,000 population; the surveillance case definition for congenital syphilis changed in 1989.

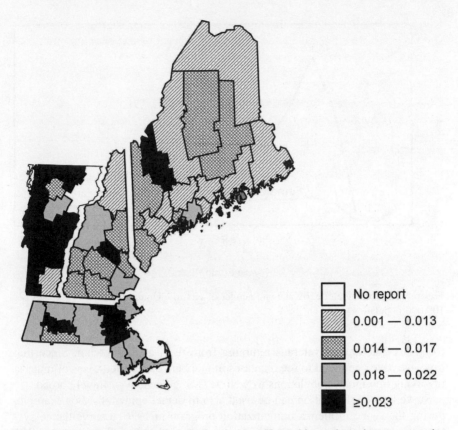

No report

0.001 — 0.013

0.014 — 0.017

0.018 — 0.022

≥0.023

Figure 1–2 Rates of *Salmonella* infection in New Hampshire and contiguous states, by county. Cases per 100,000 population.

three contiguous states. Mapping these data illustrates the pattern of the spread of disease across state boundaries (Figure 1–2). The examination of death certificates for data on homicide identifies high-risk groups and shows that the problem has reached epidemic proportions among young adult men (Figure 1–3).

Uses

The uses of surveillance are shown in Table 1–1. Portrayal of the natural history of disease can be illustrated by the surveillance of malaria rates in the United States since 1930 (Figure 1–4). In the 1940s, malaria was still an endemic health problem in the southeastern United States to the degree that persons with febrile illness were often treated for malaria until further tests were available. After the Malaria Control in the War Areas Program led to the virtual elimination of endemic malaria from the United States, rates of malaria decreased until the early 1950s, when military personnel involved in the conflict in Korea returned to the United States with malaria. The general downward trend in reported cases of malaria continued into the 1960s until, once again, numbers of cases of malaria

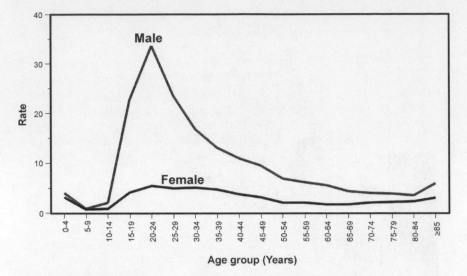

Figure 1-3 Homicide rate, by age and gender of victim—United States, 1997. Cases per 100,000 population.

rose, this time among veterans returning from the war in Vietnam. Since that time, we have continued to see increases in numbers of reported cases of malaria involving immigrant populations as well as U.S. citizens who travel abroad.

Surveillance information can be used also to detect epidemics. For example, during the swine influenza immunization program in 1976, a surveillance system was established to detect adverse sequelae related to the program (26). Working with state and local health departments, CDC was able to detect an epidemic of Guillain-Barré syndrome, which led rapidly to the termination of a program in which 40 million U.S. citizens had been vaccinated. However, most epidemics are not detected by such analysis of routinely collected data but are identified through the astuteness and alertness of clinicians and public health officials of the community. From a pragmatic point of view, the key point is

Table 1-1 The Uses of Surveillance

- quantitative estimates of the magnitude of a health problem
- portrayal of the natural history of disease
- detection of epidemics
- documentation of the distribution and spread of a health event
- facilitating epidemiologic and laboratory research
- testing of hypotheses
- evaluation of control and prevention measures
- monitoring of changes in infectious agents
- monitoring of isolation activities
- detection of changes in health practice
- planning

Source: (Reference 25)

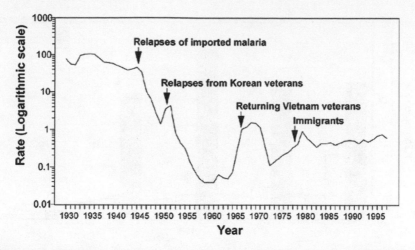

Figure 1–4 Malaria rates, by year—United States, 1930–1997. Cases per 100,000 population.

that when someone does note an unusual occurrence in the health picture of a community, the existence of organized surveillance efforts in the health department provides the infrastructure for conveying information to facilitate a timely and appropriate response.

The distribution and spread of disease can be documented from surveillance data, as seen in the county-specific data on salmonellosis (Figure 1–2). Cancer mortality statistics in the United States have also been mapped at the county level to identify several geographic patterns that suggest hypotheses on etiology and risk (*27*). Recognition of such clusters can lead to further epidemiologic or laboratory research, sometimes using persons identified in surveillance as subjects in epidemiologic studies. The association between the periconceptual use of multivitamins by women and the development of neural tube defects by their children was documented using children identified in a surveillance system for congenital malformations (*28*).

Surveillance information can also be used to test hypotheses. For example, in 1978 the U.S. Public Health Service announced a measles elimination program that included an active effort to vaccinate school-age children. Because of this program and the state laws that excluded from school students who had not been vaccinated, CDC anticipated a change in the age pattern of persons reported to have measles. Before the initiation of the program, the highest reported rates of measles were for children 10 through 14 years of age. As predicted, almost immediately after the school exclusion policy was implemented, there was not only a general decrease in the number of cases but also a shift in peak occurrence from school-age to preschool-age children (Figure 1–5). By 1979, the measles incidence was even lower, and age-specific patterns had been altered.

Surveillance information can be used in evaluating control and prevention measures. With information derived from routinely collected data, one can examine—without special studies—the effect of a health policy. For example, the in-

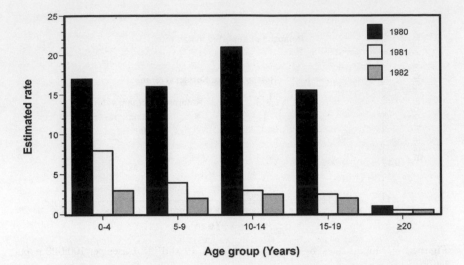

Figure 1–5 Reported cases of measles, by age group—United States, 1980–1982. Reported cases per 100,000 population. Note: Rates were estimated by extrapolating age from the records of case-patients with known age.

troduction of inactivated poliovirus vaccine in the United States in the 1950s was followed by a decrease in the number of reported number of cases of paralytic poliomyelitis, and the subsequent introduction in the 1960s of oral poliovirus vaccine was followed by an even greater decline (Figure 1–6).

Efforts to monitor changes in infectious agents have been facilitated by the use of surveillance data. In the late 1970s, antibiotic-resistant gonorrhea was in-

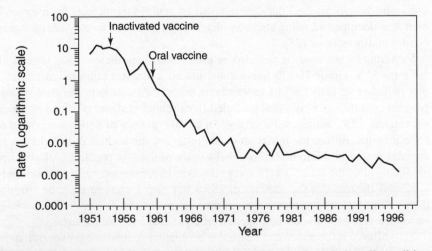

Figure 1–6 Logarithmic-scale line graph of reported cases of paralytic poliomyelitis—United States, 1951–1997. Reported cases per 100,000 population.

troduced into the United States from Asia. Laboratory- and clinical-practice-based surveillance for cases of gonorrhea enabled public health officials to monitor the rapid diffusion of various strains of this bacterium nationally and facilitated prevention activities, including notifying clinicians of proper treatment procedures (Figure 1–7). Similarly, the National Nosocomial Infections Surveillance System, a voluntary, hospital-based surveillance system for hospital-acquired infections, has been used to monitor changes in antibiotic-resistance patterns of infectious agents associated with hospitalized patients.

As noted earlier, the first use of surveillance was to monitor persons with a view of imposing quarantine as necessary. Although this use of surveillance is now rare in the United States, in 1975—with the introduction of a suspected case of Lassa fever—approximately 500 potential contacts of the patient were monitored daily for 2 weeks to ensure that secondary spread of this serious infection did not occur (29).

Surveillance information can also be used to good effect for detecting changes in health practice. The increasing use of various technologies in health care has become an issue of growing concern during the past decade; surveillance information can be useful in this area (30). For example, since 1965, the rate of cesarean delivery in the United States has increased from fewer than 5% to nearly 25% of all deliveries (Figure 1–8). This kind of information is useful both in planning research to learn the causes of these changes and in monitoring the impact of such changes in practice and procedure on outcomes and costs associated with health care.

Finally, surveillance information is useful for planning. With knowledge about changes in the population structure or in the nature of conditions that might af-

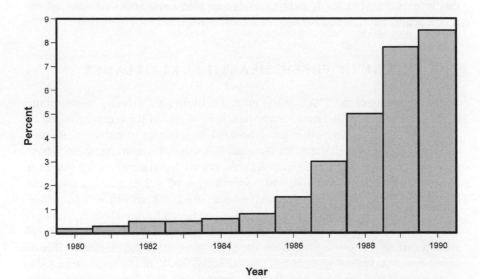

Figure 1–7 Percentage of reported cases of gonorrhea caused by antibiotic-resistant strains—United States, 1980–1990.

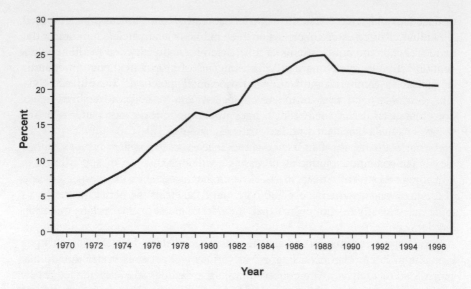

Figure 1–8 Cesarean deliveries as a percentage of all deliveries in U.S. hospitals—1970–1996.

fect a population, officials can, with more confidence, plan for optimizing available resources. For example, information about refugees who entered the United States from Southeast Asia in the early 1980s was broadly applicable; it told where people settled, described the age and gender structure of the population, and identified health problems that might be expected in that population. With this information, health officials were able to plan more effectively the appropriate health services and preventive activities for this new population.

THE FUTURE OF PUBLIC HEALTH SURVEILLANCE

At the beginning of the 21st century, several activities are expected to contribute to the evolution of public health surveillance. First, use of the computer—particularly the microcomputer—has revolutionized the practice of public health surveillance. In the United States, the National Electronic Telecommunications System for Surveillance (NETSS) links all state health departments by computer for the routine collection, analysis, and dissemination of information on notifiable health conditions (*31*). Over the next several years, the growth will be within states, with state health departments being linked to county departments, and possibly even to health-care providers' offices for routine surveillance. The Minitel system currently in use in France has already demonstrated the essential utility of office-based surveillance of various conditions of public health importance (*32*).

A distributed system of coordinated, timely, and useful multisource public health surveillance and health information can be readily developed. Integration of independently developed, disease–specific, or source-specific surveillance systems is a critical element in the implementation of such a system. This integration requires three essential elements: uniform data standards, a communications infrastructure, and policy agreements on data access, sharing, and burden reduction (33). Similar systems are used today in finance, travel, and retail marketing, but no such system is used routinely in public health practice in the United States. The technology and many of the necessary data are available; however, to make these data useful, our society must have sufficient commitment to develop and maintain such a distributed system for public health. This commitment must be underscored by the recognition and acceptance of the needs for both community health and individual confidentiality (34).

The second area of renewed activity associated with surveillance is that of epidemiologic and statistical analysis. A by-product of the use of computers is the ability to make more effective use of sophisticated tools to detect changes in patterns of occurrence of health problems. In the 1980s, applications and methods of time series analysis and other techniques have enabled us to provide more meaningful interpretation of data collected in surveillance efforts (35). More sophisticated techniques will no doubt continue to be applied in the area of public health as they are developed.

Until recently, surveillance information was disseminated as written documents published periodically by government agencies. Although paper reports will continue to be produced and the use of print media will continue to be refined, public health officials are also beginning to use electronic media such as the *MMWR* for the dissemination of surveillance information (36). More effective use of the electronic media and all the other tools of communications should facilitate the use of surveillance information for public health practice. At the same time, ready access to detailed information on individuals will continue to provide ethical and legal concerns that may constrain access to data of potential public health importance.

The 1990s have seen surveillance concepts applied to new areas of public health practice such as chronic disease (37), environmental (38) and occupational health (39), emerging infectious diseases (40) and injury control (41). In 1998, recognition of the importance of surveillance in the prevention of intentional injuries was underscored by the publication of a special issue of the *American Journal of Preventive Medicine* devoted to firearm-related injury surveillance (42). The evolution and development of methods for these programmatic areas will continue to be a major challenge in public health. In addition, changes in the organization of medical practice such as the emergence of managed care in the United States will affect the way data are collected and used in public health (43). A more fundamental principle that will underlie the ongoing development of surveillance is the increasing ability of people to view public health surveillance as a scientific endeavor (44). A growing appreciation of the need for high standards in the practice of surveillance will improve the quality of surveillance programs and will therefore facilitate the analysis and use of surveillance information. An important result of this more vigorous approach to surveillance practice will be the increased frequency and quality of the evaluation of the practice of surveillance (45).

Finally, and probably most important, surveillance needs to be used more consistently and thoughtfully by policymakers. Epidemiologists not only need to improve the quality of their analysis, interpretation, and display information for public health use, they also need to listen to persons who are empowered to set policy in order to understand what stimulates the policymakers' interests and actions. This assessment allows surveillance information to be crafted so that it is presented in its most useful form to the appropriate audience and in the necessary time frame. In turn, as we maximize the utility of the concept of "data for decision making" and better understand what is essential to that process, we will raise the area of public health surveillance to a new and higher level of importance.

The critical challenge in public health surveillance today, however, continues to be the assurance of its usefulness. In this effort, we must have rigorous evaluation of public health surveillance systems. Even more basic is the need to regard surveillance as a scientific endeavor. To do this properly, one must fully understand the principles of surveillance and its role in guiding epidemiologic research and influencing other aspects of the overall mission of public health. Epidemiologic methods based on public health surveillance must be developed; computer technology for efficient data collection, analysis, and graphic display must be applied; ethical and legal concerns must be addressed effectively; the use of surveillance systems must be reassessed on a routine basis; and surveillance principles must be applied to emerging areas of public health practice.

REFERENCES

1. Thacker SB, Berkelman RL. Public health surveillance in the United States. *Epidemiol Rev* 1988;10:164–90.
2. Eylenbosch WJ, Noah ND. Historical aspects. In: Eylenbosch WJ, Noah ND, (eds.). Surveillance in health and disease. Oxford: Oxford University Press, 1988:3–8.
3. Moro ML, McCormick A. Surveillance for communicable disease. In: Eylenbosch WJ, Noah ND (eds.). Surveillance in health and disease. Oxford: Oxford University Press, 1988:166–82.
4. Hartgerink MJ. Health surveillance and planning for health care in the Netherlands. *Int J Epidemiol* 1976;5:87–91.
5. Surveillance [Editorial]. *Int J Epidemiol* 1976;5:3–6.
6. Langmuir AD. William Farr: founder of modern concepts of surveillance. *Int J Epidemiol* 1976;5:13–8.
7. Hinman AR. Surveillance of communicable diseases. Presented at the 100th annual meeting of the American Public Health Association, Atlantic City, New Jersey, November 15, 1972.
8. Vital statistics of the United States, 1958. Washington, D.C.: National Office of Vital Statistics, 1959.
9. Trask JW. Vital statistics: a discussion of what they are and their uses in public health administration. *Public Health Rep* 1915;Suppl 12:30–4.
10. Bowditch HI, Webster DL, Hoadley JC, Frothington R, Newhall TB, Davis RT, Folson, LF. Letter from the Massachusetts State Board of Health to physicians. *Public Health Rep* 1915;Suppl 12:31.

11. Centers for Disease Control. Manual of procedures for national morbidity reporting and public health surveillance activities. Atlanta: Public Health Service, 1985.
12. Chapin CV. State health organization. *JAMA* 1916;66:699–703.
13. National Office of Vital Statistics. Reported incidence of selected notifiable disease: United States, each division and state, 1920–50. Vital Statistics Special Reports (National Summaries). 1953;37:1180–81.
14. Chorba TL, Berkelman RL, Safford SK, Gibbs NP, Hull HF. The reportable diseases. I. Mandatory reporting of infectious diseases by clinicians. *JAMA* 1989;262:3018–26.
15. Koo D, Wetterhall SF. History and current status of the national notifiable diseases surveillance system. *J Public Health Management Practice* 1996;2:4–10.
16. Langmuir AD. Evolution of the concept of surveillance in the United States. *Proc R Soc Med* 1971;64:681–9.
17. Langmuir AD, Nathanson N, Hall WJ. Surveillance of poliomyelitis in the United States in 1955. *Am J Public Health* 1956;46:75–88.
18. Nathanson N, Langmuir AD. The Cutter incident: poliomyelitis following formaldehyde–inactivated poliovirus vaccination in the United States during the Spring of 1955. I. Background. *Am J Hyg* 1963;78:29–81.
19. Langmuir AD. The surveillance of communicable diseases of national importance. *N Engl J Med* 1963;268:182–92.
20. Thacker SB, Gregg MB. Implementing the concepts of William Farr: the contributions of Alexander D. Langmuir to public health surveillance and communications. *Am J Epidemiol* 1996;144:523–8.
21. Raska K. National and international surveillance of communicable diseases. *WHO Chron* 1966;20:315–21.
22. Terminology of malaria and of malaria eradication. Report for drafting committee. Geneva: World Health Organization, 1963.
23. National and global surveillance of communicable disease. Report of the technical discussions at the Twenty-First World Health Assembly. A21/Technical Discussions/5. Geneva: World Health Organization, May 1968.
24. *Int J Epidemiol.* 1976;5:3–91.
25. Thacker SB. Les principes et la practique de la surveillance en santé publique: l'utilisation des données en santé publique. *Santé Publique* 1992;4:43–9.
26. Retailliau HF, Curtis AC, Starr G, Caesar G, Eddins DL, Hattwick MA. Illness after influenza vaccination reported through a nationwide surveillance system, 1976–1977. *Am J Epidemiol* 1980;111:270–8.
27. Pickle LW, Mungiole M, Jones GK, White AA. An atlas of United States mortality. Hyattsville, Md.: U.S. Department of Health and Human Services, National Center for Health Statistics, 1996.
28. Mulinare J, Cordero JF, Erickson D, Berry RJ. Periconceptional use of multivitamins and the occurrence of neural tube defects. *JAMA* 1988;260:3141–5.
29. Zweighaft RM, Fraser DW, Hattwick MAW, Winkler WG, Jordan WC, Alter M, Wolfe M, Wulff H, Johnson KM. Lassa fever: response to an imported case. *N Engl J Med* 1977;297:803–7.
30. Thacker SB, Berkelman RL. Surveillance of medical technologies. *J Pub Health Pol* 1986;7:363–77.
31. Centers for Disease Control. National electronic telecommunications systems for surveillance—United States, 1990–1991. *MMWR* 1991;40:502–3.
32. Valleron AJ, Bouvet E, Garnerin P, Ménarès J, Heard I, Letrait S, Lefaucheux J. A computer network for the surveillance of communicable diseases: the French experiment. *Am J Public Health* 1986;76:1289–92.

33. Morris G, Snider D, Katz M. Integrating public health informatics and surveillance systems. *J Public Health Management Practice* 1996;2:24–7.
34. Thacker SB, Stroup DF. Future directions for comprehensive public health surveillance and health information systems in the United States. *Am J Epidemiol* 1994;140: 383–97.
35. Stroup DF, Wharton M, Kafadar K, Dean AG. An evaluation of a method for detecting aberrations in public health surveillance data. *Am J Epidemiol* 1993;137: 373–80.
36. Centers for Disease Control and Prevention. Update: availability of electronic *MMWR* on Internet. *MMWR* 1995; 44:757–9.
37. Thacker SB, Stroup DF, Rothenberg RB, Brownson RC. Public health surveillance for chronic conditions: a scientific basis for decisions. *Stat Med* 1995;14;629–41.
38. Thacker SB, Stroup DF, Parrish RG, Anderson HA. Surveillance in environmental public health. *Am J Public Health* 1996;86:633–8.
39. Baker EL, Melius JM, Millar JD. Surveillances of occupational illness and injury in the United States. *J Public Health Pol* 1988;9:198–221.
40. Centers for Disease Control and Prevention. Preventing emerging infectious disease: a strategy for the 21st century. Overview of the updated CDC plan. *MMWR* 1998; 47(No. RR-15):1–14.
41. Graitcer PL. The development of state and local injury surveillance systems. *J Safety Res* 1988;18:191–8.
42. Ikeda RM, Mercy JA, Teret SP. Firearm-related injury surveillance. *Am J Preventive Med* 1998;15:1–124.
43. Rutherford GW. Public health, communicable diseases, and managed care: will managed care improve or weaken communicable disease control? *Am J Prev Med* 1998;14: 53–9.
44. Thacker SB, Berkelman RL, Stroup DF. The science of public health surveillance. *J Public Health Pol* 1989;10:187–203.
45. Centers for Disease Control. Guidelines for evaluating surveillance systems. *MMWR* 1988;37(Suppl No. S-5):1–20.

2

Considerations in Planning a Surveillance System

STEVEN M. TEUTSCH

[William Farr had] abiding faith that natural laws govern the occurrence of a disease, that these laws can be discovered by epidemiologic inquiry and that, when discovered, the causes of epidemics admit to a great extent of remedy.
Alexander D. Langmuir

Surveillance systems evolve in response to ever-changing needs of society in general and of the public health community in particular. In order to understand and meet those needs, an organized approach to planning, developing, implementing, and maintaining surveillance systems is imperative. In the sections below, approaches to the planning and evaluation processes to be presented in more detail elsewhere in this book are discussed. A description of a single surveillance system is provided in Appendix 2A. The steps in planning a system are shown in Table 2–1.

OBJECTIVES OF A SURVEILLANCE SYSTEM

Planning a surveillance system begins with a clear understanding of the purpose of surveillance, i.e., the answer to the question, What do you want to know? In the context of public health, surveillance may be established to meet a variety of objectives, including assessment of public health status of a health condition, establishment of public health priorities, evaluation of programs, and conduct of research. Surveillance data can be used in all of the following ways (see also Chapter 1):

- to estimate the magnitude of a health problem in the population at risk
- to understand the natural history of a disease or injury
- to detect outbreaks or epidemics
- to document the distribution and spread of a health event
- to test hypotheses about etiology
- to evaluate control strategies
- to monitor changes in infectious agents

Table 2–1 Steps in Planning a Surveillance System

1. Establish objectives.
2. Develop case definitions.
3. Determine data source or data-collection mechanism (type of system).
4. Develop data-collection instruments.
5. Field-test methods.
6. Develop and test analytic approach.
7. Develop dissemination mechanism.
8. Ensure use of analysis and interpretation.

- to monitor isolation activities
- to detect changes in health practice
- to assess the quality of health care
- to assess the safety of drugs or procedures
- to identify research needs and to facilitate epidemiologic and laboratory research
- to facilitate planning

Surveillance is inherently outcome-oriented and focused on various outcomes associated with health-related events or their immediate antecedents. These include the frequency of an illness or injury, usually measured in terms of numbers of cases, incidence, or prevalence; the severity of the condition, measured as a case-fatality ratio, hospitalization rate, mortality rate, or disability rate; and the impact of the condition, measured in terms of cost. Where risk factors or specific procedures are incontrovertibly linked to health outcomes, it is often useful to measure them because they are often more frequent (and hence more precisely ascertainable for small populations) than the health outcomes and may be linked to public health interventions. For example, mammography with suitable follow-up is the major prevention strategy for reducing mortality associated with breast cancer. The level of utilization of mammography by women can be regularly monitored and should be a more timely indicator of the impact of public health prevention programs than measurement of mortality from breast cancer. Surveillance data should also provide basic information on the utilization of mammography services by age and race/ethnicity of recipient, allowing better targeting of prevention efforts on the population sectors with the lowest utilization. In addition, over-utilization by some parts of the population (e.g., women under 35 years of age, who do not have other risk factors) might stimulate efforts to reduce unnecessary procedures.

High-priority health events clearly should be under surveillance. However, determining which events should be considered high-priority events can be a daunting task. Both quantitative and qualitative approaches can be used in a selection process. Some quantitative factors are shown in Table 2–2. In addition, criteria based on a consensus process to identify high-priority problems may identify emerging issues or problems that might otherwise not be considered. The consensus process leading to the Year 2000 and now the Year 2010 Health Promotion and Disease Prevention Objectives in the United States is an example of a

Table 2–2 Criteria for Identifying High-Priority Health Events for Surveillance

---

- Frequency
   incidence
   prevalence
   mortality
- Severity
   case-fatality ratio
   hospitalization rate
   disability rate
   years of potential life lost
   quality-adjusted life years lost
- Cost
   direct and indirect costs
- Preventability
- Communicability
- Public interest

---

mechanism for identifying high-priority conditions, types of behavior, and interventions that require ongoing monitoring (*1*).

Because public health surveillance in the United States is driven by the public health need to be cognizant of diseases and injuries in the community and to respond appropriately, surveillance is inherently an applied science. Therefore, as surveillance has evolved, it is generally undertaken only when there is reasonable expectation that appropriate control measures will be taken. For many conditions the link between surveillance and action is obvious (e.g., meningococcal meningitis prophylaxis for contacts of patients diagnosed as having meningitis). For emerging conditions, such as eosinophilia-myalgia syndrome, there is a compelling public health need to identify cases (delineate the magnitude of the problem), identify the mode of spread, and take appropriate action. For indicators of health-care quality, surveillance can be used to identify services that need improvement and also to guide the purchase of health care.

Surveillance data are usually augmented by additional studies to determine more precisely the causes, natural history, predisposing factors, and modes of transmission associated with the health problem. Yet undertaking surveillance exclusively for research purposes is rarely warranted. Research needs are often better served by other, more precise (and often more costly) methods of case identification (e.g., registries), which facilitate more detailed data collection and tracking of cases. For example, registries of type I diabetes may have value for surveillance, but are justified primarily because they fill research needs. The ongoing public health application of these data is more limited. Scarce public health resources and the efforts of health-care providers to report cases need to be focused on problems for which the public health importance and the need for public health action can be readily recognized.

A primary role of surveillance is the assessment of the overall health status of a community. One approach to this issue is the development and identification of a set of indicators that measure major components of health status. Such a set has been developed in the United States to be used at national, state, and local levels (2). Another approach is to examine the most frequent, severe, costly, and preventable conditions in the community by examining most frequent causes of death, hospitalization, injury, disability, infection, worksite-associated illness and injury, and major risk factors for all the preceding items. This information can be obtained in most communities in terms of age, race/ethnicity, gender, and temporal trends. Regular assessments of the information can form the basis for educating the community about its major health problems and for identifying specific conditions that merit more intensive surveillance and intervention.

METHODS

Once the purpose of and need for a surveillance system have been identified, methods for obtaining, analyzing, disseminating, and using the information should be determined and implemented (see also Chapters 6, 7, and 16).

Because surveillance systems are ongoing and require the cooperation of many individuals, careful consideration must be given to issues of evaluation discussed in Chapter 8. The system adopted must be feasible and acceptable to those who will contribute to its success; it must be sensitive enough to provide the information required to do the job at hand, while having a high predictive value positive to minimize the expenditure of resources on following up false-positive cases. A surveillance system should be flexible enough to meet the continually evolving needs of the community and to accommodate changes in patterns of disease and injury. It must provide information that is timely enough to be acted upon. All of these considerations must be carefully balanced in order to design a system that can successfully meet identified needs without becoming excessively costly or burdensome.

Case Definitions

Practical epidemiology is heavily dependent on clear case definitions that include criteria for person, place, and time and that are potentially categorized by the degree of certainty regarding diagnosis as "suspected" or "confirmed" cases (3). These have been recently documented for notifiable diseases (4).

While high sensitivity and specificity are both desirable, generally one comes at the expense of the other. A balance must be struck between the desire for high sensitivity and the level of effort required to track down false-positive cases. In addition, case definitions evolve over time. During periods of outbreaks, cases epidemiologically linked to the outbreak cases may be accepted as cases, whereas in non-epidemic periods, serologic or other more specific information may be required. Similarly, when active surveillance is used, such as in measles control programs, numbers of cases identified tend to rise.

As our understanding of a disease and its associated laboratory testing improves, alterations in case definitions often lead to changes in sensitivity and specificity. As new systems complement old ones (e.g., as a morbidity system supplements a mortality system for injury surveillance), the reported frequency and patterns of conditions change. These changes must be taken into account in analysis and interpretation of secular trends in the frequency of reporting. It is all too easy to define cases of various conditions with such different criteria that it is difficult to compare the essential descriptors of person, place, or time. For example, in surveillance of diabetes, one could determine the frequency of diabetes from surveys (self-reported), from surveys using glucose determination (laboratory-confirmed), or from reviews of ambulatory or hospital records (physician-diagnosed). Each method provides a different perspective on the problem. Self-reports are subject to vagaries of recall and variation in interpretation (patient may be under treatment, may have "a touch of diabetes"—or impaired glucose tolerance—or may have a history of gestational diabetes). Determinations of glucose levels allow detection of previously undiagnosed diabetes. Medical records identify only patients who are currently receiving medical care.

Case definitions should include criteria for person, place, time, clinical or laboratory diagnosis, and epidemiologic features.

Data Collection

Information on diseases, injuries, and risk factors can be obtained in many ways. Each mechanism has characteristics that must be balanced against the purpose of the system (see also Chapter 3). Time is of the essence for frequently fatal acute conditions such as plague, rabies, or meningococcal meningitis. Rapid provider-based disease reporting systems are most appropriate for such potentially catastrophic conditions with high and urgent preventability requirements. Conversely, detailed information on influenza strains or *Salmonella* serotypes must come from laboratory-based systems. Long-term mortality patterns are available through vital records systems.

Often, existing data sets can provide surveillance data. Such sets include vital records, administrative systems, and risk-factor or health-interview surveys. Some examples of administrative systems that can provide needed data are hospital-discharge data, medical-management-information and billing systems, police records for violence, and school records for disabilities or injuries among children. In addition, with some modification, an existing system might provide needed data more economically or efficiently than a newly initiated system. While existing data sets can be used for surveillance, they are not surveillance systems in and of themselves. Surveillance is a larger process that requires analysis, interpretation, and use of the data. These steps are not components of most data systems.

Existing registries or surveys may collect information on defined populations. To the extent that the condition of interest is uniformly distributed, the population under study is reasonably representative, and the information collected is available on a timely basis, such systems can be valuable data sources. Although many registries are established for research purposes, they often provide valuable data for surveillance purposes. In particular, cancer registries have been widely used (5).

Sentinel providers can also constitute a network for collecting data on common conditions, such as influenza; more specialized providers can provide data on less common conditions, e.g., ophthalmologists who provide information on treatment of patients for diabetic retinopathy.

Standardization

Data-collection instruments should use generally recognized and, where suitable, computerized formats for each data element to facilitate analysis and comparison with data collected in other systems, e.g., census and other surveillance data. Careful consideration should be given to using identifiers (see also Chapters 4 and 10). Although additional assurances of confidentiality and privacy considerations will be required, the ability to link data to other systems, such as through the National Death Index, may enhance the value of the system.

Active and Passive Systems

Primary surveillance systems have traditionally been classified as passive or active. For example, most routine notifiable-disease surveillance relies on passive reporting. On the basis of a published list of conditions, health-care providers report notifiable diseases on a case-by-case basis to the local health department. This passive system has the advantage of being simple and not burdensome to the health department, but it is limited by variability and incompleteness in reporting. Although the completeness of reporting may be augmented by efforts to publicize the importance of reporting and by continued feedback to communications media representatives, passive reporting systems may still not be representative and may fail to identify outbreaks. To obviate these problems, more active systems are often used for conditions of particular importance. These systems involve regular outreach to potential reporters to stimulate the reporting of specific diseases or injuries. Active systems can validate the representativeness of passive reports, assure more complete reporting of conditions, or be used in conjunction with specific epidemiologic investigations. Since resources are often limited, active systems are often used for brief periods for discrete purposes such as the measles elimination efforts.

Limited Surveillance Systems

Some surveillance efforts may not require ongoing systems. Surveillance to deal with specific problems may be needed to address problems for which all cases must be identified in order to assess the level of risk. Such programs can be conducted to resolve specific problems and then be terminated (6). Similarly, for logistic and economic reasons, it may not be feasible to mount a surveillance system across large geographic areas, and representative populations may need to be selected. Sentinel providers can also provide information on common conditions or conditions of particular interest to them.

Field Testing

The careful development and field testing of surveillance systems and procedures is important to facilitate the implementation of feasible systems and to minimize making changes as systems are implemented on a broad scale. The frustration engendered by a new and poorly executed system may undermine efforts to improve or use existing systems for the same or other conditions. As new surveillance systems or new instruments and procedures are developed, field tests of their feasibility and acceptability are appropriate. These field-test projects can demonstrate how readily the information can be obtained and can detect difficulties in data-collection procedures or in the content of specific questions. Analyses of this test information may also identify problems with the information collected. Model surveillance systems may facilitate the examination and comparison of a variety of approaches that would not be feasible on too large a scale and may identify methods suitable for other conditions or other settings.

The data to be collected by a surveillance system, the data sources and collection methods, and the procedures for handling the information should be developed and tested.

Data Analysis

A determination of the appropriate analytic approach to data should be an integral part of the planning of any surveillance system. The data needed to address the salient questions must be assessed to assure that the data source or collection process is adequate. Analyses may prove to be as simple as an ongoing review of all cases of rare but potentially devastating illnesses, such as plague. For most conditions, however, an assessment of the crude number of cases and rates is followed by a description of the population in which the condition occurs (person), where the condition occurs (place), and the period over which the condition occurs (time). These basic analyses require decisions as to the kind of information that needs to be collected. The level of detail required varies substantially from condition to condition. For instance, one may need more detailed information regarding the population that is not receiving prenatal care than on the one that is exposed to meningococcal disease, because the nature of the intervention for the former is likely to be more complex and to require an understanding of socio-economic factors. Similarly, how one will collect data on geographic areas may depend on whether the data will be examined at the county, state, or census-tract level.

Most contemporary surveillance systems are maintained electronically (see also Chapters 5 and 11). Highly integrated computer systems and networks are widely available. Surveillance systems can be operated on personal computers and over the Internet. Software to meet most basic analytic needs for surveillance, including mapping and graphing, is now widely available. The analytic approach often suggests a basic set of analyses that are performed on a regular basis. These analyses can be designed early in the development of the system and incorporated into an automated system, which can then be run by support personnel.

The adequacy of the data collection system and the processing mechanisms should be assured.

Interpretation and Dissemination

Data must be analyzed and presented in a compelling manner so that decision makers at all levels can readily see and understand the implications of the information. Knowledge of the characteristics of the audiences for the information and how they might use it may dictate any of a variety of communications systems. Routine, public access to the data—consistent with privacy constraints—should be planned for and provided. This access can be facilitated with various electronic media, ranging from systems with structured-analysis features suitable for general users to files of raw data for persons who can do special or more detailed analyses themselves. The advent of the Internet and easily used graphic and mapping techniques should rapidly enhance the availability of readily understood information.

The primary users of surveillance information, however, are public health professionals and health-care providers. More and more health-care purchasers and consumers look for information on quality of care and surveillance information to enhance management of the health-care system. Information directed primarily to those individuals should include the analyses and interpretation of surveillance results, along with recommendations that stem from the surveillance data. Graphs and maps should be used liberally to facilitate rapid review and comprehension of the data. Communications media represent a valuable secondary audience that can be used to amplify the messages from surveillance information. The media play an important role in presenting and reinforcing health messages. Innovative methods for presenting information that capitalize on current audiovisual technology should be explored (see also Chapters 7 and 16).

Evaluation

Planning, like surveillance itself, is an iterative process requiring the regular reassessment of objectives and methods (see also Chapter 8). The fundamental question to be answered in evaluation is whether the purposes of the surveillance system have been met. Did the system generate needed answers to problems? Was the information timely? Was it useful for planners, researchers, health-care providers, and public health professionals? How was the information used? Was it indeed worth the effort? Would those who participated in the system wish to (or be willing to) continue to take part? What could be done to enhance the attributes of the system (timeliness, simplicity, flexibility, acceptability, sensitivity, predictive value positive, and representativeness)?

Answers to these questions will direct subsequent efforts to revise the system. Changes might be minor (e.g., the addition of data elements to existing forms), or major (e.g., the need to obtain information from entirely different data sources). For example, a system to determine utilization of mammography might be based on administrative billing systems, yet problems with reports of multiple mammography examinations for the same individual might require the addition of unique patient identifiers, or the addition of questions on mammography use from self-reports on health-interview surveys. If access emerges as a critical factor in mammography utilization, then ongoing monitoring of the quantity and location of mammography facilities, or monitoring for appropriate medical care coverage for mammography might be indicated.

Periodic rigorous evaluation assures that surveillance systems remain vibrant. Systems that assess problems whose only interest is historical should be discontinued or simplified to reduce the burden. Contemporary systems should take advantage of the emergence of new technology for information collection, analysis, and dissemination. They should capitalize on new information systems. For example, sentinel surveillance systems have become more flexible to allow the inclusion of an array of topics. Electronic medical records and standardized clinical data bases all provide opportunities to obtain data that have been burdensome or difficult to secure (7). These information sources may also provide data in a more timely fashion and may allow individuals to be tracked, an option that would be virtually impossible without such electronic systems.

INVOLVEMENT OF INTERESTED PARTIES IN SURVEILLANCE

Virtually all surveillance systems involve networks of organizations and individuals. Surveillance of notifiable disease (see Appendix 2A) relies on healthcare providers, including clinicians, hospitals, and laboratories, to report to local health departments, who have the initial responsibility for responding to reports and amassing data. In many states, epidemiologists in the state health departments are responsible for surveillance and control of notifiable diseases in their states. In larger states, other organizational units—such as those dealing with sexually transmitted disease, immunization, or tuberculosis control—often have primary responsibility for surveillance and control of specific diseases or injuries. The state epidemiologist is responsible for the ongoing quality control, collection, analysis, interpretation, dissemination, and use of notifiable-disease data within that state. Data are subsequently forwarded each week to the national level where they are again analyzed, interpreted, and disseminated.

Programs for injuries and chronic and environmental diseases also may have complex organizational structures and may involve a wide array of external professional and voluntary interest groups whose needs must be addressed. Some basic surveillance information can be gleaned from such ongoing information systems as vital records, hospitalization programs, and registries. Although some of these conditions are part of state notifiable-disease lists, many require surveillance systems to be established in unique places (e.g., rehabilitation units and emergency medical services for spinal-cord injuries or radiology centers for mammography). The support and interest of these groups of constituents are valuable in establishing the systems; these groups can provide key input regarding purposes of systems and users of systems, as well as assistance in developing the systems themselves.

The complex relationships among these organizational units and their constituents requires open communication to establish priorities and methods consistent with the needs and resources of each group. The conflicting desire for more detailed information must be balanced against the associated burden and cost, as well as against the utility of collecting extensive amounts of data. For example, electronic systems that may facilitate higher–quality, more complete, and more timely data also involve the commitment of equipment, training, and changes in day-to-day activities that may permeate all levels of the system. One must understand the needs of each recipient group for the information and assess and assure their commitment to the system. It is also critical to be attentive to how components of the system can best be integrated into the day–to–day operation of the overall system.

The Council of State and Territorial Epidemiologists (CSTE) has the authority in the United States to recommend which health conditions should be notifiable. After this list has been agreed upon, it is then up to each state to determine whether and how the conditions should be made reportable. Although most states report all those conditions considered to be nationally notifiable, a wide range of additional conditions is reportable in only a few states (3). States may exercise their authority through regulations, boards of health, or legislative procedures. The diversity of these methods is described more fully in Chapter 12. Each of these mechanisms entails the involvement of groups with an array of medical, administrative, public health, and policy interests.

The success of surveillance depends heavily on the quality of the information entered into the system and on the value of the information to its intended users. A clear understanding of how policymakers, voluntary and professional groups, researchers, and others might use surveillance data is valuable in garnering the support of these audiences for the surveillance system.

Appendix 2A
The National Notifiable Disease Surveillance
System in the United States

Purpose

The National Notifiable Diseases Surveillance System (NNDSS) collects information on 56 notifiable diseases and conditions that are nationally reportable in the United States for the purpose of controlling those conditions (8,9). The reportable diseases are primarily infectious.

Legal Basis

Diseases and injuries are reportable to state and local health departments as indicated by relevant laws and regulations. The legal basis varies by state, as does the authority for determining which conditions are notifiable. Some are legislatively mandated, others are declared notifiable by the state health officer, state epidemiologist, or board of health (3).

The CSTE determines which conditions should be nationally reportable to the CDC. Reporting from states to CDC is voluntary, except for reports of quarantinable diseases (plague, cholera, and yellow fever), which are required by international regulation.

Reporting Mechanism

Health-care providers, including laboratories, transmit reports of notifiable conditions to their state or local health departments within specified time frames.

Data Collection

Basic demographic information, date of onset, county of report, and similar data are collected for all conditions. Health department personnel obtain additional information as needed on a case-by-case basis. Data are entered into electronic formats, usually at the state level. Data are edited for accuracy and validity.

Data Transfer

Data are sent to the appropriate state health department, which in turn forwards the information electronically to CDC primarily via the National Electronic Telecommunication System for Surveillance (NETSS) (9,10).

Analysis

Reports are reviewed on a case–by–case basis at the local level to determine the need for action on individual cases. More complete analysis by person, place, and time is performed at the state or local level to detect unusual patterns in reported conditions. Data are tabulated and graphed weekly by CDC and published. Maps with rates, by county, are prepared for selected conditions annually.

Annual summaries are prepared and published as the last issue of each volume of the *Morbidity and Mortality Weekly Report (MMWR)*.

Interpretation

On the basis of the analyses, an assessment of the characteristics of the conditions by person, place, and time are reviewed and additional investigations or actions are suggested.

Dissemination

Data are disseminated through state and local newsletters, and nationally through the MMWR. Reports include tables, graphs, and maps. National data are also available electronically. Information is transmitted directly to state and local health departments when necessary. The media often disseminate the information more widely.

Use

The data are used at the local level most directly for controlling conditions when direct action is possible and necessary. Such actions include therapy for patients, prophylaxis for contacts, initiation of research, program evaluation, and control of outbreaks.

At a state and national level, broader patterns of these conditions are assessed, such as historical trends and geographical clustering, and appropriate actions are initiated (e.g., outbreak investigations, control activities, or development of guidelines).

Evaluation

The NNDSS is evaluated every 3 years at the national level, including assessments of completeness of reporting of race and ethnicity, data flow, and management of the system. Annually, the CSTE and CDC examine the reportable conditions for importance, reporting burden, and preventability. The CSTE also provides recommendations for the data to be collected and the data-handling systems. The frequency of reviews in the states varies. Evaluations have led to changes in the graphical presentation of information, the list of reportable conditions, the data to be collected, and the computer systems used in collection and analysis.

REFERENCES

1. Healthy People 2000. National health promotion and disease prevention objectives, 1991. DHHS Pub. No. (PHS) 91-50212. Washington, D.C.: U.S. Department of Health and Human Services, Public Health Service, 1991.
2. Centers for Disease Control. Consensus set of health status indicators for the general assessment of community health status—United States. *MMWR* 1991;40:449–51.
3. Chorba TL, Berkelman RL, Safford SK, Gibbs NP, Hull HF. Mandatory reporting of infectious diseases by clinicians. *JAMA* 1989;262:3018–26.
4. Centers for Disease Control and Prevention. Case definitions for infectious conditions under public health surveillance. *MMWR* 1997;46(No. RR-10)1–55.
5. American Cancer Society. Cancer facts and figures—1991. American Cancer Society, 1991.
6. Teutsch SM, Herman WH, Dwyer DM, Lane JM. Mortality among diabetic patients using continuous subcutaneous insulin infusion pumps. *N Engl J Med* 1984;310: 361–8.
7. Ellwood PM. Outcomes management. A technology of patient experience. *N Engl J Med* 1988;318:1549–56.
8. Roush SW, Birkhead GS, Koo D, Cobb AN, Fleming DW. Mandatory reporting of diseases and conditions by health-care providers and laboratories. *JAMA* (in press).
9. Koo D, Wetterhall SF. History and current status of the national notifiable diseases surveillance system. *J Public Health Management Practice* 1996;2:4–10.
10. Centers for Disease Control. National Electronic Telecommunications System for Surveillance—United States, 1990–1991. *MMWR* 1991;40(29):502–3.

3

Sources of Health-Related Information

R. GIBSON PARRISH II
SHARON M. MCDONNELL

*Finagle's three laws on information: 1) The information you have is not what
you want. 2) The information you want is not what you need. 3) The information you need is not what you can obtain.*

J. H. Murnaghan (1)

The determinants of the health of individuals and populations are many and they
have complex inter-relationships. In this chapter we use the term *determinant* to
refer to both proximal (direct, immediate) and distal (indirect, remote, underlying) causes of health status as well as other factors that are associated with health
status, but for which a definite causal relationship may not yet be established (2).
Thus, causes are a subset of determinants. Last defines *determinant* as "any factor, whether event, characteristic, or other definable entity, that brings about
change in a health condition, or other defined characteristic" (3). A number of
models and conceptual frameworks for health and its determinants have been developed to aid in our understanding of this complex issue (4–8). These determinants include the physical, social, economic, and political environment, the
biological constitution and behavior of individuals and populations, and the availability and effectiveness of individual and population health services (Table 3–1).
(Last defines *health services* as "services that are performed by health-care professionals, or by others under their direction, for the purpose of promoting, maintaining, or restoring health" (3). In addition to personal health care, health services include measures for health protection and health education (9)). The goal
of individual and population-based health programs and services is the improvement of health, which is accomplished in various ways, including clinical
and community-based preventive services, environmental monitoring and protection programs, educational programs, behavioral interventions, and the treatment of individual patients (9,10).

Information is essential to the health of individuals and populations. In particular, information is needed concerning *a*) the *health status* of individuals and
populations (i.e., What is the general condition of their health and what are the

Table 3–1 Measures and Determinants of Individual and Population Health Status and Strategies and Capacities for Improving Health

---

1. **Health Status**
   - mortality (overall and cause-specific for various geographical areas and population groups)
   - morbidity (overall and cause-specific for various geographical areas and population groups)
   - life expectancy
   - functional status and capacity (activity limitation; activities of daily living)
   - quality of life (self-assessed health; well being)
2. **Determinants of Health Status**
   Natural environment
   - climate
   - weather
   - geology and topography
   - vegetative cover (type and distribution of vegetation)
   - water resources (surface and underground)
   Human modification of the natural environment
   - air quality
   - water supply and quality
   - waste disposal
   - land use and soil fertility and quality
   Social, economic, and political environment
   - level of economic development (income, GNP per capita)
   - employment, occupation, and workplaces
   - food production and quality
   - housing and recreational facilities
   - education and schools
   - transportation and communication infrastructures
   - population size and density
   - fertility and natality
   - urbanization
   - racial and ethnic composition
   - religion
   - form of government and stability
   Biological composition
   - genetic endowment
   - age and sex distribution
   - immune status
   Individual behavior
   - diet and nutrition
   - sanitary practices
   - food handling and preparation
   - physical activity
   - sexual behavior
   - substance abuse tobacco; alcohol; other substances
3. **Strategies and Processes to Improve Health**
   Protecting the physical environment
   - environmental controls
   - laws and regulations
   Providing a healthful economic and social environment
   - education
   - jobs
   - family planning
   - laws and regulations

(continued)

Table 3–1 Measures and Determinants of Individual and Population Health
Status and Strategies and Capacities for Improving Health (Continued)

Enhancing population's biological composition
- genetic screening and early intervention
- immunization
- chemoprophylaxis
- disease screening and early treatment

Promoting healthy population behavior
- health education
- health communication
- counseling (clinical patient education)
- behavior modification to prevent problem
- self-care to treat existing health condition

Providing effective health care
- home care
- ambulatory care
- inpatient care
- health-care personnel
- health-care facilities
- laboratory and other diagnostic methods
- national and local health-care expenditures

4. **Capacity and Resources**

Human resources
- health: skills; management and supervision
- nonhealth: community members and groups; community services (e.g., police, fire, schools)

Health programs and services

Public and private organizational and administrative capacities

Physical facilities, equipment, and consumable supplies
- health-care facilities
- laboratories
- computers
- cars

Infrastructure
- transportation
- communication
- logistical capabilities

Financial resources

Note: See Table 3–6 for examples of available information systems for each of these categories. See also the "Summary of district health profile" in reference *12*, pages 146–153.

major diseases, injuries, and disabilities that afflict them?), *b*) the *determinants* of poor and good health in individuals and populations (e.g., smoking, diet, poverty, behavior), *c*) *strategies and processes* for improving health (e.g., What strategies are available for preventing or treating health problems in individuals or populations and are these strategies effective?), and *d*) the *capacity and resources* for providing these strategies (i.e., What human, material, organizational, and financial resources are available to implement these strategies in a given setting?) (Table 3–1) (*9*).

The purpose of this chapter is to provide the reader with basic principles and practical guidelines for selecting appropriate sources of and methods for gathering information needed to assess and improve health in a particular setting.

PRINCIPLES

Health information system (HIS) is the term we shall use to refer to an organized set of activities and programs whose purpose is to gather, maintain, and provide health-related information in order to improve individual or population health. (Last defines a health information system as "a combination of vital and health statistical data from multiple sources, used to derive information about the health needs, health resources, costs, use of health services, and outcomes of use by the population of a specified jurisdiction" (*3*)). The relationship of a health information system (and its staff or agents who collect, manage, analyze, and disseminate data) to its source(s) of information can be simple or very complex (Figure 3–1). An HIS can consist of a single program to gather information on a health problem in a community, or a group of surveys, registries, and monitoring systems to gather information on all health problems in a whole country. (Many groups gather health-related information. In most jurisdictions or geographic areas, some entity is usually responsible for monitoring health and for gathering population-level, health-related information. This entity is often a government agency, but it may also be a publicly—or privately—supported nongovernmental health-care organization, or in some settings a set of health-care providers or health-care facilities.) A national or local survey whose staff contacts and questions individuals directly is conceptually quite simple. On the other hand, a national system for obtaining and reviewing health-care records from multiple sites may involve millions of patients, thousands of health-care providers and their records, hundreds of health-care facilities, tens of health-care organizations, and a multitude of agents of the system. Additional national and international levels of reporting may be involved for selected health conditions and may further increase the complexity.

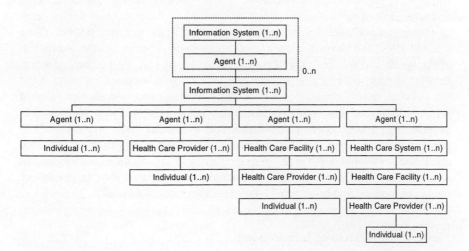

Figure 3–1 Model of the entities and relationships that constitute a health information system.

Purpose of Collecting Information

The first, and most important, consideration in selecting a source of health-related information is to determine the uses for the information (Table 3–2). These uses typically fall into the following categories and may relate to either individuals or populations:

1. Identify, characterize, and monitor the patterns and trends of health status.
2. Identify, characterize, and monitor the patterns and trends of the determinants of health status.
3. Determine strategies to prevent or treat health problems (applied research and evidence-based clinical and public health practice).
4. Develop policies and plans that support individual and community health efforts.
5. Implement prevention and treatment (control) programs for individuals and populations.
6. Monitor health programs and capacity—assure adequate capacity to prevent and treat health problems.
7. Evaluate the effectiveness, accessibility, and quality of health services and other interventions.

Too often information is collected without clear objectives, and the result is complicated reporting or data collection programs with no link to public health action (14,15).

Sources of Health-Related Information

There are three sources of health-related information: a) individuals (or their surrogates, e.g., spouse, daughter, co-worker, and neighbor); b) health-care providers; and c) other entities that collect intersectoral information through the observation or monitoring of the activities of individuals or populations, or of the environment (e.g., air pollution monitoring, observation of traffic patterns, tax records on tobacco sales, and alcohol sales) (13,16). (Intersectoral refers to the interaction of the health and non-health sectors to promote health (17,18). For lack of a better term, we use intersectoral information to refer to information gathered about the physical, social, economic, and political environments and the activities of people within these environments that are not directly related to health care.) In general, the primary source of information on the health status of individuals or populations, or the prevalence of behavioral determinants of health, is individuals. Health-care providers are the primary source of information on diseases and injuries. Other entities collecting intersectoral information are the primary source for environmental and other non-behavioral determinants of health.

Methods of Obtaining Information

There are three methods for obtaining health-related information from these sources: a) interview, b) observation, and c) the review of records or other documentation. Information is usually obtained from individuals by asking them questions (e.g., personal interview, printed questionnaires or forms, and electronically administered questionnaires) and less frequently by observing them. Various tools are available to aid this interviewing process, including specialized forms and computer-assisted personal or telephone interviewing tools (CAPI and CATI, respectively).

The first two methods (interview and observation) are sometimes referred to as *primary* because they usually involve the collection of information through

Table 3–2 Principal Uses of Individual and Population-Based Health-Related Information

1. **Identify, characterize, and monitor the patterns and trends of health status**
   a. Characterize and monitor health status
      i. Individual
         (1) Routine general examinations of individuals (screening for problems)
      ii. Population
         (1) General health status
         (2) Rate and causes of mortality
         (3) Prevalence and causes of morbidity
   b. Identify and characterize new health problems, including outbreaks of disease
   c. Monitor specific diseases and health conditions
2. **Identify, characterize, and monitor the patterns and trends of the determinants of health status**
   a. Identify [diagnose] and monitor known determinants of health problems
      i. Individual
         (1) Perform diagnostic tests
         (2) Identify behaviors that contribute to disease or disease risk
         (3) Identify individual exposures to environmental hazards
      ii. Population
         (1) Conduct epidemiological studies and surveys to characterize and monitor known determinants of health problems in communities
         (2) Investigate outbreaks
   b. Conduct research on health conditions whose determinants are unknown or incompletely understood
      i. Basic research (e.g., molecular, genetic, environmental) to better understand the determinants of specific diseases
      ii. Individual research (clinical)
      iii. Population research (analytic epidemiological studies)
3. **Determine strategies to prevent or treat health problems (using applied research and evidence-based clinical and public health practice)**
   a. Individual [e.g., clinical trials; USPHS Clinical Preventive Services Guidelines; Cochrane collaboration]
   b. Population [e.g., identify effective population based control measures; USPHS Guide to Community Preventive Services]
4. **Develop policies and plans that support individual and community health efforts**
   a. Characterize the setting in which the health effort will take place—level of development, physical and political setting (e.g., natural disaster, civil unrest, war)
   b. Assess resources available for individual and population level prevention and control of health problems (e.g., physical facilities, diagnostic methods, consumable supplies, trained staff)
   c. Enact policies and laws needed to implement health-related programs
   d. Establish goals and develop measures (indicators) to assess progress toward those goals
   e. Identify and allocate resources to programs or other entities responsible for improving health (see also item 6)

(continued)

5. Implement prevention and treatment (control) programs
   a. Individual
      i. Prevent disease or injury through the delivery of health care or social services at the individual level
          (1) Screen for determinants of disease (e.g., serum cholesterol, genetic markers)
          (2) Counsel about healthy behavior
          (3) Provide chemoprophylaxis and immunization for infectious diseases
      ii. Treat disease or injury through the delivery of health-care services at the individual level
          (1) Provide screening for the early detection and treatment of disease (e.g., breast or cervical cancer; hypertension; childhood lead poisoning; and human immunodeficiency virus or tuberculosis infection)
          (2) Provide medical and surgical treatment of disease (e.g., diabetes, cancer, and systemic lupus erythematosus)
          (3) Provide counseling for psychological and social disorders (e.g., psychotherapy and grief counseling)
          (4) Instruct patients and families about self or home care (taking medication, preventing pressure sores, the need for follow-up care)
   b. Population
      i. Prevent disease or injury through the delivery of health services at the population level (services are principally directed at determinants of health)
          (1) Ensure a safe and healthful physical environment
              (a) Maintain the quality of environmental media (water treatment; air pollution controls)
              (b) Ensure the quality of the food supply (inspection of food production and distribution facilities; inspection of imported food)
              (c) Identify and control physical hazards (e.g., safer highway design, housing codes for fire prevention, availability of seat belts and air bags in vehicles)
              (d) Control vectors of disease (dogs, mosquitoes, rats)
              (e) Supplement food and water with nutrients or other compounds to prevent disease (fluoridation of water; vitamin fortification of grains; iodination of salt)
              (f) Enforce environmental laws, rules, regulations (pollution controls on vehicles; limits on discharges of wastes from industrial facilities)
          (2) Prevent disease or injury through the delivery of services at the population level that target individual behavior (modification of individual behavior for community good)
              (a) Provide warnings about weather and geologic hazards and facilitate evacuations (cyclones, volcanoes, floods)
              (b) Implement health promotion and education programs
              (c) Enforce individual compliance with laws, rules, regulations (traffic speed limits; mandatory vehicle inspection; ban on alcohol consumption while driving; ban on tobacco sales to young people)
      ii. Treat or control disease or injury through the delivery of health services at the population level
          (1) Investigate and control outbreaks that threaten the population. *Note: The investigation usually takes place at the population level; the control of disease may occur at the individual or population level depending on the disease and setting*
              (a) Infectious disease (measles, tuberculosis, sexually transmitted diseases)
              (b) Noninfectious (poisoning due to contamination of food with pesticides)
          (2) Eradicate disease (smallpox, polio, onchocerciasis)
          (3) Mobilize community partnerships to identify and solve health problems
6. Monitor health programs and capacity; assure adequate capacity to prevent and treat health problems
   a. Monitor supplies (number of syringes, adequate supply of vaccine)
   b. Assure a competent public health and personal health-care workforce
   c. Facilitate community involvement in health-related activities and programs
7. Evaluate effectiveness, accessibility, and quality of health services and other interventions
   a. Personal health services (Is individual patient improving?)
   b. Population-based health services (Is population health improving?)
      i. Are effective strategies reaching intended audience?

Note: See References *12* and *13* for additional discussion of the uses of information.

the direct interview or observation of a "subject" by an "agent" of the HIS to meet a specific objective of the HIS. Examples of primary information collection include the completion of a death certificate using information obtained from an interview of a member of the decedent's family, and the sampling and testing of a water supply for micro-organisms. The third method (record review) is referred to as *secondary* because it relies on existing records or information first collected by another entity for a different primary purpose; thus, the system is making *secondary* use of the information. An example is the use of data from medical records for a birth-defects registry. Another example is the use of financial records from health-care organizations to better describe the delivery of specific services. Because the information was originally collected for another purpose, its usefulness for secondary use should be carefully assessed and its limitations for this use understood (*17–19*).

We use the terms *agent, agent of the HIS,* and *agent of the system* to refer to people who act on the behalf of an HIS. They may be paid or unpaid. If the primary purpose of a person's action is to collect information for, or provide information to, an HIS, then the person is an agent of this HIS with respect to this action. Thus, a health-care provider is acting as an agent of an HIS when he or she completes and submits a form to the HIS to document a particular episode of care (e.g., a death certificate, a notification of a case of cholera). On the other hand, when a health-care provider enters information in the medical record of a patient for the primary purpose of documenting an episode of care, the provider is *not* acting as an agent of an HIS, assuming that the objective of the HIS is to track episodes of health care in a particular jurisdiction. There may, of course, be secondary use of this medical record by the HIS for tracking health care.

Information is usually obtained from health-care providers by reviewing their records (e.g., hospital discharge surveys and cancer registries) and less frequently by asking them questions through the use of printed questionnaires or reporting forms (e.g., birth and death registration, administrative health reports, reports of notifiable diseases). (These approaches usually derive their information from a review of individual health-care records by the provider or an agent of the provider. Sometimes an agent of the HIS performs this task. With the advent of electronic health-care records, it will become increasingly possible to obtain information directly from health-care records without the need to complete questionnaires or reporting forms.) The information obtained from health-care providers ultimately derives from the interaction (i.e., interview, observation, physical examination, diagnostic testing, and treatment) of health-care providers with individual patients or their family members or other surrogates.

Intersectoral information is usually obtained through the review of records or reports produced by public or private entities that: *a*) monitor the physical environment (e.g., traffic patterns, fecal coliforms in waters where shellfish are harvested, temperature, and humidity); *b*) collect financial information from businesses (e.g., alcohol and tobacco sales, sales of specific food items in stores); *c*) receive reports from businesses about the production or consumption of specific products (e.g., tons of pesticides used on a specific crop, amount of chemicals released into the environment by industrial facilities); or *d*) conduct surveys of the population on a variety of topics not directly related to health or health care (e.g., number of persons viewing a specific television program, household or neighborhood characteristics).

Factors That Influence the Quality and Usefulness of Information

Several factors influence the quality and usefulness of information that can be obtained from each of these sources.

Individuals

When interviewing individuals or asking them to complete forms, three factors are important:

- Fluency and literacy. Is the individual sufficiently fluent in the language being used to pose questions to respond reliably to them? Does the individual have sufficient verbal or written language skills to respond to the questions being asked?
- Comprehension (i.e., Does the individual understand what is being asked?), acceptability (i.e., Is there a cultural or psychological prejudice about the subject matter [e.g., death, abortion]?)
- Familiarity. If a surrogate is being questioned, does the surrogate know the individual well enough to answer questions about or for the individual?

Health-Care Providers

Factors that influence the quality and usefulness of health-care providers and their records as a source of information include

Availability and Accessibility of Health-Care Resources to Patients (Table 3–3)

- number, type, location, and quality of health-care facilities (e.g., hospitals, ambulatory health centers, laboratories, and other diagnostic facilities)
- number, training, skills, experience, location, and availability of clinical, laboratory, and public health personnel
- availability of equipment and supplies needed to diagnose and treat patients and to document episodes of health care
- physical access to health care (i.e., proximity of providers, which is influenced, by availability and cost of transportation)
- ability of the patient to travel to facility (e.g., not too sick; able to get off work; and availability of alternative child care)
- economic access (i.e., free or affordable care for those who seek it)

Utilization of Health-Care Resources by Patients

This will, in turn, be influenced by the patient's perception of the usefulness and acceptability of the health-care provider or facility for improving the patient's condition (generally this will correspond to the severity of the illness, but other cultural and social factors may also influence this perception) (*20,21*).

Nature and Availability of Records Kept by Health-Care Providers on Patients and the Ease with Which They Can Be Used by the HIS (Table 3–3)

- content and comprehensiveness of individual health-care records (e.g., demographic information, medical history, clinical notes, laboratory results, and description of procedures)
- quality (e.g., completeness; use of standard case definitions, terminology, and classification and coding schemes; reliability and validity of coding)
- format (e.g., electronic and paper-based)
- proportion of patients treated by health-care providers for whom there is a record of their care
- legal, administrative, or physical barriers to the use of the records by the HIS

The method(s) by which the HIS obtains information from individuals and health-care providers also affects its quality. For example, if data collection forms are used, have questionnaires and forms been pilot tested to assess their validity? Are forms readable and understandable and can they be completed in a reasonable amount of time? Is participation in a survey or study requested in an acceptable way? Does HIS staff conduct interviews in a professional and culturally acceptable manner? Do the agents of the HIS have adequate training and experience to accurately and reliably abstract information from health-care records?

Other Entities

Many factors influence the quality of intersectoral data as a result of the great variety of data and the large number of entities gathering them, and listing these factors is more difficult than for the factors influencing individuals and health-care providers. The various methods for collecting and analyzing environmental samples, for collecting financial information, for conducting audits, for counting occurrences of specific events, and for gathering other types of information may or may not be controlled by well-recognized standards or be subject to quality control programs or regulatory review. Some intersectoral data are collected to support regulatory or revenue-producing activities, and the data may be comprehensive and of high quality. In other settings, data may be collected haphazardly with little quality control. For all data collection efforts, particularly those that are not standardized, the skill and experience of those collecting the data, the quality of the technical methods used, and the condition and maintenance of equipment required to make measurements are important. Various methods are available to assess the quality of data and the process of collecting it. Knowledge of how the data were collected is important in assessing its appropriateness for a particular use.

Scope, Content, and Timeliness of Information

The intended use of the health-related information should guide decisions about the scope, content, and timeliness of the data collection effort and the final selection of the specific source(s) of data and the method(s) employed to gather them (*22*).

Table 3-3 Spectrum of Individual Health Care and Information Available from Health-Care System on Morbidity

Spectrum of Individual Health Care		Information Available from Health-Care System
Medical specialists with state-of-the-art clinical and laboratory diagnostic methods and medical treatment. Tertiary-care center.	**More developed**	There is a complete, electronic lifetime health and death record for each individual. Each individual has a unique, unduplicated record that is accessible by the individual and all authorized health-care providers at any time. The record's structure, content (e.g., terminology, classification), and exchange format follow accepted international and national standards (e.g., International Organization of Standards (ISO), and American National Standards Institute (ANSI) [United States]).
General medical practitioners with good, but not state of the art, clinical and laboratory diagnostic methods and medical treatment. Inpatient or outpatient primary-care center.		Each provider or facility maintains a longitudinal, completely electronic, patient-based health record for each patient. Records from different facilities not normally linked. Records can be linked with some effort via name or other identifier.
Few medically trained practitioners with basic clinical and laboratory diagnostic methods and medical care. Hospitalization may be available in primary care center with limited resources.		Each provider or facility maintains a longitudinal, partially electronic, (electronic data available from some departments, e.g., lab, radiology) patient-based health record for each patient. Records from different facilities not normally linked. Records can be linked with considerable effort via name or other identifier.
Basic medical care with limited diagnostic methods and treatment. Primarily outpatient services only.		Each provider or facility maintains a longitudinal, complete, paper, patient-based health record for each patient. Records from different facilities not normally linked. Records can be linked with some effort via name or other identifier.
Outpatient clinic with ancillary medical staff (nursing or paramedical) providing basic medical care. Primarily syndrome-based clinical diagnosis. Few or no laboratory diagnostic methods. Limited or intermittently available medications and supplies.		Each provider or facility maintains a longitudinal, partial (data available from some departments, e.g., lab, radiology), paper patient-based health record for each patient. Records from different facilities not normally linked. Records can be linked with considerable effort via name or other identifier.
Community health care by outreach of basic and voluntary health workers. Syndrome-based clinical diagnosis. No laboratory diagnostic methods. Limited or intermittently available medications and supplies. Principally supportive care with referral as available.		Each department in health-care facility maintains a separate, longitudinal, patient-based paper record for each patient. Records contain name or other identifier that allows them to be linked.
Supportive care at home by family or community members. No laboratory diagnostic methods. No formally trained health-care personnel.		Each provider or facility maintains separate disease or diagnosis-based, longitudinal records for patients with specific conditions (e.g., TB, pregnancy). Records usually contain name that allows them to be linked with considerable effort.
None	**Less developed**	Each provider or facility maintains an encounter-based register with patient identifier that allows construction of a longitudinal record within the facility only with effort— difficult to follow patient over time.
		Each provider or facility maintains an encounter-based register with no consistent patient identifier.
		Not possible to construct longitudinal record for most patients.
		Providers and facilities do not maintain any records.

Scope (Where, When, Who, and How Much?)

What geographic area should be covered (e.g., country, rural districts in a country, urban areas with a population greater than 2 million)? What time period should be included (e.g., last 5 years and January through June 1995)? Who or what should be assessed (e.g., women living within this area and time period who became pregnant, motor vehicle crashes resulting in an injury requiring hospitalization)? Should all subjects or events of the universe defined by the three parameters above, or only a sample, be included (e.g., population sampling, temporal sampling, geographic sampling)?

One may attempt to gather information on the entire population or on all occurrences of a health condition(s) affecting it (e.g., census of a population, comprehensive mortality registration, cancer registration, and reports of certain—mainly infectious—diseases), or only part of the population or some occurrences of a health condition, by using a sampling strategy. Samples may be drawn so that they are representative of the population (i.e., probabilistic sample), or they may attempt to obtain information on easily identified individuals or occurrences with little or no effort to ensure that the sample is representative (i.e., a non-probabilistic, "grab," or "convenience" sample (3). The use of sentinel physicians or sentinel practices is an example of this latter strategy, although in some settings there may be an effort to achieve some semblance of a representative sample of physicians or practices.

The decision of whether to gather information on all members (or events) of a population (i.e., a census) or on a sample of the population depends on the time, resources and personnel available, and thus, to the "value" placed on complete information. A census usually requires more time, more staff, and greater cost than sampling. Some programs that attempt to gather information on all events (e.g., vital registration, disease notifications) rely on reporting by members of the population or by health-care providers, and thereby shift the burden from paid agents of the HIS to unpaid agents in the community (a.k.a., "passive reporting"). These require less effort and cost on the part of the HIS, but are usually less complete unless significant incentives (or penalties) are provided (e.g., large payments for identifying cases of smallpox during final phases of eradication) (24). In contrast, sampling usually requires less effort for the same amount of information on each subject or event because fewer subjects are questioned or fewer events are observed. It is usually cost-prohibitive to obtain the level of detail on each person or event in a population census that is possible for a sample of the population. Thus, if detailed information is needed, a sampling strategy is usually selected rather than a census. Sampling may, however, miss rare events, be susceptible to bias, and not allow estimates for small geographic areas or subgroups of the population. Complex sampling strategies have been devised to deal with some of these issues. Sometimes gathering information on all individuals, conditions, or events in a sample of jurisdictions (e.g., Surveillance, Epidemiol-ogy, and End Results [SEER], Drug Abuse Warning Network [DAWN]) may provide sufficiently detailed information for action.

Content (What Information Should Be Collected?)

What basic information and use-specific information should be collected about or from each subject or event? (Gather all the information you need, but gather *only* the information you need.) Abramson (*16*) suggests that consideration be given to gathering information on three types of variables in all data collection efforts: universal variables, measures of time, and variables that delineate the individuals, populations, or events under study. *Universal variables* (i.e., sociodemographic) include sex, age, parity, ethnic group, religion, marital status, social class (or indicators of class, e.g., education, occupation, income), place of birth, and place of current residence. *Measures of time* refer to the dates and times of specific events, including dates of injury, onset of disease, treatment, and death. *Variables that delineate individuals, populations, and events* are those that are used to select and characterize the people or events about which information is gathered and to compare them with those not included. These variables are important for assessing the generalizability of the information that is gathered. In addition to these three types of variables, one must identify the use-specific information that is needed and develop questions and variables that capture this information (e.g., assess the use of a specific toy in order to assess its relationship to a particular kind of injury in children, identify foods consumed at a dinner followed by an outbreak of gastroenteritis, determine the presence and type of disabilities in individuals in order to determine their prevalence within a population).

Once the information of interest and the variables have been selected, one needs to develop operational definitions for the variables. This includes the specific wording of questions, observational approaches, and environmental sampling methods that will be used to gather information on the selected variables. Numerous books on survey and questionnaire design and monitoring methods address this issue. If information will be collected on diseases, it is important to establish clear definitions for diseases and what criteria must be met for a person to be considered a case of a disease (*13,23*).

Timeliness (How Quickly Is the Information Needed?)

How quickly do those who need to use it need the information? (Consider multiple levels of data use and collection. Consider the actions taken or programs designed to address the health problem.) How frequently does information need to be collected (continuously, weekly, yearly, once)?

How frequently information is gathered by the system and how long the delay can be between the occurrence of an event; the collection, recording, or registration of the event by the system; and the dissemination of information by the system (a day, a month, a year) should be determined by the use to which the data will be put. Put another way, how frequently does information need to be updated and disseminated to ensure timely action (Figure 3–2)?

In the case of epidemic infectious diseases, the sum of intervals 1–5 should not exceed the incubation period of the disease or the period required to interrupt the cycle of secondary transmission (Figure 3–2). For environmental hazards, the sum of the intervals should not exceed the time required to remove or

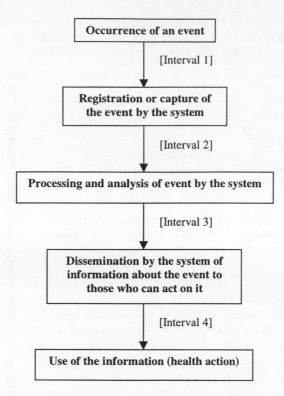

Figure 3–2 Sequence of actions needed to gather and use health-related information.

clean up the hazard or to evacuate potentially exposed populations before further exposures occur. The optimal frequency and timeliness is often tempered by the operational constraints of the HIS, including its infrastructure and resources. When the HIS is not able to provide timely information on important health problems to those needing it, the design and operation of the HIS may need to be modified and improved, or more timely methods of obtaining the information may need to be established. Periodic evaluations of the HIS should be conducted to ensure that it is meeting its objectives.

Balancing Effort, Burden, and Importance

The effort required by an HIS to gather information, the burden placed on individuals or populations under observation (the "subjects"), and the importance of the information for specific health actions are important factors in the selection of the source of information and of the method for collecting it. The literature on public health surveillance often uses the terms *active* and *passive* to describe the collection of information (*17,26*). We prefer to describe the level of effort that an HIS and its agents, and subjects must expend to produce the information (Table 3–4). In general, as the level of effort on the part of an HIS increases, the level of effort required by subjects decreases and vice versa. One exception to

Table 3–4 Hypothetical Model of Surveillance That Depicts Available Methods That Can Be Used by an Observer to Obtain Information about a Subject, Showing the Level of Effort Expended by Each Party

Method of Obtaining Information	Effort by Subject	Effort by Observer
The subject—without her knowledge—is under constant surveillance by the observer. The observer keeps detailed records of the subject's activities	**Less**	**Greater**
The subject—without her knowledge—is under periodic (e.g., weekly, monthly) surveillance by the observer. The observer keeps detailed records of the subject's activities		
The subject is periodically visited and interviewed by the observer about her activities or the occurrence of specific events. The observer keeps ongoing records of these visits and interviews. There is independent verification of the accuracy and completeness of the subject's responses through occasional, direct observation of the subject		
The subject is required to keep ongoing records of her activities or the occurrence of specific events. The observer periodically visits the subject, reviews the subject's records, and questions the subject about her records, as needed. There is independent verification of the accuracy and completeness of the reports through infrequent, direct observation of the subject		
The subject is required to keep ongoing records of her activities or the occurrence of specific events. The observer periodically visits the subject, reviews the subject's records, and questions the subject about her records, as needed. There is no independent verification of the accuracy and completeness of the reports		
The subject is required to keep ongoing records of her activities or the occurrence of specific events and to visit the observer on a regular basis to provide the records and to answer questions about her records and activities		
The subject is required to keep ongoing records of her activities or the occurrence of specific events and to report these on a regular basis by mail or by telephone to the observer. The observer verifies compliance with the reporting requirement through regular review of the reports		
The subject is required to report specific activities or the occurrence of specific events to the observer whenever they occur. There is no requirement for reporting if the specific activity or event does not occur. (Note: Depending on the frequency of occurrence of the activity or event of interest, this method of reporting may require more effort on the part of the observer than the previous method)	**Greater**	**Less**

this occurs when the agents of the system directly question or physically examine subjects; this may entail substantial effort on the part of both parties.

Agents who are employed by an HIS are usually paid for their efforts. In some settings, community members or health-care providers may be asked to act as agents of an HIS. In ideal circumstances their efforts are supported through financial or managerial incentives. In other settings, health-care providers are required by law or regulation to act as its agents (e.g., they are required to complete a death certificate for their patients who die, or to notify health authorities of cases of cholera) and may even be threatened with fines or other sanctions for not participating. Depending on the incentives or the severity and extent of the enforcement of sanctions, the perceived importance of the health problem (e.g., rabies versus seasonal upper respiratory infections), or the perceived ability of the system or others to control the problem, the completeness and quality of reporting by health-care providers may vary considerably. Too often, an HIS places the greatest burden of reporting on the health-care provider at the health-service level where the information that is collected is least used. These health-care providers are asked or required to act as agents of the HIS, but they receive little or no benefit for their efforts. In addition, in less developed health systems the majority of reporting falls to health-care providers who have few skills and little interest in population-health-related activities (15,20,24). Finally, to encourage participation in HIS activities, subjects may be paid (e.g., members of a community are paid to participate in a community survey that includes a physical examination and laboratory testing).

Approaches and Terminology

Various approaches have been developed for gathering population-level information needed to meet health-related objectives, including censuses, surveys, registries, and disease notifications (Table 3–5). Environmental monitoring is also important and includes programs to inspect agricultural products and restaurants, and to monitor disease vectors, air quality, and water quality (25). In the first edition of this book, Stroup, Zack, and Wharton comprehensively describe the use of routinely collected health data (e.g., disease notifications, vital statistics, surveys, disease registries, and administrative reports) for public health surveillance and include many examples of the application of these data to public health practice (27). Thacker and Stroup discuss the relationship of surveillance systems to health information systems, disease notifications, sentinel notifications, surveys, registries, and administrative data systems (11). Thacker and Wetterhal describe many of these same approaches and present four case studies illustrating the application of these approaches to a) monitor the health of a community (cardiovascular disease), b) advocate for health programs (breast cancer control program), c) evaluate program outcomes (prevention of teen pregnancy), and d) evaluate programs (prevention of influenza) (28). Simoes and Brownson list data sources that provide information concerning health indicators (29). Abramson describes several types of "documentary" sources for studying populations or their members (14). Otten (30) and Chapter 13 in this book describe approaches to gathering data that are particularly useful in developing countries.

These approaches to gathering population-level information can be classified in several ways, such as frequency of data collection and method of sampling. Using level of effort expended by the HIS to gather information (i.e., low vs. high) as the basis for classification, most approaches can be seen as either reg-

Table 3–5 Approaches to Gathering Public-Health-Related Data Described by Various Authors

Approach	Thacker and Stroup[†]	Stroup, Wharton, and Zack (27)	Thacker and Wetterhall (28)	Otten (30)	Simoes Brownson[‡]	Abramson[§]
Registration systems						
Vital-event registration		■	■	■		■
Disease notifications	■	■				■
Sentinel notifications	■					
Studies						
Surveys	■	■	■	■	■	
Registries	■	■				■
Epidemic investigations						
Population and house census					■	
Research			■			

Shading indicates that author described the approach.

[†]See reference *11*. We have excluded health information system from this list because it does not fit with the content of this table.

[‡]See reference *29*, page 175. We have excluded the following categories because they do not fit with the content of this table: routine health services records, health programs delivery records, and hospital discharge data.

[§]See reference *14*, pages 193–207. We have excluded the following categories because they do not fit with the content of this table: clinical records, medical audit, hospital statistics, health diaries and calendars, other documentary sources, and record linkage.

Table 3-5 (Continued)

Approach	Thacker and Stroup[1]	Stroup, Wharton, and Zack (27)	Thacker and Wetterhall (28)	Otten (30)	Simoes Brownson[2]	Abramson[3]
Other						
Administrative data systems	▨	▨				
Program evaluations			▨			
Public health surveillance			▨	▨		
Exit interviews and focus groups				▨		
Alternative data sources			▨			
Other data banks from programs outside the health sector					▨	

Shading indicates that author described the approach.

[1]See reference *11*. We have excluded health information system from this list because it does not fit with the content of this table.

[2]See reference *29*, page 175. We have excluded the following categories because they do not fit with the content of this table: routine health services records, health programs delivery records, and hospital discharge data.

[3]See reference *14*, pages 193–207. We have excluded the following categories because they do not fit with the content of this table: clinical records, medical audit, hospital statistics, health diaries and calendars, other documentary sources, and record linkage.

istration systems or studies. Registration systems usually rely on primary reporting by health-care providers to a health agency (i.e., the HIS) using either a paper or electronic form. Although they generally attempt to gather all occurrences or instances of a specific event, disease, or other factor, relatively little effort is expended by the HIS to gather information and, as a result, the ascertainment of events by these systems is usually incomplete (except for systems with significant rewards or penalties associated with reporting, or the lack thereof). The HIS usually compiles and analyzes the data and produces reports. Registration systems include vital registration, disease notifications, reports from laboratories, and sentinel provider systems. *Studies,* in contrast, usually gather information on a sample of occurrences, require significant effort by the HIS to gather information from individuals or health-care records, and make an effort to achieve high response rates. Studies include epidemiological studies, disease registries, population surveys, and surveys of health records. *Surveillance* is not a specific data-gathering approach, but rather the use of data derived from either of these basic approaches in order to contain and control disease. (See comment under *Surveillance* in Appendix 3A.)

The terms (e.g., *survey, surveillance,* and *registry*) used for these various approaches, however, are inconsistent and at times confusing. Because many of the approaches share certain characteristics (e.g., source of data; population coverage; frequency of data collection), the same term has been used for different approaches, and diffeent terms have been used for the same approach. (See Appendix 3A for definitions and further discussion of terms [*3,14,19,31,32*]).

PRACTICE

The purpose of most investigations in community medicine, and in the health field generally, is the collection of information that will provide a basis for action, whether immediately or in the long run.

J. H. Abramson (*19*)

In practice, two basic types of information are needed to meet most needs in public health practice.

First, *general, population-based information on health status, health problems, and health determinants* is needed in order to identify major health problems and risk factors in the population, (population can be at any level of geography or political organization [e.g., entire country or community]) to decide what health programs to develop and implement, and to allocate resources to these programs. In order of priority the information needed includes (Table 3–6):

- setting (physical, social, economic, and political environments)
- health status of the population under study
- health-care resources and gaps
- determinants of health status in the setting under study
- available and feasible strategies and processes for improving health in the setting

Table 3–6 Health-Related Information Needed to Support Population-Based Health Programs, Typical Approaches for Gathering This Information, and Examples of Programs That Gather Information or Other Sources of Information in the United States, Philippines, and Uganda

Type of Information	Typical Approaches for Gathering Information; Sources of Information	Programs That Gather Information, United States (10)	Programs That Gather Information, Philippines*	Programs That Gather Information, Uganda[†]
Natural environment				
Climate and weather	Weather monitoring stations; satellite data	National Oceanographic and Atmospheric Administration and National Weather Service data files	PAGASA (Philippine Weather Bureau)	Uganda Meteorological Service
Geology, topography, vegetative land cover, and water resources	Land surveys; satellite images; aerial photographs	U.S. Geological Survey	PHILVOLCS (Philippine Volcanology Institute)	
Animal vectors	Field surveys			
Human modification of the natural environment				
Land Use	Land surveys; satellite images; aerial photographs	U.S. Department of Agriculture		Ministry of Agriculture
Air quality, water supply and quality, waste disposal	Environmental monitoring systems; sentinel surveys and special studies of vectors	Environmental Protection Agency; Aerometric Information Retrieval System (EPA); WATSTORE	Department of Energy and Natural Environment	

(continued)

*Source: Mark H. White, Director, Division of International Health, Centers for Disease Control and Prevention, personal communication, August 1999.
[†]Source: Peter Nsubuga, Epidemic Intelligence Service Officer, Division of International Health, Centers for Disease Control and Prevention, personal communication, August 1999.

Table 3–6 Health-Related Information Needed to Support Population-Based Health Programs, Typical Approaches for Gathering This Information, and Examples of Programs That Gather Information or Other Sources of Information in the United States, Philippines, and Uganda (Continued)

Type of Information	Typical Approaches for Gathering Information; Sources of Information	Programs That Gather Information, United States (10)	Programs That Gather Information, Philippines*	Programs That Gather Information, Uganda[†]
Socioeconomic determinants (e.g., income, employment, housing)	Population surveys;	Decennial census; Current Population Survey; Bureau of Labor Statistics; Dept of Housing and Urban Development	Decennial census; National Demographic and Health Survey (NDHS)	Decennial census; World Bank reports
Social, economic, and political environment				
Population (number, geographic distribution, and demographic characteristics)	Census and periodic surveys of population	Decennial census; Current population survey	National Demographic and Health Survey (NDHS) conducted every 5 years	Decennial census
Fertility and natality (number, geographic and demographic distribution, and temporal trends)	Vital registration; health-care records; periodic surveys of population or health-care providers	National Vital Statistics System; CDC Abortion Surveillance System	National Demographic and Health Survey (NDHS)	Demographic and Health Survey (DHS)
Urbanization (location and extent) and housing	Population surveys; land surveys; satellite images; aerial photographs	Decennial census; Department of Housing and Urban Development	Department of Science and Technology (DOST); Philippine decennial census	Ministry of Housing
Economic development (e.g., income, employment)	National financial records; World Bank; International Monetary Fund	Department of Commerce; Department of Labor	National Economic Development Authority (NEDA) World Bank; International	Monetary Fund

*Source: Mark H. White, Director, Division of International Health, Centers for Disease Control and Prevention, personal communication, August 1999.
[†]Source: Peter Nsubuga, Epidemic Intelligence Service Officer, Division of International Health, Centers for Disease Control and Prevention, personal communication, August 1999.

Table 3-6 Health-Related Information Needed to Support Population-Based Health Programs, Typical Approaches for Gathering This Information, and Examples of Programs That Gather Information or Other Sources of Information in the United States, Philippines, and Uganda (Continued)

Type of Information	Typical Approaches for Gathering Information; Sources of Information	Programs That Gather Information, United States (10)	Programs That Gather Information, Philippines*	Programs That Gather Information, Uganda[†]
Transportation infrastructure	Land surveys; satellite images; aerial photographs	U.S. Department of transportation		Ministry of Transportation and Communication
Communication infrastructure	Population surveys; government agencies and private organizations	Federal Communications Commission; Bureau of Census; private companies		Ministry of Transportation and Communication
Health status				
Mortality (number, geographic and demographic distribution, temporal trends, causes) and life expectancy	Vital registration; health-care records; periodic surveys of population or health-care providers; "verbal autopsy"	National Vital Statistics System; medical examiners and coroners	Department of Health	Periodic surveys conducted by the Ministry of Health

(continued)

*Source: Mark H. White, Director, Division of International Health, Centers for Disease Control and Prevention, personal communication, August 1999.
[†]Source: Peter Nsubuga, Epidemic Intelligence Service Officer, Division of International Health, Centers for Disease Control and Prevention, personal communication, August 1999.

Table 3-6 Health-Related Information Needed to Support Population-Based Health Programs, Typical Approaches for Gathering This Information, and Examples of Programs That Gather Information or Other Sources of Information in the United States, Philippines, and Uganda (Continued)

Type of Information	Typical Approaches for Gathering Information; Sources of Information	Programs That Gather Information, United States (10)	Programs That Gather Information, Philippines*	Programs That Gather Information, Uganda†
Morbidity (number, nature and severity, geographic and demographic distribution, temporal trends, causes). Note: Type of health-care facility visited is often used as a surrogate for severity. • Hospitalizations (inpatient visits) • Ambulatory care (outpatient visits; general practice) • Specific diseases	General: registers of visits to health-care facilities; electronic health-care records; administrative or financial data derived from health-care records (e.g., insurance claims, data collected by payers from health-care providers in order to process payment for providing health care, and reports required by government and regulatory agencies); population surveys Hospitalizations: hospital records; hospital discharge surveys Specific diseases: disease notifications; reporting of sentinel disease by health-care providers; Required reporting of epidemic diseases ("disease notifications"); registries of patients with specific diseases kept by health-care providers or facilities, or health agencies	General: databases maintained by Managed Care Organizations; MEDSTAT research databases and other commercial health-care data sets; Medicaid data files; Medicare data files Hospitalizations: National Hospital Discharge Survey (NCHS‡); State hospital discharge surveys; Medicaid data files; Healthcare Cost and Utilization Project; Medical Expenditure Panel Survey Ambulatory: National Ambulatory Medical Care Survey (NCHS) Specific diseases: NNDSS; National System of Cancer Registries; State birth defects registries; Drug Abuse Warning Network; National Electronic Injury Surveillance; Annual Survey of Occupational Injuries and Illnesses	General: Field Health Services Information System (FHSIS); National Demographic and Health Survey (NDHS) Hospitalizations: Hospital Information System Specific diseases: National Epidemic Sentinel Surveillance System (timely, but incomplete geographic and population coverage of 12 epidemic diseases and causes of diarrhea); treatment and control programs for tuberculosis, sexually transmitted diseases (STD), and other diseases	General: Demographic and Health Survey (DHS) Hospitalizations: Health Management Information System Specific diseases: treatment and control programs for tuberculosis, sexually transmitted diseases [STD], and other diseases

*Source: Mark H. White, Director, Division of International Health, Centers for Disease Control and Prevention, personal communication, August 1999.

†Source: Peter Nsubuga, Epidemic Intelligence Service Officer, Division of International Health, Centers for Disease Control and Prevention, personal communication, August 1999.

‡NCHS = National Center for Health Statistics.

Table 3–6 Health-Related Information Needed to Support Population-Based Health Programs, Typical Approaches for Gathering This Information, and Examples of Programs That Gather Information or Other Sources of Information in the United States, Philippines, and Uganda (Continued)

Type of Information	Typical Approaches for Gathering Information; Sources of Information	Programs That Gather Information, United States (10)	Programs That Gather Information, Philippines*	Programs That Gather Information, Uganda†
Functional status and quality of life	Population surveys (self-reported health status)	National Health Interview Survey; State Behavioral Risk Factor Surveys; National Health and Nutrition Examination Survey	National Demographic and Health Survey (NDHS)	
Health-care resources				
Number and types of persons and facilities, geographic distribution, type of care given, number of people that can be served; utilization of health care	Ministry of health reports; licensure of health professionals; surveys of health facilities and health-care providers	National Health Provider Inventory; Annual Survey of Hospitals; Physician Masterfile; National Medical Expenditure Survey Office of Hospitals; LGAM	(Local government systems)	Ministry of Health statistical abstracts
Determinants of health status				
Behavior (prevalence, geographic and demographic distribution)	Population surveys (e.g., behaviors, activities); observations of behavior; health examination surveys (e.g., body fat, nutritional status)	National Health Interview Survey; State Behavioral Risk Factor Surveys	HIV and STD population surveys; proposed behavior survey	

(continued)

*Source: Mark H. White, Director, Division of International Health, Centers for Disease Control and Prevention, personal communication, August 1999.

†Source: Peter Nsubuga, Epidemic Intelligence Service Officer, Division of International Health, Centers for Disease Control and Prevention, personal communication, August 1999.

Table 3–6 Health-Related Information Needed to Support Population-Based Health Programs, Typical Approaches for Gathering This Information, and Examples of Programs That Gather Information or Other Sources of Information in the United States, Philippines, and Uganda (Continued)

Type of Information	Typical Approaches for Gathering Information; Sources of Information	Programs That Gather Information, United States (10)	Programs That Gather Information, Philippines*	Programs That Gather Information, Uganda†
Biological composition (e.g., genetic endowment, immune status)	Health-care records; health examination surveys (e.g., hypertension, immune status)	Human genome project; research studies; outbreak investigations; National Health and Nutrition Examination Survey		
Strategies and processes to improve health				
Protecting the environment	Environmental laws and regulations; specific programs doing cleanup; locations of major sources of pollution; research studies of pollutants and their effects	Environmental Protection Agency; Aerometric Information Retrieval System (EPA); WATSTORE	Programs of the Department of Energy and Natural Environment; programs of the Department of Health	Ministry of Environment and Natural Resources
Promoting healthy population behavior	Qualitative research; behavioral risk factor surveys; exit surveys; focus groups	National Health Interview Survey; State Behavioral Risk Factor Surveys	Programs of the Department of Health; activities of social groups	
Providing effective health care	Population surveys; regulations; Studies of health-care quality and access to care; accreditation and licensing of health-care providers and facilities	Clinical Laboratory Improvement Act; Joint Commission on the Accreditation of Health Care Organizations; Clinical Preventive Services Guidelines	Department of Health; private sector	

*Source: Mark H. White, Director, Division of International Health, Centers for Disease Control and Prevention, personal communication, August 1999.
†Source: Peter Nsubuga, Epidemic Intelligence Service Officer, Division of International Health, Centers for Disease Control and Prevention, personal communication, August 1999.

The frequency of collecting and the timeliness of this information should depend on the frequency of planning and budgeting. Typically, data should be collected every 1 to 3 years and be available within 1 year of collection to allow for changes in strategies and budgets for national, regional, and local health agencies. Information of this type is usually collected via population surveys, periodic reviews of health records, or vital or disease registrations.

The second basic type of information needed is *specific, timely information on selected health conditions and risk factors* in order to investigate and characterize these conditions, or to plan and manage programs to prevent or treat them. Typically, the data should be collected and available within a time frame that facilitates managing a program, treating patients, implementing prevention or control measures, and assessing the effectiveness of each of these efforts. The time frame will, in turn, depend on

- importance of the health conditions (e.g., incidence, prevalence, and severity)
- availability of effective interventions
- feasibility and accessibility of those interventions in a particular setting, and how quickly one must act

Actions include preventing spread of disease (e.g., meningococcal meningitis; cholera; polio), the occurrence of additional injuries resulting from a hazard (e.g., unsafe roadway), exposure of additional individuals to an environmental hazard (e.g., exposure to food contaminated with lead or pesticides; exposure to high levels of air pollutants), and progression of disease within affected individuals (e.g., screening for phenylketonuria, cervical cancer, and treatment of tuberculosis).

Information of this second type is usually collected via active, targeted case finding; review of laboratory tests for specific health conditions; and active monitoring of environmental media or vectors.

Systems that are established to obtain information of the first type are not usually able to provide sufficiently detailed and timely information for the second need. Conversely, information systems of the second type are too detailed and too limited in coverage (i.e., they provide data only for one or a few diseases or risks factors that are covered by the program) to provide the information to meet the first need. Using information from either of these systems to assess a population's health status will not provide a comprehensive picture. There is a tendency to try to make an information system serve both of these purposes, when, in fact, it makes more sense to recognize the need for separate systems and to design or operate them so that the information from the two systems is complementary and comparable.

Sixteen Steps to Health-Related Information

Having described various principles concerning the collection and use of health-related information, we now present a practical, step-wise approach to gathering health-related information (*19,29*). See Table 3–7 for other examples of how to

Table 3–7 Steps in Designing and Conducting an Investigation, Survey, or Surveillance System to Gather Health-Related Information as Described by Various Authors

Stages of an Investigation*	Steps in Designing a Surveillance System†	Steps in Designing and Conducting a Survey‡
1. Identifying of problem	1. Problem statement	1. Thinking about topics for health surveys
2. Preliminary steps	2. Objectives	2. Matching the survey design to survey objectives
a. Clarifying the purpose	3. Definition of the event	3. Defining and clarifying the survey variables
b. Formulating the topic	4. Sources of data	4. Planning the analysis of the survey data
3. Planning phase	5. Other characteristics	5. Choosing the methods of data collection
a. Formulating study objectives	a. Passive, active, or combination	6. Drawing the sample
b. Planning methods	b. Census or sample	7. Formulating the questions
i. Study population	c. Continuous or intermittent	8. Formatting the questionnaire
(1) Selection and definition	6. Frequency of reporting	9. Monitoring and carrying out the survey
(2) Sampling	7. Case reporting form	10. Preparing the data for analysis
(3) Size	8. Method of data recording and transmission	11. Implementing the analysis of the survey data
ii. Variables	9. Who will receive the information and who will edit (clean up) the data and enter it into the computer	12. Writing the research report
(1) Selection	10. Data analysis	
(2) Definition	11. Reports	
(3) Scales of measurement	12. Evaluation	
iii. Methods of collecting data		
iv. Methods of recording and processing		
4. Preparing for data collection		
5. Collecting the data		
6. Processing the data		
7. Interpreting the results		
8. Writing a report		

*Based on reference *14*, pages 1–4, 29–35. Abramson does not include "Reviewing the literature" as a separate stage in his scheme because he views it as vitally important throughout the investigation.

†CDC, unpublished document, stepdesc.doc, July 1986.

‡Based on reference *42*.

approach this issue. Step-by-step approaches developed by various authors for designing and conducting an investigation, a survey, and a surveillance system are presented in Table 3–7. We illustrate the application of our 16-step approach to three settings in Table 3–8 on pages 63–68.

The Steps
1. State the problem.
2. Understand the setting.
3. Clarify the purpose and use of the information.
4. Formulate the topic and content.
5. Define the scope.
6. Determine what specific information is needed about each individual, health-care provider, or event.
7. Determine how quickly information is needed.
8. Identify the resources available for gathering health-related information or utilizing existing information.
9. Select the source of information and the method of collection based on purpose, content, scope, and setting.
10. Conduct pilot test to determine whether source and method can provide needed information.
11. Collect the data.
12. Compile, process, and analyze the data.
13. Interpret the data.
14. Write report and disseminate findings.
15. Ensure that those who need the information receive it.
16. Evaluate usefulness of data that are collected to those who use it.

Steps 1 through 10 are discussed in more detail below. Steps 11 through 16 are outside the scope of this chapter but are covered in numerous places elsewhere in this book.

1. State the Problem

What is the problem, action, or decision for which information is needed? For example,

- Cost of health care is too high.
- Maternal mortality is too high.
- Women are not receiving mammography.
- Too many women are dying of breast cancer.
- Is tuberculosis in our country becoming resistant to standard therapy?
- Should we increase the resources devoted to preventing smoking?
- How can we make our diarrheal disease program work better?
- An outbreak of plague has occurred in two western states.

The problem may be defined or perceived differently by local health officials than by national officials or external donors, and by policymakers versus scientists or program officials. In some instances there may be agreement about the problem but different reasons for, or means to, solve it. It is important to state the problem clearly and in such a way that there is a shared understanding by all involved in addressing the problem. It is also important to describe what is known. For example, if there is an excessive number of deaths from breast cancer, is the problem a high ratio of fatalities to cases among certain groups, the lack of access to early prevention (i.e., mammography), a combination of the two, or something else?

2. Understand the Setting

What are the physical, social, economic, and political environments in which information will be gathered and used (e.g., level of development, climate, geographic distribution of population, transportation, communication, political situation, security, language, and literacy)? What is the type and organization of the health-care system? What information is available from the system and can anyone use it?

3. Clarify the Purpose and Use of the Information

Why is information being collected? For what purpose will the information be used (Table 3–2)? Will the information be used to address a health problem, direct action, or make decisions? Who will use the information to make decisions and implement the strategies or actions? Define the target audience(s) and, if necessary, interview them in order to determine what will be the most useful and persuasive information for addressing the health problem under consideration (see also Chapters 7 and 16).

4. Formulate the Topic and Content

What specific information is needed for the use identified in Step 3?
  Examples:

  • mortality rate from tuberculosis for all districts in country
  • leading costs of health care in Provinces A and B in Country X
  • principal reasons that women die during pregnancy or childbirth
  • completeness of reporting of infectious diseases to district and national health officials
  • number of districts using injury data to guide control programs
  • characteristics and location of persons at high risk for contracting a specific disease in order to take preventive action
  • cultural practices in weaning and principal barriers to breast-feeding

5. Define the Scope

For what specific geographic area, population, and time period is information needed?
  Examples:

  • Determine the causes of *infant* mortality *in District A over the past 5 years.*
  • Compare different approaches for educating *mothers* about oral rehydration therapy for the control of diarrheal disease *among persons without a supply of clean drinking water in sub-Saharan Africa.*
  • Identify the principal factors contributing to smoking among *teenagers in urban areas in the United States from 1990 through 1995.*

6. Determine What Specific Information Is Needed About Each Individual, Health-Care Provider, or Event

Three products are needed to accomplish this step:

- selection of the specific content or variables to address the objectives of the system (e.g., name, address, weight, medical diagnosis, concentration of coliforms in drinking water, and date of onset of disease)
- selection of existing, or development of new, operational definitions of variables, including what constitutes a case of a disease (e.g., a confirmed case of chancroid consists of painful genital ulceration, inflammatory inguinal adenopathy, and isolation of Haemophilus ducreyi from a clinical specimen) (*23*); the presence of a risk factor (e.g., a smoker is a person who has smoked at least 1 cigarette per day in the past month), or event of interest (e.g., the maximum daily carbon monoxide level is the highest measured concentration of carbon monoxide in ambient outdoor air during an 8-hour period from 0800 to 1600 hours; a neonatal death is the death of an infant under 28 days of age)
- selection or development of categories, classification schemes, and scales of measurement for variables (e.g., age in years versus 5-year age groups, ICD for disease classification, Glasgow coma scale for severity of head injury)

7. Determine How Quickly Information Is Needed

How much time do you have to complete the process (includes planning, gathering, analyzing, and presenting information) before a decision or action is needed? The information-gathering process may be sequenced by first addressing questions that must be answered immediately and following this with a system to gather other needed, but less time-sensitive, information over a longer period of time (e.g., number of cases of measles in a refugee setting versus census of refugee population to determine denominator for calculating rates of measles).

8. Identify the Resources Available for Gathering Health-Related Information or Utilizing Existing Information

This consists of a complete inventory of human resources, community organizations and activities, communication infrastructure, transportation system, physical facilities, and supplies that will be available to gather, analyze, present, and use the information, and the financial resources to pay for each of these (*43*). Will resources be available for the duration of the information-gathering effort? What kinds of staff and skill level of staff are available? How might local resources be integrated to better use information for action? The level of resources required will be dependent on the level of development of the area under study and its existing health, communication, and transportation infrastructure. It is important to identify gaps in resources because they may adversely affect the sustainability of the information-gathering effort.

9. Select Source of Information and the Method of Collection Based on Purpose, Content, Scope, and Setting

Assess the Ability of Existing HIS to Provide Needed Information

In selecting source and method, it must first be determined if an existing system for collecting health-related information can provide the information you need in a timely, useful, and cost-effective way. This determination requires that two questions are posed.

First, *Can existing information be used?* Many developed countries have established ongoing, fairly comprehensive programs or systems to gather health-related information from individual members of the population, health-care providers, and other entities for many of the uses listed in Table 3–2). Most developing countries also have existing systems, but their scope and coverage may be limited. Even in developed countries the coverage of certain subpopulations and small geographic areas may be quite limited. Types of health-related information, types of systems typically providing it, and examples of health information systems for the United States, Philippines, and Uganda are shown in Table 3–6. Thus, depending on the setting, systems may be available already or may need to be developed. Guidelines have been developed to evaluate existing systems (see also Chapter 8) (*44–47*).

Second, *Can existing information or HIS be modified to meet your information needs?* An existing system, with modification, may be able to provide the needed information. Adapting an existing system has the advantage of using *a*) staff already familiar with data collection procedures, forms, and health-care providers, *b*) existing manuals, procedures, and software, *c*) existing organizational relationships, and *d*) existing communication systems.

Establish New System for Collecting Needed Information
If it is determined that existing information and HIS cannot provide the needed information, it may be necessary to establish a system to do so. Because of the expense and time required, this decision should not be taken lightly. Adequate planning and consultation with others knowledgeable about a country's or area's physical and social environment, population, health-services systems, and existing health information systems should be done before establishing a new system. Others may be able to provide resources or share the development of a new system by serving multiple needs.

The source and method used to obtain information will depend on the intended use of the information and the setting: the physical and social environment; demographic characteristics of the population, including literacy; the communication and transportation infrastructure; the nature of the system for providing individual and population-based health services, including the type and quality of health records; and the resources available to gather the information. For example, in some settings because of available resources or concerns about physical safety (e.g., civil war), the use of periodic population-based surveys may be preferable to establishing a comprehensive vital registration system. Some general guidelines follow; first, for the selection of the source:

- For information on the *health status* of individuals or populations or the prevalence of *behavioral determinants* of health, the primary source of information is individual *members* of the population.
- For information on *diseases and injuries* affecting the population, *health-care providers* serve as the primary source of information.

- For *environmental and other nonbehavioral determinants,* intersectoral information from *other entities* is used.
- Consider the use of multiple sources of information to provide a more complete perspective.

Guideline for the selection of method include:

- Decide whether to sample. (Sampling may be able to provide enough information to meet the objectives of the system and usually requires considerably less time, effort, and expense than a census or monitoring or observing all occurrences of a condition or event. It may also be more accurate. Sampling is most useful when the health problem, event, or determinant is common and a sample can provide a representative view of the frequency, magnitude, and relative importance of the problem or determinant.)
- Decide whether a sample of the population, health conditions, or events of interest is sufficient or if a census is necessary. If a sample is used, determine what size the sample should be to provide accurate and reliable estimates for the population, geographic area, and time period of interest (i.e., power calculations).
- Decide whether to continuously or intermittently collect information on the population or events. If intermittently, decide the frequency (e.g., weekly, monthly, and yearly).
- Select method of obtaining information from the source.
- For information on the *health status* of individuals or populations or the prevalence of *behavioral determinants* of health, the primary method to obtain information is *interviewing* members of the population, followed by *observation* of individuals and *review* of administrative and financial records.
- For information on *diseases and injuries* affecting the population, the best way to obtain information is *reviewing the records* of health-care providers, followed by *interviewing* health-care providers. (Because the likelihood that a person with a disease or injury will visit a health-care provider and that the health-care provider will keep a record that documents the visit and injury increases with the severity of the disease or injury, the coverage and usefulness of the records of health-care providers are related to the severity of the disease or injury.) Both of these methods are very labor intensive; if complete and accurate electronic records are available, this may reduce the burden on both health-care providers and the HIS. If neither reviewing records nor interviewing providers is feasible, requesting health-care providers to report specific disease and injuries can be tried, but reporting is usually very incomplete.
- For *environmental and other nonbehavioral determinants, observation* or monitoring the environment is the best method, followed by review of intersectoral information from other entities.
- Select method of recording information (e.g., disease notification form, CATI, self-completed questionnaire, form for abstracting health records, and electronic transmission of laboratory test results).

*10. Conduct Pilot Test to Determine Whether Source and Method
Can Provide Needed Information*

Discuss usefulness, reliability, and acceptability of this source with decision makers who will use or pay for the data. If the initial approach to gathering information, including the source of information and methods, cannot provide needed
information, return to Step 9 and start again (e.g., consider members of community instead of health-care providers). Repeat selection and pilot testing cycle
until an adequate approach is found.

11. Collect the data

See Chapters 2, 5, and 6.

12. Process and analyze the data

See Chapter 6.

13. Interpret the data

See Chapter 6.

14. Write report and disseminate findings

See Chapters 7 and 16.

15. Ensure that those who need the information receive it

See Chapters 7, 8, and 16.

*16. Evaluate usefulness of disseminated information for those who
use it*

See Chapters 7 and 16.

Examples of Application of Steps to Health Problems

Table 3–8 illustrates the application of these steps to the following three settings:

> *Example 1.* It is 1999, and you have been hired by the Ministry of Health
> (MOH) of a Central American country to assess the health of the coun-
> try's people and to provide recommendations on how the MOH should
> allocate its resources for health services for the next 5 years.
> *Example 2.* It is 1989, and you are the head of the Asian bureau of a non-
> governmental organization and have been asked to characterize and de-
> velop a program to address high maternal mortality in Province A of
> Afghanistan.
> *Example 3.* It is 1952, and you are the head of the new Epidemiology Ser-
> vice at the National Communicable Disease Center and have been given
> responsibility for assessing current efforts to eradicate malaria in the
> United States and to propose additional actions as needed.

The authors wish to acknowledge Jim Mendlein, Wayne Brown, Peter Nsubuga, Steve Thacker, and Mark White for their contributions to this chapter.

Table 3–8 Steps in Gathering Information to Meet a Health-Related Objective* and Their Application to Three Health Issues

Step	Example 1: Allocation of Health-Care Resources in Country X, 1999	Example 2: Reduction of Maternal Mortality in Afghanistan, 1987†	Example 3: Eradication of Malaria in the United States, 1930–60‡
1. State the problem	How should country X allocate its health-care resources over the next 5 years?	Maternal mortality is very high in province A of Afghanistan	In the 1930s, malaria was a deeply rooted endemic problem in rural sections of the Atlantic and Gulf coastal plains and of the Mississippi Delta area of the United States.
2. Understand the setting			
General physical, social, economic, and political environment		Poor, semiarid, mountainous, insecure, travel difficult and worse during certain times of the year, electricity is unreliable. Population is dispersed in many small villages and isolates farms. Very low literacy. Two local languages are spoken. Security for civilian population poor with fighting between rival factions and land mines important causes of morbidity and mortality. No phones. Hospital with radio. Electricity erratic or nonexistent Most maternal death within 2–12 hours of delivery. Most births are not attended by trained worker but by female family member. Women reluctant to request birth assistance from male health workers Even though "high" maternal mortality the event is relatively rare (2–3/1000 births)	Subtropical, heavily forested area of the southeastern United States with many rivers, lakes, and swampy areas. Population lives in 13 states (population approximately 50 million) in both urban and rural areas and is relatively poor compared to rest of the United States. In the mid- to late 1940s, large numbers of veterans of World War II, who had served in areas elsewhere in the world with endemic *Plasmodium vivax*, returned to the United States. Good transportation and communication infrastructure. Numerous national and local programs to control malaria have been undertaken: 1933–1944—TVA Malaria Control Program (water management, antilarval, and antimaginal) 1935–1942—WPA Malaria Control Drainage Program (antilarval measures) 1942–1945—War Areas Program (to protect military trainees from malaria—antilarval measures) 1945–1947—Extended Program (to prevent spread of malaria from returning troops—DDT) 1947–1951—Malaria Eradication Program (DDT and treatment) 1950–1952—Malaria Surveillance and Prevention 1952—Primaquine treatment of servicemen on transports returning from malarious areas

(continued)

Table 3-8 Steps in Gathering Information to Meet a Health-Related Objective* and Their Application to Three Health Issues (Continued)

Step	Example 1: Allocation of Health-Care Resources in Country X, 1999	Example 2: Reduction of Maternal Mortality in Afghanistan, 1987†	Example 3: Eradication of Malaria in the United States, 1930–60‡
Type and organization of health-care system		Isolated health posts (hospitals and clinics) run primarily by different NGOs located in villages. One government hospital. Some physicians. No labs. Few female health workers. Referral system poor and depends on personal resources to get transport. Voluntary health workers not part of socio-cultural history	Urban and rural private and public clinics and hospitals. Availability and quality of health care vary for different population groups. Long established but poorly funded state and local health departments responsible for environmental and clinical health services
Information available from health-care system(s)	Vital records system in place with data sent to regional (or national level)	Patient registers are kept in local language at hospital and clinics with patient name and sometimes address, date of visit, reason for visit, diagnosis, and treatment. No longitudinal records for individual people in clinics. Hospital has patient charts. In the government hospital data are supposed to be summarized and sent to regional and national level monthly. Compliance with these reporting requirements very low (<40%). No formal check of data quality or validity has been done. Assume sensitivity and positive predictive value are low as female population access is low and case definitions for maternal mortality unclear to health workers and used haphazardly.	Basic paper medical records. Prior to 1947 state health departments in the three states with the highest reported incidence of malaria requested weekly reports from health-care workers of the total number of cases seen rather than by name of individual patient

*Based on reference 19, pages 1–4 and 23–27.
†Source: Sharon McDonnell.
‡Based on reference 37.

Table 3–8 Steps in Gathering Information to Meet a Health–Related Objective* and Their Application to Three Health Issues (Continued)

Step	Example 1: Allocation of Health-Care Resources in Country X, 1999	Example 2: Reduction of Maternal Mortality in Afghanistan, 1987†	Example 3: Eradication of Malaria in the United States, 1930–60‡
3. Clarify the purpose and use of the information	1. Identify major health problems for Country X 2. Identify feasible interventions for these leading causes for Country X 3. Prioritize health programs on the basis of prevalence and feasible interventions	To define maternal mortality and assist in monitoring trends To investigate each maternal death and describe leading causes and contributing factors Develop effective programs for: • training women to attend births • train male health workers to provide education and referral • hospital staff Fundraising and donor reports (MOH, NGOs, UNICEF, WHO)	To evaluate the presence of malaria in the southeastern United States To direct prevention and control activities
4. Formulate the topic and content	Identify leading causes of mortality and morbidity for the entire population of Country X last year	Of known interventions (from previous studies and literature), which are most appropriate and feasible for this province (i.e., determine literacy; cultural practices; type, sex, and training of health workers; access to care within the province in order to determine which intervention to use) Baseline rate of maternal mortality so that effectiveness of intervention can be determined	Identify cases of malaria in the 13-state region on a on-going basis Adopt new criteria for evaluating the presence of malaria that are based on clinical findings and laboratory confirmation Gather sufficient demographic and geographic information about cases to determine epidemiological relationship of cases and, thereby, to assess endemic presence of malaria

(continued)

Table 3–8 Steps in Gathering Information to Meet a Health-Related Objective* and Their Application to Three Health Issues (Continued)

Step	Example 1: Allocation of Health-Care Resources in Country X, 1999	Example 2: Reduction of Maternal Mortality in Afghanistan, 1987†	Example 3: Eradication of Malaria in the United States, 1930–60‡
5. Define the scope (geographic area, population[s], and time period to be covered)	Entire population of Country X last year	Last and current year, Province A in Afghanistan, all women of childbearing age. Calculated by estimates based on NGO survey data from 5 years ago with adjustments for population mobility and demographic trends	Thirteen states in the southeastern United States thought to have endemic malaria. Entire population with focus on rural population. Weekly reporting of cases and deaths from malaria, starting in 1947 using new criteria
6. Determine what specific information is needed about each individual, health-care provider, or event		Number of deaths in women of childbearing age. Number of deaths associated with maternity. If birth attended and by whom. If patient under medical care at or prior to death. Associated medical factors (age, number of previous births, cause of death)	Weekly reporting of cases and deaths from malaria, starting in 1947 using new criteria. Name and address and demographic characteristics of each case, name of health-care provider, basis for diagnosis (clinical, laboratory)
7. Determine how quickly information is needed	Within 6 to 12 months so that annual planning and budgeting can respond to changes in mortality and morbidity	Baseline information needed in one month to obtain funding from donor. To be used to monitor situation and adjust program data needed in 1–2 years. To respond to each death data needed within 1 month to allow re-interview of health workers and family	Data needed at local and state level within 1–4 weeks to ensure follow-up, epidemiological investigation, and treatment of cases. Data needed at local level quarterly to adjust treatment and control programs. Data needed at national level every 6 months to monitor effectiveness of treatment and control programs at local level and to allocate resources to local, state, and national control programs

Table 3–8 Steps in Gathering Information to Meet a Health-Related Objective* and Their Application to Three Health Issues (Continued)

Step	Example 1: Allocation of Health-Care Resources in Country X, 1999	Example 2: Reduction of Maternal Mortality in Afghanistan, 1987[†]	Example 3: Eradication of Malaria in the United States, 1930–60[‡]
8. Identify the resources available for gathering health-related information or utilizing existing information	Moderate	Low level	High level of resources available, given the perceived importance of malaria
9. Select source of information and the method of collection based on purpose, content, scope, and setting	Existing information system can be used. Local personnel need to learn how to analyze and get access	Two sources selected to meet variety of objectives: 1. Community survey using expatriate female health workers and local staff 2. Sentinel sites (clinics and hospitals) selected based on % of female patients seen	Ongoing reporting by health-care providers of cases to local or state health department using standard form Application to these reports of standard case definition that includes results of laboratory tests to ensure that reports represent true cases of malaria Epidemiological investigation of every confirmed case by local, state, or national health department to identify the source of infection
10. Conduct pilot test to determine whether the source and method can provide needed information	Planned		Conducted in one state in 1947. Reports of new cases of malaria dropped from 17,764 in 1946 to 914 in 1947. Epidemiological investigation of reported cases revealed that only a very few could be verified Based on success of pilot, the new criteria to evaluate the presence of malaria were adopted and used for reporting elsewhere

(continued)

Table 3–8 Steps in Gathering Information to Meet a Health-Related Objective* and Their Application to Three Health Issues (Continued)

Step	Example 1: Allocation of Health-Care Resources in Country X, 1999	Example 2: Reduction of Maternal Mortality in Afghanistan, 1987†	Example 3: Eradication of Malaria in the United States, 1930–60‡
11. Collect the data		By survey staff and sentinel sites	States adopted and use the approach described in Step 9
12. Process and analyze the data		By survey staff and sentinel sites	By state and national staff
13. Interpret the data		By survey staff and sentinel sites	By state and national staf
14. Write report and disseminate findings		Provide to NGOs, MOH, donors (UNICEF, WHO, others)	Number of cases reported weekly by the National Communicable Disease Center and summarized annually
15. Ensure that those who need the information receive it			Accomplished through ongoing exchange of data and reports between local, state, and national disease control agencies
16. Evaluate the usefulness of data that is collected to those who use it		Continued program monitoring using process indicators • Improvements in % of assisted deliveries • Quality of care with delivery • Reporting compliance and quality from sentinel sites • Follow changes in contributing factors (literacy, access to care)	Periodic evaluations of the data and its use by control programs are conducted

*Based on reference *19*, pages 1–4 and 23–27. †Source: Sharon McDonnell. ‡Based on reference *37*.

Appendix 3A
Glossary

See Chapter 2, references *14* and *19,* for further discussion of several of these terms.
†Definitions preceded by "OED" are taken from reference *31.*
‡Definitions preceded by "Last" are taken from reference *3.* For brevity, examples and other explanatory text have been omitted from some definitions.
§Definitions preceded by "MTID" are taken from reference *32.* See also *Merriam Webster Online Dictionary* (http://www.m-w.com).

Census

- OED: "an official enumeration of the population of a country or district, with various statistics relating to them."
- *Merriam Webster Online Dictionary:* "a usually complete enumeration of a population; specifically: a periodic governmental enumeration of population."
- Last: "an enumeration of a population, originally intended for the purposes of taxation and military service."

Community diagnosis

- Last: "the process of appraising the health status of a community, including assembly of vital statistics and other health-related statistics and of information pertaining to determinants of health, such as prevalence of tobacco smoking, and examination of the relationships of these determinants to health in the specified community." (See Morris JN. *Br Med J* 1955; 2:395–401.)

Experiment

- Comment: Abramson (*19,* page 5) defines experiment as "an investigation in which the researcher, wishing to study the effects of exposure to or deprivation of a defined factor, himself decides which subjects (persons, animals, towns, etc.) will be exposed to, or deprived of, the factor."

Health statistics

- Last: "aggregated data describing and enumerating attributes, events, behaviors, services, resources, outcomes, or costs related to health, disease, and health services. The data may be derived from survey instruments, medical records, and administrative records."

Information system

- Last: "a combination of vital and health statistical data from multiple sources, used to derive information about the health needs, health resources, costs, use of health services, and outcomes of use by the population of a specified jurisdiction."

Monitoring

- MTID: "to watch, observe, or check esp. for a special purpose"
- Last: "the performance and analysis of routine measurements, aimed at detecting changes in the environment or health status of populations. Not to be confused with 'surveillance.' To some, monitoring also implies intervention in the light of observed measurements."

Register, registry

- OED: "a book or volume in which regular entry is made of particulars or details of any kind which are considered of sufficient importance to be exactly and formally recorded."
- MTID: "a book or system of public records; a roster of qualified or available individuals ⟨a civil service register⟩"
- Last: "a file of data concerning all cases of a particular disease or other health-relevant condition in a defined population such that the cases can be related to a population base. . . . A register requires that a permanent record be established, including identifying data. . . . The register is the actual document, and the registry is the system of ongoing registration."

Research

- OED: "a search or investigation directed to the discovery of some fact by careful consideration or study of a subject."
- Last does not define "research."

Sentinel health event

- OED defines "sentinel" as "one who or something which keeps guard like a military sentry."
- Last: "a condition that can be used to assess the stability or change in health levels of a population, usually by monitoring mortality statistics."
- Rutstein *et al.* (*33–35*): a "preventable disease, disability, or untimely death whose occurrence serves as a warning signal that the quality of preventive and /or therapeutic medical care may need to be improved." Conditions were originally selected because they were (a) relatively easily recognized by the practicing physician; (b) appeared as an unnecessary disease, an unnecessary disability, and/or an unnecessary untimely death, i.e. a condition that was either preventable and/or manageable; and c) the recognition of a single case raises the question, "Why did this happen?" and justifies a careful search for remediable underlying causes.

Sentinel reporting

- Last defines "sentinel physician, sentinel practice" as "in family medicine, a physician, practice, that undertakes to maintain surveillance for and report certain specific predetermined events, such as cases of certain communicable diseases, adverse drug reactions."

- Comment: Sandiford (*13*) provides the following cautionary note concerning sentinel sites: "Unfortunately, information systems based on sentinel sites depend largely upon the sites being and remaining representative of the population at large. Selecting representative sites is in itself problematic, but perhaps a bigger worry is that if actions are taken on the basis of the information generated (and one hopes that they well be), those actions, for one reason or another, will often be most vigorously undertaken in the sentinel sites where the problem was identified in the first place. This results in a tendency for sentinel sites to become progressively less typical of the populations that they are intended to represent."

Statistics

- OED "...collection, classification, and discussion of facts (especially of a numerical kind) bearing on the condition of a state or community."
- Last: "the science and art of collecting, summarizing, and analyzing data that are subject to random variation."

Study

- OED: "...careful examination or observation of (an object, a question, etc.)"; "examine in detail, seek to become minutely acquainted with or to understand (a phenomenon, a state of circumstances, a series of events, a person's character, etc); to investigate (a problem)"
- Last defines various types of studies, e.g., cohort, case control

Surveillance

- OED: "watch or guard kept over a person, etc. especially over a suspected person, prisoner, or the like."
- MTID: "the close and continuous observation of one or more persons for the purpose of direction, supervision, or control."
- Last: "ongoing scrutiny, generally using methods distinguished by their practicability, uniformity, and frequently their rapidity, rather than by complete accuracy. Its main purpose is to detect changes in trend or distribution in order to initiate investigative or control measures."
- Comment: Initially surveillance was used in public health to describe the close monitoring of individuals who, because of an exposure, were at risk of developing highly contagious and virulent infectious diseases that had been controlled or eradicated in a geographic area and population (e.g., cholera, plague, and yellow fever in the United States in the later 1800s). These individuals were monitored so that they could be quarantined if they developed evidence of disease to prevent its spread to others.

  In 1952, the U.S. Communicable Disease Center described its effort to redirect its large-scale control programs for several infectious diseases, which had achieved their purpose, "toward the establishment of a continuing surveillance program. The objective of this redirected program is to maintain constant vigilance to detect the presence of serious infectious diseases anywhere in the country, and when necessary, to mobilize all available forces to control them" (*36*).

In 1962 at the Cutter Lecture on Preventive Medicine, Langmuir applied the term surveillance to diseases rather than individuals: "Surveillance, when applied to a disease, means the continued watchfulness over the distribution and trends of incidence through the systematic collection, consolidation and evaluation of morbidity and mortality reports and other relevant data. Intrinsic in the concept is the regular dissemination of the basic data and interpretations to all who have contributed and to all others who need to know. The concept, however, does not encompass direct responsibility for control activities. These traditionally have been and still remain with the state and local health authorities" (*37*). He illustrated its application to four diseases: malaria, poliomyelitis, influenza, and hepatitis.

In 1968 at the 21st World Health Assembly *surveillance* was defined as "the systematic collection and use of epidemiological information for the planning, implementation, and assessment of disease control"(*38*). In 1976, an entire issue of the International Journal of Epidemiology was devoted to surveillance, especially its role in the eradication of smallpox (*39*). In the 1980s and 1990s, Thacker and others, including one of the authors of this chapter (RGP), expanded the term to encompass not just disease, but any outcome, hazard, or exposure* (*12,25,40–41*). In fact, the term *surveillance* is often applied to almost *any* effort to monitor, observe, or determine health status, diseases, or risk factors within a population. This is unfortunate because surveillance as originally conceived is a very useful and important concept and is still needed for those situations in which there is the need to rapidly identify and monitor (observe) individuals and problems that pose an immediate threat to the health of the public for the purpose of implementing measures to control the problems. Second, to apply the term *surveillance* to virtually any program for, or method of, gathering information about a population's health muddies our thinking about other approaches, supplants the use of more appropriate terminology, and leads to disagreement and confusion on the part of public health policy makers and practitioners. For these reasons, some prefer to use the term *monitoring* to refer to the entire set of efforts to gather information about a population or its environment for health-related purposes and to restrict the use of the term *surveillance* to rapidly identifying and monitoring individuals and problems that pose an immediate threat to the health of the public.

---

*Vaugh and Morrow describe two different uses for the term surveillance: (a) "continuous scrutiny of the factors that determine the occurrence and distribution of disease and other conditions of ill health. . . . Such a broad definition almost equates surveillance with routine health information systems and the two can therefore be considered together," (b) "special reporting system which is set up for a particularly important health problem or disease . . . Such a surveillance system is often organized for a limited period and is closely integrated with the management of a health intervention programme" (*12*).

Survey

- OED: "the act of viewing, examining, or inspecting in detail, esp. for some specific purpose."
- *Merriam Webster Online Dictionary:* "to query (someone) in order to collect data for the analysis of some aspect of a group or area" (*http://www.m-w.com*)
- Last uses Abramson's definition of a survey as "an investigation in which information is systematically collected, but in which the experimental method is not used"(*19*). (See definition of *experiment* above.) Abramson goes on to add, "Surveys are not necessarily brief operations; they may involve the long-term *surveillance* [emphasis added] of the status of a group or population."

REFERENCES

1. Murnaghan JH. Health-services information systems in the United States today. *N Engl J Med* 1974;290(11):603–10.
2. Lerer LB, Lopez AD, Kjellstrom T, Yach D. Health for all: analyzing health status and determinants. *World Health Stat Q* 1998;51(1):7–20.
3. Last JM. A dictionary of epidemiology. Second edition. New York: Oxford University Press, 1988.
4. Evans RG, Stoddart GL. Producing health, consuming health care. In: Evans RG, Baker ML, Marmor TR (eds.). Why are some people healthy and others not? The determinants of the health of populations. New York: Aldine DeGruter, 1994.
5. National Academy of Science, Committee on Leading Health Indicators for Healthy People 2010. Health indicators for healthy people 2010, final report. Chrvala CA, Bulger RJ (eds.). Washington, D.C.: National Academy Press, 1999.
6. National Academy of Sciences, Committee on Using Performance Monitoring to Improve Community Health. Improving health in the community: a role for performance monitoring. Durch S, Bailey LA, and Stoto MA (eds.). Washington, D.C.: National Academy Press, 1997.
7. Office of Disease Prevention and Health Promotion, U.S. Department of Health and Human Services. Leading indicators for Healthy People 2010: a report from the HHS Working Group on Sentinel Objectives. Washington, D.C.: DHHS, March 1998.
8. Roemer MI. Analysis of a national health system. In: Detels R, Holland WW, McEwen J, Omenn, GS (eds.). Oxford Textbook of Public Health. Volume 2. New York: Oxford University Press, 1997: 1539–51.
9. National Research Council, Panel on Performance Measures and Data for Public Health Performance Partnership Grants. Assessment of performance measures for public health, substance abuse, and mental health. Washington, D.C.: National Academy Press, 1997:5–12.
10. Pearce ND. Information resources in the United States. In: Detels R, Holland WW, McEwen J, Omenn GS (eds.). Oxford textbook of public health. Volume 2. New York: Oxford University Press, 1997:435–50.
11. Thacker SB, Stroup DF. Future directions for comprehensive public health surveillance and health information systems in the United States. *Am J Epidemiol* 1994;140:383–97.
12. Bettcher DW, Sapirie S, Goon EHT. Essential public health functions: results of the international Delphi study. *World Health Stat Q* 1998;51(1):44–54.

13. Public Health Functions Steering Committee. Essential public health services. Washington, D.C.: American Public Health Association, 1994.
14. Vaugh JP, Morrow RH. Manual of epidemiology for district health management. Geneva: World Health Organization, 1989.
15. Sandiford P, Annett H, Cibulskis R. What can information systems do for primary health care? An international perspective. *Soc Sci Med* 1992;34(10):1077–87.
16. Abramson JH. Survey methods in community medicine. Fourth edition. Edinburgh: Churchill Livingston, 1990.
17. Buehler JW. Surveillance. In: Rothman KJ, Greenland S (eds.). Modern epidemiology. Second edition. Philadelphia: Lippincott Williams & Wilkins, 1998:435–7.
18. Kreisel W, von Schirnding Y. Intersectoral action for health: a cornerstone for health for all in the 21st century. *World Health Stat Q* 1998;51(1):75–8.
19. Abramson JH. Survey methods in community medicine. Third edition. Edinburgh: Churchill Livingston, 1984.
20. Henderson DA. Surveillance of smallpox. *Int J Epidemiol* 1976;5(1):19–28.
21. Rifkin SB, Muller F, Bichmann W. Primary health care: on measuring participation. *Soc Sci Med* 1988;26(9):931–40.
22. Devine O, Parrish RG. Monitoring the health of a population. In: Stroup DF, Teutsch SM (eds.). Statistics in public health. New York: Oxford University Press, 1998:60–6.
23. Centers for Disease Control and Prevention. Case definitions for infectious conditions under public health surveillance. *MMWR* 1997;46(No. RR-10).
24. Foege WH *et al.* Surveillance projects for selected diseases. *Int J Epidemiol* 1976; 5(1):29–37.
25. Thacker SB, Stroup DF, Parrish RG, Anderson HA. Surveillance in environmental public health: issues, systems, and sources. *Am J Public Health* 1996;86:633–8.
26. Centers for Disease Control. Principles of epidemiology. Second edition. Atlanta: CDC, 1992.
27. Stroup NE, Zack MM, Wharton M. Sources of routinely collected data for surveillance. In: Teutsch S, Churchill E (eds.). Principles and practice of public health surveillance. New York: Oxford University Press, 1994:31–85.
28. Thacker SB, Wetterhall SF. Data sources for public health. In: Stroup DF, Teutsch SM (eds.). Statistics in public health. New York: Oxford University Press, 1998:39–57.
29. Simoes EJ, Brownson RC. Implementing and managing programs. In: Stroup DF, Teutsch SM (eds.). Statistics in public health. New York: Oxford University Press, 1998:165–92.
30. Otten M. Important surveillance issues in developing countries. In: Teutsch S, Churchill E (eds.). Principles and practice of public health surveillance. New York: Oxford, 1994:235–55.
31. Oxford English Dictionary. Glasgow: Oxford University Press, 1971.
32. Webster's Third New International Dictionary. G & C Merriam Co., 1976. See also Merriam Webster Online Dictionary (http://www.m-w.com).
33. Rutstein DD, Berenberg W, Chalmers TC, Child CG, Fishman AP, Perrin EB. Measuring the quality of medical care: a clinical method. *N Engl J Med* 1976;294:582–8.
34. Rutstein DD, Berenberg W, Chalmers TC, Fishman AP, Perrin EB, Zuidema GD. Measuring the quality of medical care: a second revision of tables and indexes [letter to the editor]. *N Engl J Med* 1980;302:1146.
35. Rutstein DD, Mullan RJ, Frazier TM, Halperin WE, Melius JM, Sestito JP. Sentinel health events (occupational): a basis for physician recognition and public health surveillance. *Am J Public Health* 1983;73(9):1054–62.

36. Communicable Disease Center. Communicable Disease Center Activities 1952–1953. Public Health Service Publication Number 391. Atlanta: Department of Health, Education, and Welfare, 1953.
37. Langmuir AD. The surveillance of communicable diseases of national importance. *N Engl J Med* 1963:268(4):182–92.
38. World Health Organization. Report of the technical discussions at the Twenty-First World Health Assembly on national and global surveillance of communicable diseases. Geneva: WHO, 1968:A21.
39. *International Journal of Epidemiology* 1976;5(1). The editorials and articles from that issue and cited below addressed surveillance:

Editorial: Surveillance: pages 3–4.

Editorial: Epidemiological surveillance: pages 4–6.

Editorial: Smallpox eradication: pages 6–7.

Langmuir AD. William Farr: founder of modern concepts of surveillance: pages 13–8.

Henderson DA. Surveillance of smallpox: pages 19–28.

Foege WH *et al.* Surveillance projects for selected diseases: pages 29–37.

Lucas AO. Surveillance of communicable diseases in tropical Africa: pages 39–43.

Miller DL. Monitoring communicable disease: vaccination programmes: pages 45–50.

Morley D. Nutritional surveillance of young children in developing countries: pages 51–5.

Irwig LM. Surveillance in developed countries with particular reference to child growth: pages 57–61.

Styblo K. Surveillance of tuberculosis: pages 63–8.

Griffith GW. Cancer surveillance with particular reference to the uses of mortality data: pages 69–76.

Fejfar Z. Surveillance and monitoring of cardiovascular disease: assessment of trends: pages 77–81.

McLachlan G. Monitoring health services: pages 83–6.

Hartgerink MJ. Health surveillance and planning for health care in the Netherlands: pages 87–91.
40. Thacker SB, Berkelman RL. Public health surveillance in the United States. *Epidemiol Rev* 1988;10:164–90.
41. Wegman DH. Hazard surveillance. In: Halperin W, Baker E, Monson R (eds.). Public health surveillance. New York: Van Nostrand Reinhold, 1992:62–5.
42. Aday LU. Designing and conducting health surveys: a comprehensive guide. San Francisco: Jossey-Bass, 1989.
43. National Association of County Health Officials. Assessment protocol for excellence in public health (APEXPH). Washington, D.C.: National Association of County Health Officials, 1991.
44. Feinleib M. From information to knowledge: assimilating public health data. *Am J Public Health* 1993;83(9):1205–7.
45. Klaucke DN, Beuhler JW, Thacker SB, Parrish RG *et al.* Guidelines for evaluating surveillance systems. *MMWR* 1988;37(No. S-5):1–18.
46. Thacker SB, Parrish RG, Trowbridge FL *et al.* A method for evaluating systems of epidemiological surveillance. *World Health Stat Q* 1988;41:11–8.
47. World Health Organization. Protocol for the evaluation of epidemiological surveillance systems. Geneva: WHO, 1997.

4

The Changing Health-Care Information Infrastructure in the United States: Opportunities for a New Approach to Public Health Surveillance

DENISE KOO
R. GIBSON PARRISH II

It is change, continuing change, inevitable change, that is the dominant factor in society today. No sensible decision can be made any longer without taking into account not only the world as it is, but the world as it will be.

Isaac Asimov

The medical system in the United States has changed considerably over the last 10 to 15 years, primarily because of the growth of organized health-care delivery systems, including health-maintenance organizations. By 1997, nearly 70 million Americans were enrolled in health maintenance organizations, a ten-fold increase from 1978 (*1*). These figures include mounting numbers of Medicare and Medicaid beneficiaries who have moved or been shifted into managed care to control costs and improve access to care. These figures do not include preferred-provider organizations, another form of managed care that is rapidly expanding but for which enrollment is more difficult to measure. Continuing mergers and acquisitions among hospitals and medical practices along with wider variability in the insurance products offered has also led to fluidity in the size and composition of health-care organizations. These changes provide important opportunities for public health, as managed-care organizations and the general medical community have become increasingly concerned with costs and provision of cost-effective health care, especially prevention and population-based health (see Chapter 14). For example, some health plans have implemented practices geared toward improving the level of immunization and cancer screening among their enrollees (*2*). Another important change is the shift of public health from direct delivery of certain health-care services toward ensuring (through purchase, regulation, or negotiation) that appropriate health services are available and accessible.

This interdependence of public health and health care is also reflected in current thinking about medicine and medical education. Recent reports by the American Association of Medical Colleges and the Pew Health Professions Commission acknowledged that in the next century understanding and application of the principles of population-based health, i.e., "the epidemiology of common maladies within a defined population, and the systematic approaches useful in reducing the incidence and prevalence of such maladies" will be a critical competency for health professionals (3,4). In addition to the changes described above, these reports cite the evolving and necessary shift to a focus on health, rather than medical care, in an era of cost-cutting and accountability. The economic benefits of prevention have been increasingly recognized (5).

This increasing and appropriate acknowledgment of the interdependence of the public health and health-care systems provides the opportunity for a paradigm shift in the approach to public health surveillance, away from an independent disease-based orientation toward a more comprehensive, cross-cutting one. Such efforts would entail access of data from key sources for multiple health-related uses, including public health. Such a shift could improve dramatically the quality and quantity of information routinely collected on diseases or conditions of public health importance, as well as on behavioral and other risk factors that play a role in causing these diseases. Concurrent advances in information technology and processing also facilitate this opportunity to transform the practice of public health. Public health, therefore, is attempting to take advantage of these opportunities by moving away from independent disease-based systems to collect data toward a more comprehensive approach that involves capture of data that are already electronic, especially from, although not limited to, the health-care system. Such an approach acknowledges the interdependence especially of public health and health-care delivery, and should improve the efficiency of systems to support both. It requires new partnerships with other federal, state, and local government agencies, as well as private organizations such as managed care, standards development organizations, laboratories, and medical informaticians. This chapter briefly reviews the traditional approach to public health surveillance, describes a future vision for public health surveillance (focused especially on its relationship to the health-care system), portrays the current environment, outlines barriers and facilitating factors in the path toward this long-term vision, and relates various activities under way in the United States.

THE TRADITIONAL APPROACH TO PUBLIC HEALTH SURVEILLANCE

In 1963 Langmuir described the surveillance of diseases, and in particular, the surveillance of infectious diseases, which at the time were a major focus of public health programs (6). Traditionally, surveillance for infectious diseases has involved the reporting of individual cases of disease or isolates of microorganisms by individual health-care providers or laboratories to local or state health departments. This reporting is generally passive; that is, it relies on health-care providers or laboratories to report to public health authorities. Submission of reports by mail, telephone, or facsimile were—and remain—the most common means of reporting to the health department. Public health officials at state health departments and the CDC collaborate in determining which infectious diseases should be reported (i.e., "notifiable") particularly on a national basis, although reporting by providers and laboratories is mandated only at the state level (by state legislation or regulation). State health departments, in turn, accumulate these reports from local health departments and on a weekly basis report them to CDC, who coordinates and publishes national data in preliminary form weekly in the *MMWR,* and in final form at year end in the annual *Summary of Notifiable Diseases, United States (7,8).*

This emphasis on infectious diseases has persisted, but starting in the late 1970s and continuing through the 1980s, interest in and approaches to surveillance for other health outcomes and risk factors for these outcomes were developed, including surveillance for behavioral risk factors, occupational exposures and injuries, drug abuse–related mortality, and transportation–related deaths. In the 1990s, the number of outcomes and risk factors expanded even further. Various environmental hazards are also under surveillance, including air pollutants, and biological and chemical water contaminants (9). In part because the data sources and needs for each of these problems are different and also because the U.S. Congress funds individual public health programs for disease prevention and control (e.g., sexually transmitted diseases, tuberculosis, cancer, occupational illness), most of these programs have independently developed methods to gather information for a specific health problem, which has limited the breadth of their applicability and their efficiency for public health as a whole (see Chapter 3). For example, programs with responsibility for monitoring the occurrence of birth defects and determining their causes cannot easily access data from infectious disease surveillance systems (which are located in another program), data which might be useful for evaluating the causal association between birth defects and certain infectious diseases. Or, persons responsible for control of occupational diseases such as tuberculosis do not have ready access to surveillance data about the incidence of tuberculosis among different worker populations. In part this also reflects the fact that, compared to other health-related activities at the local, state, and federal levels, surveillance—setting up an efficient, coordinated system for gathering information—has received few resources, in spite of its crucial role in monitoring health problems (10–12). The lack of critical funding for the infrastructure for public health surveillance has resulted in this fragmented approach to surveillance, one that was initially magnified rather than ameliorated by the use of information technology.

Use of Information Technology in Surveillance

Starting in the mid- to late 1980s with the widespread availability of personal computers, the ways in which surveillance, particularly for infectious diseases, was conducted and information transmitted among public health agencies began to change. Personal computers provided the means for automating this process and the potential for improving the type, timeliness, quantity, and accuracy of the data for surveillance. The first attempt to integrate various systems developed for surveillance was the National Electronic Telecommunications System for Surveillance (NETSS), operated by CDC (7,13). To achieve this NETSS, which supported the National Notifiable Diseases Surveillance system, provided a standard record format and variables for reporting all individual cases of disease, and did not require the use of a specific software application. In addition to the common format and variables, NETSS also incorporated disease-specific data elements at the end of the standard record, for certain infectious diseases (e.g., hepatitis, meningitis). Some states developed their own NETSS applications using dBase, Foxpro, or other application development software, while the majority used a customized version of a NETSS application built with *Epi Info*™ software by CDC. The NETSS standard record allowed the continued use or development of distinct state systems, while facilitating the creation of an aggregated, integrated national data base for notifiable diseases.

Despite the initial promise of this model for standardized reporting of data to CDC, other CDC programs provided with funding by Congress for the surveillance, study, and control of specific diseases (e.g., tuberculosis, sexually transmitted diseases [STDs], acquired immunodeficiency syndrome [AIDS], lead exposure) independently developed disease-specific computer applications for use at the state (and sometimes local) level for the collection, entry, and analysis of surveillance data. The distinct funding streams, mechanisms for delivering clinical care and health services, partners, and data sources (e.g., STD program managers and clinics for STDs, TB program managers and clinics for TB, and clinical laboratories for blood lead levels) promoted such independence. Examples of these systems for infectious diseases include the Human Immunodeficiency Virus/AIDS Reporting System (HARS), the Sexually Transmitted Disease Management Information System (STD-MIS), and the Surveillance System for Tuberculosis (SURVS-TB, now replaced by the Tuberculosis Information Management System, TIMS). Examples of these systems for other conditions include the Adult Blood Lead Epidemiology and Surveillance program (ABLES) and the Childhood Blood Lead Surveillance System.

These systems played an important role in standardizing reporting across the nation for their respective diseases. As such, they provided, and continue to provide, information that is crucial to public health practice. However, a crucial shortcoming of these systems is that they were not horizontally integrated. Variables common to multiple systems, classification and coding schemes, user interfaces, data-base formats, and methods for transmitting or analyzing data were unit modifier not standardized. Most of these applications did not allow the import or export of data. Personnel at local and state health departments were required to use multiple, incompatible applications to enter and analyze data; data could not easily be exchanged, linked, or merged by different programs (e.g., notifiable disease reports and laboratory reports of isolates). As the sophistication of local and state health departments in computing and information management and the need to exchange and use electronic data increased, the shortcomings of the initial, uncoordinated, and unstandardized efforts to computerize surveillance (and the delivery of certain public health clinical services, e.g., STD and TB control) became apparent.

The Need for a Comprehensive Approach

This disease-based approach to prevention and control, with its accompanying disease-specific surveillance information systems, makes it more difficult for state and local health departments to efficiently assess the diseases and health problems in their communities. In order to evaluate the overall health of their jurisdictions, local and state health officials must use and access multiple information systems. In addition, these distinct approaches to prevention and control of various conditions impede the development of unified strategies for delivery of individual health-care services and public health interventions. For example, separate programs for STDs and hepatitis B hampered development of integrated approaches to controlling the spread of diseases that are all transmitted sexually (*14*), and maternal and child health programs cannot easily access data in the independent surveillance information systems for childhood lead poisoning and vaccine-preventable diseases. It was clear by the mid-1990s that a change in the approach to conducting public health surveillance and building information systems to support these activities was needed (*12,15*).

THE FUTURE OF PUBLIC HEALTH SURVEILLANCE

Public health continues to expand the variety and sources of data for surveillance in order to monitor more completely both old and new public health problems (*16–23*). We have already noted that public health officials are generally interested in surveillance data on hazardous agents (whether chemical or biological), behaviors, exposures, health events/conditions, and deaths.

Information on the health-care system and its effects on health are also important: service delivery and information on public health programs, including coverage of preventive services. Because the most appropriate data source varies for a given problem or disease, public health professionals frequently must combine information from multiple, usually incompatible systems and sources to obtain a more inclusive and accurate depiction of the problem—e.g., an accurate estimate of its incidence, the prevalence of behavioral or environmental risk factors, and the availability and use of preventive services related to the disease or condition. As was also described above, such efforts are usually undertaken independently, that is, individual public health programs at the federal or state level gather data from state or local health departments, laboratories, and other federal or state agencies in a different way, using resources that are often duplicative. For improved efficiency, a more comprehensive and better coordinated approach to public health surveillance and to gathering and disseminating data is needed.

Rethinking public health surveillance in a more comprehensive fashion can provide not only increased efficiency, but also increased effectiveness. A more coherent approach would support efficient data collection from multiple sources, such as computerized medical and laboratory records as well as sources of data outside the health arena (e.g., environmental monitoring systems, highway traffic crash data). It would use standards for data elements and transmission of data, and ensure appropriate linkage and integration of systems. Public health officials would be able in a more timely and effective fashion to access and use data to depict current disease trends or to detect outbreaks and to document new or emerging problems missed by the current myriad, fragmented surveillance systems. They would be able to make public health policy and implement interventions that are comprehensive, such as designing a prevention program for all childhood diseases and conditions, rather than separate programs for vaccine-preventable diseases, lead poisoning, nutrition, violence, etc. But the complexity of taking an integrated approach to surveillance cannot be underestimated.

An essential and immediate area of focus for these efforts, given the substantial reliance of public health on data originating from health-care providers, is at the interface of public health and the health-care system. In the integrated public health and health-care information system of the future, "health-related data and information is [sic] generated automatically, as a by-product of delivering and paying for medical care and carrying out essential public health services" and such data are captured electronically by public health (24). This desired endpoint will require increased collaboration among agencies and organizations traditionally responsible for health-care provision and reimbursement and those responsible for public health. Public health officials will need to ensure that evolving standards for a computer-based patient record (25) facilitate its use by public health, e.g., the exchange of clinically relevant data for public health surveillance.

Future Scenarios

Imagine a scenario from this future: a public health computer system would alert public health officials in real time of a substantial increase in the incidence of an uncommon neurologic syndrome, distributed across the country. This increase would have been detected because the computer was automatically searching health-care data bases across the country, and was programmed to note increases above "baseline" in any problem. The public health official requests and evaluates the data, and notes that the syndrome is indeed an unusual one, and that the increase has taken place over the last few months. Upon further query of medical data bases for any common characteristics among those affected, the official learns that many patients were recorded as having had a new outpatient procedure, X. This procedure usually involved treatment with anesthetic A. A quick query about this anesthetic reveals other procedures (Y, Z) during which the drug is used, and it is noted that all patients ill with this uncommon problem had either procedure X, Y, or Z. In addition, through a query of health-care data bases for all patients receiving anesthetic A in the last few months, the public health official finds that several of them have also suffered from a condition similar to the one of interest, but were diagnosed with a variant of the uncommon syndrome (which was not picked up by the computer as it is even more rare). At this point the official is very concerned and calls the Food and Drug Administration (FDA), as well as the company that manufactures the drug, to find out more. Through these and other inquiries of drug, chemical, and medical procedure data bases, it is learned that this anesthetic was newly on the market and had not been used previously in this procedure, and that the procedure involves use of a dye that mixes, at least in the laboratory, with the solvent for the anesthetic to form a dangerous neurotoxic compound. Upon notification of these findings, the FDA immediately issues a moratorium on the use of the anesthetic in procedures involving the dye, pending further investigation.

In a simpler scenario, the computer tracks the rate of drug resistance among isolates of various bacteria, and flags increasing resistance to antibiotic P. Through a query of pharmaceutical data bases across the country, the public health official notes an increase in utilization/sales of this antibiotic in the period over the last several years, prior to and concurrent with the increase in resistance. Regardless of whether this is cause or effect, the official drafts a notice to health-care providers for these areas of the country, pointing out the likely decreased effectiveness of drug P. In addition, the official makes plans to step up the campaign for the judicious use of antibiotics.

Barriers and Facilitating Factors for the Future

The 1995 report of the U.S. Public Health Service entitled *Making a Powerful Connection: The Health of the Public and the National Information Infrastructure* highlighted the opportunity to integrate public health and health-care delivery and argued that in order to move in this direction, "health-care organizations and the public health community will need to coordinate not only their roles and responsibilities, but also their information systems" (24). The report described several requirements for the development of "logically integrated health information systems, in which information collected once can serve multiple purposes." They cited the need for nationally uniform policies for data standards, privacy and security, unique identifiers, and data sharing. They also mentioned organizational and financial barriers as well as a lack of informatics training in public health as impediments to the development of such policies. Below, we describe some of these barriers and factors that will facilitate overcoming them.

Standards for Health Information

The Health Insurance Portability and Accountability Act

Standards for exchanging electronic data are the critical glue for improving the sharing and use of health information systems of all kinds. In 1996, the U.S. Congress passed the Health Insurance Portability and Accountability Act (HIPAA) (P.L. 104-191), which at the request of health-care providers and the industry that finances health-care contained provisions for administrative simplification, i.e., it mandated the development, implementation, and use of standards for exchanging financial and administrative data related to health care. In order to increase the administrative efficiency of health care, these provisions required the Secretary of the Department of Health and Human Services (DHHS) to adopt by February 1999 national uniform standards for electronic transactions related to health insurance enrollment and eligibility, health-care encounters, and health insurance claims; for identifiers for health-care providers, payers and individuals, as well as code sets and classification systems used in these transactions; and for security of these transactions. An approach to standards for the electronic exchange of medical record data must also be recommended by August 2000. (For up-to-date information about the status of these standards, see http://aspe.os.dhhs.gov/admnsimp.) Anyone who conducts these transactions electronically will be required to use these national standards, which include input from standards development organizations, the health-care industry, and state and local government. However, agreement on standards is particularly challenging because of the diverse needs of the groups who record and use health information, including providers, payers, administrators, researchers, and public health officials. Most of the coding systems or standards currently in use have not previously taken into account public health data needs, and public health's interests are not uniformly regarded as compatible with the business needs of other organizations (26).

However, HIPAA has provided the impetus for various standards development organizations (SDOs) and terminology and coding groups to work collaboratively to harmonize their separate systems (27). For example, both the American National Standards Institute–accredited SDO the Accredited Standards Committee (ASC) X12N (http://www.x12.org), which has dealt in the past principally with standards for health insurance transactions, and Health Level Seven (HL7, http://www.hl7.org), which has dealt with standards for clinical messaging and exchange of clinical information within health-care institutions (e.g., hospitals), have collaborated on a standardized approach for providing supplementary information to support health-care claims (the draft Notice of Proposed Rulemaking for Claims Attachments, Health Care Financing Administration). The payers, billing and clinical arenas, and their respective organizations had traditionally remained separate. In the area of the classification and coding of diseases and other medical terms, the National Library of Medicine has traditionally provided the Unified Medical Language System, a metathesaurus for clinical coding systems that allows terms in one coding system to be mapped to another (28,29). The passage of HIPAA and the anticipated adoption of standards for electronic medical records has increased the level of efforts directed toward the integration of clinical terminologies such as the U.S. College of American Pathologists' Systematized Nomenclature of Medicine (SNOMED) and the British Read codes, the National Health Service thesaurus of health-care terms in Great Britain; as of March 1999, it was agreed that these two clinical terminologies would be merged (30).

Until recently, public health agencies had not worked closely with SDOs such as ASC X12 or HL7, or with clinical coding systems. Thus, neither health-care information systems nor public health information systems took into account issues such as electronic transmission of laboratory data directly to public health agencies, using medical codes designated by public health as relevant, or capture and coding of behavioral or environmental risk factors in the medical record, or even simply the capture of race and ethnicity or educational background with the enrollment of a patient. Development of integrated data systems for public health requires clear definition of public health data needs and the sources for these data, consensus on data and communications standards—to facilitate comparability and exchange of data—along with policies to support data sharing, and generation of mechanisms and tools for accessing and disseminating such data in a useful manner. Below we describe some public health activities directed toward ensuring the utility and re-usability of data captured in clinical systems for population-based health.

Privacy of Health Information

Of course, having similar standards and coding for data will not be useful if it is not permissible to share the data, and maintaining the privacy of a person's health information is a key requirement for allowing the sharing of data with others. Health information privacy refers to "an individual's claim to control the circumstances in which personally identifiable health information is collected, used, and disclosed" (*31*). Current privacy protection of health information is based on a patchwork of state laws and regulations that predate the electronic age and do not provide adequate protection for either paper or electronic health information; no federal statute currently exists that protects the confidentiality of all personally identifiable health data (*32,33*). Consumers have many apprehensions about sharing electronic health records with outsiders in this dawning era of computerized medical records, and health information privacy is, therefore, a hotly debated topic. Several bills introduced in the U.S. Congress in recent years were intended to provide privacy protection while still permitting critical analytic uses of data. These bills generally include the following: a definition of protected health information, description of disclosures that may occur only with consent, and disclosures that may occur without consent, such as to public health for surveillance purposes. None of these bills has yet become law, but HIPAA requires that the Secretary of Health and Human Services promulgate privacy standards by regulatory authority if privacy legislation is not enacted by Congress.

Security

Lost in the discussion about health information privacy and amid concerns about electronic medical records is the recognition that use of electronic information systems can actually result in *improved* security of medical data (*34*). Security includes technological, organizational, and administrative processes designed to ensure that data systems are accessed only by authorized persons. It is widely acknowledged that the technology exists for markedly improved security and protection of electronic health information, and the National Research Council (NRC) has made recommendations for how to ensure such security (*35*). Several institutions have collaborated to demonstrate the feasibility and efficacy of an approach that incorporates these recommendations (*36*). Nationally, security standards for health information systems that closely follow the NRC recommendations are under development as part of HIPAA. In addition, given aforementioned concerns about privacy and confidentiality, CDC has developed agency-wide Internet security standards and a secure Internet pipeline for transmission of data that are consistent with the NRC recommendations for security of health-related data. It is hoped that these standards will eventually facilitate electronic exchange of data between public health and the health-care system.

Unique Health Identifier

Related to the immediately preceding issue of privacy and security is that of unique health identifiers, especially for individuals. One of the standards mandated by HIPAA is that of a unique health identifier for individuals, which would allow for longitudinal and geographic links among a patient's health-care records. Unique health identifiers for individuals (in addition to those for providers, health plans, and employers) would not only increase the availability and quality of information for improved clinical care of the patient, but would also facilitate the exchange and linkage of health data for population-based functions like public health surveillance. However, in part due to fears about privacy, and because there is as yet no overarching federal law protecting health information privacy, the United States still has not defined a mechanism for assigning unique health identifiers to individuals.

Organizational Issues

As should be apparent from the discussion in the immediately preceding section, integration of public health and health-care delivery systems is not primarily a technical problem, but rather a political and an organizational one. The DHHS is organized into 11 operating divisions, of which CDC/ATSDR is only one (Table 4–1). Clearly, other DHHS agencies have responsibilities for and collect data from the public and various parts of the health-care delivery system. Some of these data are also useful for public health surveillance. However, each of these agencies operates independently and develops partnerships with its own programmatic contacts, not unlike the partnerships developed by CDC's disease-specific programs with their state-based counterparts (e.g., HCFA with state Medicaid or Medicare directors; FDA with state food agencies). The organizational and managerial challenges of coordinating the efforts of these DHHS agencies cannot be understated and similar challenges have already been recognized in the medical informatics field (37–39).

Acknowledging the need for increased coordination around data issues, the DHHS formed the Data Council in August 1995. The Data Council coordinates all health and non-health data collection and analysis activities of the DHHS. These activities include developing an integrated health data collection strategy, coordinating health data standards, and dealing with health information and privacy issues. The Data Council is also the focal point for the DHHS interactions with the National Committee on Vital and Health Statistics (NCVHS), an external advisory committee to the Secretary of the DHHS in the areas of health data policy, data standards, privacy concerns related to health information, and population-based data.

Together with the National Center for Health Statistics (part of CDC) and the Data Council, the NCVHS is developing a vision for health statistics for the 21st

Table 4–1 U.S. Department of Health and Human Services: Operating Divisions

Division	Mission/Overview
National Institutes of Health (NIH)	The NIH mission is to uncover new knowledge that will lead to better health for everyone. The NIH works toward that mission by conducting research in its own laboratories; supporting the research of nonfederal scientists in universities, medical schools, hospitals, and research institutions, throughout the country and abroad; helping in the training of research investigators; and fostering communication of biomedical information. The NIH comprises 24 separate institutes, centers, and divisions which include the National Library of Medicine and the National Center for Human Genome Research. The NIH has 75 buildings on more than 300 acres in Bethesda, MD. Established: 1887, as the Hygienic Laboratory, Staten Island, N.Y. Headquarters: Bethesda, MD
Food and Drug Administration (FDA)	The FDA assures the safety of foods and cosmetics, and the safety and efficacy of pharmaceuticals, biological products, and medical devices. The FDA is charged with protecting American consumers by enforcing the federal Food, Drug, and Cosmetic Act and several related public health laws. To carry out this mandate of consumer protection, the FDA has some 1100 investigators and inspectors who cover the country's almost 95,000 FDA-regulated businesses. These employees are located in district and local offices in 157 cities across the country. Established: 1906. Headquarters: Rockville, MD
Centers for Disease Control and Prevention (CDC)	The CDC's mission is to promote health and quality of life by preventing and controlling disease, injury, and disability. Working with states and other partners, the CDC provides a system of health surveillance to monitor and prevent outbreak of diseases, and maintains national health statistics. The CDC also guards against international disease transmission, with CDC personnel stationed in more than 25 foreign countries and supports research into disease and injury prevention. Established: 1946, as the Communicable Disease Center. Headquarters: Atlanta, GA
Agency for Toxic Substances and Disease Registry (ATSDR)	Working with states and other federal agencies, the ATSDR seeks to prevent exposure to hazardous substances from waste sites. The agency conducts public health assessments, health studies, surveillance activities, and health education training in communities around waste sites on the U.S. Environmental Protection Agency's National Priorities List. The ATSDR also has developed toxicological profiles of hazardous chemicals found at these sites. Established: 1980. Headquarters: Atlanta, GA
Indian Health Service (IHS)	The IHS provides a comprehensive health services delivery system for American Indians and Alaska Natives with opportunity for maximum tribal involvement in

Table 4–1 U.S. Department of Health and Human Services: Operating Divisions (Continued)

Division	Mission/Overview
	developing and managing programs to meet health needs. The mission of the IHS, in partnership with American Indian and Alaska Native people, is to raise their physical, mental, social, and spiritual health to the highest level. The IHS provides health services to 1.4 million American Indians and Alaska Natives, with 37 hospitals and more than 100 other health facilities in 27 states. Established: 1924 (mission transferred from the Interior Department in 1955). Headquarters: Rockville, MD
Health Resources and Services - Administration (HRSA)	The HRSA directs national health programs which improve the health of the nation by assuring quality health care to underserved, vulnerable, and special-needs populations and by promoting appropriate health professions workforce capacity and practice, particularly in primary care and public health. The HRSA helps provide health resources for medically underserved populations. A nationwide network of 643 community and migrant health centers, plus 144 primary care programs for the homeless and residents of public housing, serve 8.1 million Americans each year. The HRSA also works to build the health-care workforce and maintains the National Health Service Corps and provides services to people with AIDS through the Ryan White CARE Act programs. Established: 1982, bringing together several already-existing programs. Headquarters: Rockville, MD
Substance Abuse and Mental Health Services Administration (SAMHSA)	The SAMHSA's mission within the nation's health system is to improve the quality and availability of prevention, treatment, and rehabilitation services in order to reduce illness, death, disability, and cost to society resulting from substance abuse and mental illnesses. The SAMHSA's mission is accomplished in partnership with all concerned with substance abuse and mental illnesses. The SAMHSA provides funding through block grants to states for direct substance abuse and mental health services, including treatment for over 340,000 Americans with serious substance abuse problems; helps improve substance abuse treatment through its Knowledge Development and Applications grant program; monitors prevalence and incidence of substance abuse and mental illness. Established: 1992 (a predecessor agency, the Alcohol, Drug Abuse and Mental Health Administration, was established in 1974). Headquarters: Rockville, MD
Agency for Healthcare Research and Quality (AHRQ) formerly Agency for Health Care Policy and Research (AHCPR)	The AHRQ was established in December 1989 under Public Law 101-239 (Omnibus Budget Reconciliation Act of 1989). The AHRQ is the lead agency charged with supporting research designed to improve the quality of health care, reduce its cost, and broaden access to essential services. The agency's broad programs of *(continued)*

87

Table 4–1 U.S. Department of Health and Human Services: Operating Divisions (Continued)

Division	Mission/Overview
	research bring practical, science-based information to medical practitioners and to consumers and other health-care purchasers. Established: 1989. Headquarters: Rockville, MD
Human Services Operating Divisions	
Health Care Financing Administration (HCFA)	The HCFA administers Medicare, Medicaid, and the Child Health Insurance Program, which provide health-care coverage to about one in every five Americans. Medicare provides health insurance for 37 million elderly and disabled Americans. Medicaid, a joint federal-state program, provides health coverage for 36 million low-income persons, including 17.6 million children. Medicaid also pays for nursing home coverage for low-income elderly, covering almost half of total national spending for nursing home care. In addition to providing health insurance, the HCFA also regulates all laboratory testing (except research) in the United States through the Clinical Laboratory Improvement Amendments (CLIA) program. Established: 1977. Headquarters: Baltimore, MD
Administration for Children and Families (ACF)	The ACF, within the DHHS, is responsible for federal programs which promote the economic and social well-being of families, children, individuals, and communities. ACF administers the new state-federal welfare program, Temporary Assistance to Needy Families, providing assistance to an estimated 12.2 million persons, including 8.4 million children; a national child support enforcement system, collecting some $11.8 billion in 1996 in payments from non-custodial parents; and the Head Start program, serving about 800,000 preschool children. ACF also provides funds to assist low-income families in paying for child care, and supports state programs to provide for foster card adoption assistance; and funds programs to prevent child abuse and domestic violence. Established: 1991, bringing together several already-existing programs. Headquarters: Washington, DC
Administration on Aging (AA)	The mission of the AA is to enable the DHHS to respond the diverse needs of our aging population. The AA has the charge of serving the nation's 43 million seniors. The AA has a network of 670 Area Agencies on Aging, 57 Territorial and State Units on Aging, 270 tribes and native organizations, and over 27,000 service providers, and supports some 240 million meals for the elderly each year, including home-delivered "Meals on Wheels"; helps provide transportation and at-home services; supports ombudsman services for the elderly; and provides policy leadership on aging issues

century, one that is supportive of the concept of integration of public health and health-care delivery systems (*40*). It is intended that the vision reflect all manifestations of health and health-care delivery, and encompass population health, health-care delivery systems, and the interactions between the two. This vision will integrate and coordinate public and private data sets, and national, state, and locally collected and maintained data. The NCVHS also recommends building and integrating the health information infrastructure through a set of technologies, standards, and applications that support communication and information, into a National Health Information Infrastructure. They have described three component types of computer-based health records: patient (clinical care), personal (consumer), and population, for monitoring the health of the public and outcomes. They have recommended that this infrastructure be driven by patient care and health status, and not by reimbursement. This comprehensive view is consistent with the long-term direction in which public health needs to go.

ACTIVITIES IN THE PUBLIC HEALTH ARENA

The CDC and many of its partner public health organizations have acknowledged that our "national" system to gather public health information is a fragmented patchwork of multiple systems, and each has described a vision for a more unified future (*41–44*). Each of these visions acknowledges the key role of information for public health decision making, and implicitly or explicitly states that the development of integrated and comprehensive public health information systems requires the ongoing cooperation, collaboration, and contributions of public and private organizations. These include but are not limited to state and local health department epidemiologists, public and private medical and public health laboratories, state and federal vital statistics programs, federal agencies (e.g., in addition to the DHHS agencies, the Department of Transportation, the Environmental Protection Agency, and the Department of Labor), managed-care organizations, professional organizations, and national standards development organizations.

One step taken at CDC was the formation of a high-level policy board to oversee and coordinate activities directed toward its vision of integrated health information and surveillance systems. The CDC Health Information and Surveillance Systems Board (HISSB) met for the first time in January 1996, and its membership includes several public health partner organizations. Activities conducted under the auspices of or adopted as policy by the HISSB fall into several overlapping categories (see http://www.cdc.gov/od/hissb):

- policies to support integration of public health surveillance and information systems
- development of standards for data and security
- activities to strengthen the public health information infrastructure through increased connectivity and training of the work force
- collaborative projects with parts of the health-care system

Examples of the latter include connectivity to the Internet, such as that provided through the Information Network for Public Health Officials (INPHO) (45). Collaborative projects with parts of the health-care system (e.g., private laboratories, emergency departments, managed-care organizations, standards-development organizations) are described in detail in the Web site listed above.

Through the HISSB, CDC is undertaking an effort to integrate several of its major surveillance systems as a first step toward full integration of public health surveillance activities into a network of systems that are "coordinated, interconnected, comparable, and easy to use" (15). A key component of this project includes elucidating a data architecture or framework, based on a conceptual data model for public health surveillance with categories and properties of data needed for surveillance (e.g., persons, health-related activities, case definitions, risk factors), and relationships between them (e.g., a person can have many episodes of illness but each episode can only have one date of onset, with many dates for multiple specimens), as well as detailed standards for data elements (including variable definition, with valid values for possible responses, as well as standards for how to collect, code, calculate, store, and transfer the variable). These efforts will rely heavily on data standards currently under development (e.g., HIPAA, HL7 version 3, Common Request Broker Architecture for health care, CORBAMed: see http://www.omg.org/homepages/corbamed/), clinical terminologies and classification schemes (e.g., SNOMED, Read, International Classification of Diseases, version 10) that may play a role in the computerized medical record, and the next generation of the Internet and standards developed for it (e.g., XML—extensible markup language, see http://www.w3.org/XML/ and JAVA, see http://java.sun.com). Through these and other standards-related activities with its public health partners, health-care partners, and SDOs (e.g., defining electronic messaging standards for clinical laboratory data, and for immunization and cancer registries, developing electronic birth and death certificates, and standardizing Data Elements for Emergency Department), CDC is defining standards for data important to public health, in order to ensure representation of the public health perspective (46–52).

In exploring these new partnerships particularly with standards development organizations, public health has recognized the need for new skills among the public health workforce. These skills require an understanding of the role of data modeling and standards and the use of increasingly sophisticated information technology. Public health informatics is the "systematic application of information and computer science to public health practice, research, and learning" (53). In order to develop integrated systems for sharing data electronically with the health-care information infrastructure, it will be essential for all public health workers to have a basic understanding of public health informatics, and for some workers to develop a deeper understanding of the application of informatics to gathering data for public health. The CDC has made some initial efforts to develop the needed educational programs through a one-week general overview course in public health informatics for public health program managers (54) and a 2-year public health informatics fellowship for training persons interested in a career in public health informatics (see http://www.cdc.gov/epo/dphsi/informat.htm). It is hoped that through expansion of these programs and through partnerships with the National Library of Medicine, which sponsors training programs in medical informatics at academic medical centers across the country, the numbers of public health workers trained in informatics will steadily increase. These efforts are critical for assembling the pool of workers that will build and maintain our public health information systems in the future.

CONCLUSIONS

The continuing changes in the health-care system in the United States, the increased emphasis on standardization of health-care transactions, and the advent of the Internet and other advances in information technology are converging with a strong and growing interest in capturing health-related data electronically. Together these forces provide exciting opportunities to transform many of public health's monitoring functions, and to integrate them more closely with the health-care information infrastructure. To be most effective, the public health community must be able to use data from many different sources both within and outside of public health, with rapid dissemination of data to those who need to take action to protect the health of the public. The United States is well behind other countries such as Australia (55), Great Britain (56), and Canada (57), where efforts are well under way to integrate public health and health information systems and activities. To catch up, the United States needs to take a more proactive, integrated, and creative approach to monitoring and providing health-related services to its people.

We are grateful to Dr. Meade Morgan for his insightful comments.

REFERENCES

1. National Center for Health Statistics. Health, United States 1998, with socioeconomic status and health chartbook. Hyattsville, Md.: Centers for Disease Control and Prevention, 1998.
2. Stoto MA, Abel C, Dievler A (eds.). Healthy communities: new partnerships for the future of public health. Washington, D.C.: National Academy Press, 1996.
3. American Association of Medical Colleges. Contemporary issues in medicine: medical informatics and population health. Washington, D.C.: AAMC, June 1998.
4. Pew Health Professions Commission. Critical challenges: revitalizing the health professions for the twenty-first century, December 1995.
5. Messonier ML, Corso PS, Teutsch SM, Haddix AC, Harris JR. An ounce of prevention . . . what are the returns? Am J Prev Med 1999;16:248–63.
6. Langmuir AD. The surveillance of communicable disease of national importance. N Engl J Med 1963;268:182–92.
7. Koo D, Wetterhall SF. History and current status of the National Notifiable Diseases Surveillance System. J Public Health Management Practice 1996;2:4–10.
8. Centers for Disease Control and Prevention. Summary of notifiable diseases, United States 1997. MMWR 1997;46(54).

9. Thacker SB, Berkelman RL. Public health surveillance in the United States. *Epidemiol Rev* 1988:10:164–90.
10. Berkelman RL, Bryan RT, Osterholm MT, LeDuc JW, Hughes JM. Infectious disease surveillance: a crumbling foundation. *Science* 1994:264:368–70.
11. Osterholm MT, Birkhead GS, Meriwether RA. Impediments to public health surveillance in the 1990s: the lack of resources and the need for priorities. *J Public Health Management Practice* 1996;2:11–5.
12. Thacker SB, Stroup DF. Future directions for comprehensive public health surveillance and health information systems in the United States. *Am J Epidemiol* 1994:140:383–97.
13. Centers for Disease Control. National Electronic Telecommunications System for Surveillance—United States, 1990–1991. *MMWR* 1991;40:502–3.
14. Centers for Disease Control and Prevention. Recommendations for prevention and control of hepatitis C virus (HCV) infection and HCV-related chronic disease. *MMWR* 1998;47(No. RR-19).
15. Morris G, Snider D, Katz M. Integrating public health information and surveillance systems. *J Public Health Management Practice* 1996;2:24–7.
16. Koobatian TJ, Birkhead BS, Schramm MM, Vogt RL. The use of hospital discharge data for public health surveillance of Guillain-Barre Syndrome. *Ann Neurol* 1991;30:618–21.
17. Huff L, Bogdan G, Burke K *et al.* Using hospital discharge data for disease surveillance. *Public Health Rep* 1996;1111:78–81.
18. Thacker SB, Stroup, DF, Parrish RG, Anderson HA. Surveillance in environmental public health: issues, systems, and sources. *Am J Public Health* 1996:86:633–8.
19. Ackman DM, Birkhead G, Flynn M. Assessment of surveillance for meningococcal disease in New York State, 1991. *Am J Epidemiol* 1996;144:78–82.
20. Chen RT, Glasser JW, Rhodes, PH, Davis RL, Barlow WE, Thompson RS *et al.* Vaccine safety data-link project: a new tool for improving vaccine safety monitoring in the United States. *Pediatrics* 1997;99:765–73.
21. Newman TB, Brown AN. Use of commercial record linkage software and vital statistics to identify patient deaths. *JAMIA* 1997;4:233–7.
22. Annest JL, Mercy JA. Use of national data systems for firearm-related injury surveillance. *Am J Prev Med* 1998;15:17–30.
23. Saltzman LE, Ikeda RM. Recommended data elements for firearm-related injury surveillance. *Am J Prev Med* 1998;15:113–9.
24. Lasker RD, Humphreys BL, Braithwaite WR. Making a powerful connection: the health of the public and the national information infrastructure. Washington, D.C.: Public Health Data Policy Coordinating Committee, U.S. Public Health Service, 1995.
25. Dick RS, Steen EB (eds.). The computer-based patient record: an essential technology for health care. Washington, D.C.: National Academy Press, 1991.
26. Harman J. Topics for our times: new health-care data—new horizons for public health. *Am J Public Health* 1998;88:1019–21.
27. Chute CG, Cohn SP, Campbell JR *et al.* A framework for comprehensive health terminology systems in the United States: development guidelines, criteria for selection, and public policy implications. *JAMIA* 1998;5:503–10.
28. Humphreys BL, Lindberg DB, Schoolman HM, Barnett GO. The unified medical language system: an informatics research collaboration. *JAMIA* 1998;5:1–11.
29. Selden CR, Humphreys BL. Unified medical language system. *Current Bibliographies in Medicine* 1997;8:96.

30. College of American Pathologists. SNOMED^R RT and READ codes to be combined in an international terminology of health. Joint development agreement by the College of American Pathologists and United Kingdom's Secretary of State for Health. Press release, March 1999. (Available at http://www.cap.org/html/public/snomed_intl.html.)
31. Gostin LO, Hodge JG. Balancing individual privacy and communal uses of health information. White paper prepared for the workshop on "The Implications of HIPAA's Administrative Simplification Provisions for Public Health and Health Services Research," November 2–3, 1998, Washington, D.C. (Available at http://www.lewin.com/hipaa)
32. Gostin LO. Health information privacy. *Cornell Law Rev* 1995;80:451–528.
33. Gostin LO, Lazzarini Z, Neslund VS, Osterholm MT. The Public Health Information Infrastructure. A national review of the law on health information privacy. *JAMA* 1996;275:1921–7.
34. Barrows RC, Clayton PD. Privacy, confidentiality, and electronic medical records. *JAMIA* 1996;3:139–48.
35. For the record: protecting electronic health information, computer science and telecommunications board, commission of physical sciences, mathematics and applications, National Research Council. Washington, D.C.: National Academy Press, 1997.
36. Halamka JD, Szolovits P, Rind D, Safran C. A WWW implementation of national recommendations for protecting electronic health information. *JAMIA* 1997;4:458–64.
37. Braude RM. People and organizational issues in health informatics. *JAMIA* 1997; 4:150–1.
38. Lorenzi NM, Riley RT, Blyth AJ, Southon G, Dixon BJ. Antecedents of the people and organizational aspects of medical informatics: review of the literature. *JAMIA* 1997;4:79–93.
39. Southon FCG, Sauer C, Dampney CN. Information technology in complex health services: organization impediments to successful technology transfer and diffusion. *JAMIA* 1997;4:112–24.
40. National Committee on Vital and Health Statistics. Assuring a health dimension for the national information infrastructure. A concept paper by the National Committee on Vital and Health Statistics. Presented to the U.S. Department of Health and Human Services Data Council. October 14, 1998. (Available at http://aspe.os.dhhs.gov/ncvhs/hii-nii.htm.)
41. Integrating public health information and surveillance systems—a report and recommendations from the CDC/ATSDR steering committee on public health information and surveillance system development. Atlanta: Centers for Disease Control and Prevention, 1995.
42. Meriwether, RA. Blueprint for a national public health surveillance system for the 21st century. *J Public Health Management Practice* 1996;2:16–23.
43. National Association for Public Health Statistics and Information Systems. Committee on Virtual State Centers Report. Virtual State Center Workgroup. Washington, D.C.: NAPHSIS, 1998. (Available at http://www.naphsis.org/HomeArt3.htm.)
44. Association of State and Territorial Health Officials and National Association of County and City Health Officials. Joint ASTHO/NACCHO Health Information Infrastructure, Integration, and Technology Meeting, July 31, 1997–August 1, 1997, Chicago. Summary of Proceedings.
45. Baker EL, Friede A, Moulton AD, Ross DA. CDC's information network for public health officials (INPHO): a framework for integrated public health information and practice. *J Public Health Management Practice* 1995;1:43–7.

46. Electronic reporting of laboratory information for public health, January 7–8, 1999. Summary of meeting proceedings. Atlanta: Centers for Disease Control and Prevention, 1999.
47. White MD, Kolar LM, Steindel SJ. Evaluation of vocabularies for electronic laboratory reporting to public health agencies. *JAMIA* 1999;6:185–94.
48. National Immunization Program. Implementation guide for immunization data transactions using version 2.3 of the Health Level Seven (HL7) Standard Protocol: Implementation guide version 2.0. Atlanta: Centers for Disease Control and Prevention, 1999. (Available at http://www.cdc.gov/nip/registry/download/hl7guide610.pdf.)
49. Centers for Disease Control and Prevention. Working toward implementation of HL7 in NAACCR information technology standards: meeting summary report. Atlants, Ga.: CDC, 1998. (Available at http://www.cdc.gov/nccdphp/dcpc/npcr/npcrpdfs/hl7mtg8.pdf.)
50. Weed JA. Vital statistics in the United States: preparing for the next century. *Population Index* 1995;61:527–39.
51. Starr P, Starr S. Reinventing vital statistics: the impact of changes in information technology, welfare policy, and health care. *Public Health Rep* 1995;110:534–44.
52. National Center for Injury Prevention and Control. Data elements for emergency department systems, release 1.0. Atlanta: Centers for Disease Control and Prevention, 1997.
53. Yasnoff WA, O'Carroll PW, Koo D, Linkins RW, Kilbourne EM. Public health informatics: improving and transforming public health in the information age. Submitted to *Am J Public Health* for its November 1999 special issue on information technology.
54. O'Carroll PW, Yasnoff WA, Wilhoite W. Public health informatics: a CDC course for public health program managers. Proceedings of the 1998 AMIA Annual Fall Symposium (formerly SCAMC). Bethesda, Md.: AMIA, 1998: on CD-ROM.
55. Ministry of Health/Australia. Agreement between the health authorities of the Commonwealth of Australia, the states and territories of Australia, the Australian Institute of Health and Welfare, and the Australian Bureau of Statistics. National Health Information Agreement, established 1993. (Available at: http:// www.aihw.gov/au/html/NHIAproc.htm.)
56. National Health Service Information Authority, United Kingdom. The background to the health-care modeling programme. Birmingham, U.K.: NHSNIA, 1999. (Available at http://www.imc.exec.nhs.uk/hcm/index.htm.)
57. Health Canada. Advisory committee on health info-structure established. August 20, 1997. (Available at http://www.hc-sc.gc.ca/main/hc/web/english/archives/96-97/97_49e.htm.)

5

Management of the Surveillance Information System and Quality Control of Data

SAMUEL L. GROSECLOSE
KEVIN M. SULLIVAN
NORMA P. GIBBS
CAROL M. KNOWLES

Are the data what they purport to be?
D. J. Finney (*1*)

This chapter describes the components of a notifiable-diseases surveillance information system and its associated activities, including data collection, entry, editing, and system maintenance. Although the health events and risk factors monitored by surveillance are diverse, including infectious diseases, injuries, environmental and occupational hazards, reproductive outcomes, and various types of behaviors, this chapter focuses on disease-reporting systems for notifiable diseases. We will emphasize the practical management and quality control of a surveillance information system. Public health surveillance encompasses more than the collection and management of health-related data, however; it also requires analysis, interpretation, and use of those data (*3*).

Notifiable-disease surveillance systems operate in city and county health departments, in state health departments, and within the federal government. It is important to note that in most health jurisdictions there are laws or regulations that specify which diseases and injuries are reportable, who is responsible for reporting, and what method and timing of reporting are to be used (e.g., by telephone within 24 hours of diagnosis or by mail within 1 week of diagnosis) (*4*). Because these reporting laws differ by geographic locale and municipal unit, the material in this chapter is restricted to a general overview of a disease-surveillance system, recognizing that some aspects may not be applicable to all areas of the country and that issues specific to jurisdiction are not covered completely. The term *state* is used in this discussion; although *state* is a geographic designation in the United States, analogous geographic units have similar functions in other countries, and much of the material presented here is also relevant to surveillance systems in other countries (see also Chapter 13).

TYPES OF REPORTS AND SURVEILLANCE SYSTEMS

There are generally three categories of notifiable-disease reports: *a*) individual case reports that include information collected on each individual with the disease or condition under surveillance; *b*) reports that present aggregated data on the total number of persons (often stratified by sex or age group) with the disease or condition; and *c*) reports of the total number of cases or syndromes if, and only if, there is judged to be an outbreak or public health emergency. Each category generally requires the collection of specific types of data, often facilitated by the use of specific forms. Once an individual case report has been received, for many conditions a public health nurse or other disease investigator may request that the reporting source provide additional information for case management or investigation.

Traditionally a surveillance system may be classified as *passive* or *active* (5). A passive surveillance system is one in which a health jurisdiction receives disease reports from physicians, laboratories, or other individuals or institutions as mandated by state law. In contrast, an active surveillance system is established when a health department regularly contacts reporting sources (e.g., once per week) to elicit reports, including negative reports (no cases). An active surveillance system is likely to provide more complete reporting but is much more labor intensive and is therefore more costly to operate than a passive system.

Most U.S. states have comprehensive, passive disease surveillance systems. For example, "...as required by law in all 50 U.S. states..." means that any health worker who has knowledge of a person with a reportable condition is obligated to report that case to the local or state health department (4). Regular contact initiated by the health department and directed to all possible reporting sources is neither feasible nor required for surveillance of some conditions. However, periodic newsletters, journal articles, or web sites that are directed toward healthcare providers and laboratorians and that include information on conditions of public health importance and their proper management, along with public health reporting requirements, may enhance disease reporting.

In most U.S.-based surveillance systems, any health worker who has knowledge of an individual with a notifiable condition may be required to report that case to the health department. Surveillance data captured through passive surveillance systems may be augmented by targeting specific sources of surveillance data. In a sentinel surveillance system, only selected physicians or facilities report specified diseases. Proponents of sentinel systems maintain that it is preferable to receive disease reports of high quality from a few sources than to receive data of unknown quality from (in theory) all potential reporting sources in a population. This, of course, presupposes *a*) that the reporters in a sentinel system will, in fact, provide high-quality information on a reliable basis and *b*) that the cases of disease identified by the sentinel system are fairly representative of the condition being monitored. However, sentinel systems are inadequate when every case of a particular condition needs to be identified, e.g., in the context of programs to eliminate specific diseases or programs monitoring diseases of public health importance.

INFORMATION TECHNOLOGY AND SURVEILLANCE INFORMATION SYSTEMS

Technologic advances in managing information have resulted in the increased availability of information, more methods to collect and disseminate data, potential for real-time access to data, and increased opportunities for sharing data and information. These advances have resulted in the need to validate the accuracy of the data, to establish and maintain data security, and to ensure that the data are available, electronically aggregated, timely, and accessible to those who need to know. Public health practitioners need to be aware of current and emerging information technologies as they implement and administer surveillance information systems.

Before the computer era, public heath workers received individual report forms for morbidity that were completed by physicians; those reports were aggregated at the local health department level before summaries were forwarded to the state health department each week or month. Depending on the condition being monitored, data might have been aggregated by single or multiple variables, e.g., age group, disease, sex, or geographic area of residence. Analyses were often hand-tallied, data were transcribed onto columnar pads, and calculations were performed by hand. As mainframe and minicomputers became available at the state and local level, morbidity data were entered into computerized data bases which often allowed better data management and more powerful analyses to be performed. For many conditions, additional information on case management, risk behavior, and health services was collected on supplemental data-collection forms in order to allow public health prevention and control programs to assess other aspects of disease epidemiology and prevention programs. These supplemental data were often not included with the computerized disease surveillance data or were included in a separate data base.

In the late 1980s, further technologic advances resulted in the widespread use of personal computers in public health and led to the development of many local, state, and federal health-information systems to support the collection, management, analysis, reporting, and dissemination of surveillance and other health-related information. These systems were often stand-alone systems—built specifically for monitoring a specific condition, e.g., tuberculosis or sexually transmitted diseases. Computerized data bases were often relational in structure and allowed multiple events to be related to a single individual. Electronic transfer of encrypted data by modem or computer diskette became feasible, which allowed health departments to securely transfer data electronically between jurisdictions.

The health-care sector is moving toward computerized entry of clinical and laboratory data at the point of service. This change increases the timeliness and accessibility of health information. As the Internet continues to develop, future surveillance information systems will likely allow data on health problems to be entered directly into or electronically-transferred via Internet-based applications by health-care practitioners, laboratories, and health department staff. Electronic data security and data integrity protocols allow data access to be limited by the use of multiple passwords and data encryption routines and allow modifications of or access to data to be monitored via electronic audit trails. Several states are currently developing Internet-based surveillance information systems which allow secure data entry by local health departments into a central data base, local health department access to their own data, and central management of a statewide morbidity data base.

Improved computer technology has allowed health records from two or more different sources that contain different types of information to be linked into a single file for an individual, thus increasing the usefulness of the information. Data linkages have identified the need to ensure computer system compatibility, availability of accurate linkage information, and procedures to resolve data discrepancies. Much of the health-care sector's experience in electronic data management has been in the area of health-care claim transactions between providers and payors and in health-care encounter reporting (6). These activities have resulted in an acute awareness of the need to adopt data standards and electronic data interchange (EDI) standards (see also Chapter 4) (6).

In order to promote integration of health information, public health surveillance systems must begin to incorporate standardized classification systems for health-related data, including those that deal with causes of morbidity or death (e.g., *International Classification of Diseases,* tenth revision [*ICD-10*], and *ICD,* ninth revision. *Clinical Modifications*) (7,8), those that relate to therapeutic and operative procedures (e.g., *Current Procedural Terminology*™) (9), those that relate to clinical laboratory results (*Logical Observation and Identifier Names and Codes* [*LOINC*]) (10), those associated with pathology findings (*Systematized Nomenclature of Medicine* [*SNOMED*]) (11), and those associated with geographic location (e.g., census tracts and U.S. postal zip codes). Additionally, the use of standard EDI protocols, such as the American National Standards Institute's (ANSI) X12, currently used for health-care claims and reimbursement, and Health Level Seven (HL7), currently used for clinical and administrative data, should enhance the accuracy and speed with which health data can be exchanged (12,13). Although these current EDI standards define the data structure necessary to facilitate communication among systems, they include numerous optional fields, and many field values are not specified (14). Ideally, core data elements and data classification systems would be incorporated into existing EDI standards to maximize the potential for integrating health information. Electronic reporting of laboratory data is one area in which the public health community is working closely with clinical laboratories to define core data elements and data and EDI standards needed to use HL7 for reporting findings suggestive of notifiable diseases (15). Electronic laboratory reporting represents an important first step in the surveillance process, but it must be coupled with appropriate data analysis and interpretation and communication of results.

The public health sector has begun to change its information management procedures as a result of advances in technology and will likely continue to adopt new practices and procedures afforded by these technologies. However, surveillance systems must also look toward process improvement, not just automation. In many settings, automation is not necessarily the answer to information management problems. In resource-poor settings, a paper record system may continue to be the most effective and flexible data management scheme for surveillance information. However, as surveillance information systems are implemented, every effort should be made to incorporate standardized processes for system connectivity and integration, protocols for data exchange and information access, core health data elements, and standard data classification schemes.

REPORTING AND COLLECTION OF DATA

Disease reporting laws at the state and local levels specify who is responsible for reporting as well as to whom the reports are to be directed. In many systems, morbidity report forms are the major data collection instrument implying that they should facilitate accurate and error-free data collection. When reporters need information on surveillance case definitions or notification procedures for proper case reporting and follow-up, placing that information on the morbidity report form may improve reporting. In the least complicated reporting situation, a physician diagnoses a reportable condition and sends the appropriate information by morbidity report form or by telephone call to the local health department, where the data on that case are added to the appropriate disease-surveillance information system. Summaries of case reports are reviewed regularly and are analyzed by staff at local health departments to identify any conditions that may require follow-up for case management or those that are being reported more frequently than expected on the basis of past experience. After disease reports have been processed at the local level, the information is forwarded to the state health department to be consolidated with reports from other local health departments, and the composite data are examined for trends. Each state health department then voluntarily reports these cases to the CDC on a weekly basis (16).

Health-care provider and laboratory reporting can be reasonably effective, but problems can arise. For example, how does one notify health-care professionals about the requirements and procedures for reporting to the health department? Who is responsible for such notification? How are new practitioners in the jurisdiction identified and notified of their responsibility to report? Who provides quality assurance for the process? How? At what frequency? Other issues include reporting of suspected cases while laboratory results are pending, the desired routing of reports, the mechanism for updating or completing reports as additional information is received, reporting of disease among transients (e.g., military personnel or migrant workers), and defining appropriate time frames for reporting a case of a specific disease (Table 5–1).

There may not be one correct answer to each of the questions formulated in Table 5–1. The answers to these questions often depend on the situation. How-

Table 5–1 Essential Questions for the Practice of Effective Disease Reporting

---

Initiation and Sources of Reports

- How and by whom are health-care practitioners (existing and newly practicing) and laboratories entered into the reporting network?
- How are practitioners and laboratories notified of changes in the list of notifiable diseases or conditions and of modifications in reporting procedures?
- By what agency are conditions reported for such temporary residents as college students, military personnel, and migrant workers?

Routing and Timing of Reports

- How should "suspected case, laboratory results pending" be handled?
- Should the local or the state health department update a case report when additional information is received?
- Should case reports arise from the health jurisdiction in which the patient resides? In which the patient became infected? In which the patient became ill (or received treatment)?
- Under what circumstances, should a diagnostic laboratory send data on reportable conditions to local and state health departments?
- If a case occurs during one calendar year, but is not reported until early in the next calendar year, what is the year of report? What is the cut-off date for reports from the previous year? How are reports treated that are for the previous year but are received after the established deadline?
- Is there a mechanism for reporting disease across state lines, as appropriate?

Policy Issues in Reporting Disease and Injury

- What mechanisms are in place and who is responsible for placing a health outcome under public health surveillance? For removing a disease or condition from surveillance?
- How are cases to be identified and reported? What surveillance method(s) should be adopted for specific conditions under surveillance? Provider-based reporting? Laboratory-based reporting? Both? Sentinel surveillance networks?
- What information will be recorded on each case? Is it possible to reduce the amount of information collected to establish the occurrence of the event?
- Are data elements commonly defined and coded? Is there a mechanism to disseminate data collection and coding guidelines to health-care practitioners and laboratories?
- What items on the reporting form *must* be completed before a report can be forwarded? Does this vary by condition or public health jurisdiction?
- If a reportable condition has a specific case definition (such as measles and AIDS), should the case be reported before confirmation by a disease investigator (3)?
- What mechanism will be (has been) established to deal with situations in which cases must be reported in batches rather than individually because the number of reports is overwhelmingly large?
- How will the information be stored and communicated at each level of the public health sector?
- If case reports are held pending laboratory confirmation, should the "date of report" reflect the *original date* of report or the date laboratory confirmation *was received* or some other date associated with this health event?
- Are reports generated to identify records with incomplete or unconfirmed data so that follow-up can be initiated?
- Who will be responsible for producing analyses or servicing requests for data? Who will produce reports?
- How does one avoid duplicate reports of the same case?
- How are discrepancies in the information on duplicate reports resolved?

---

ever, a disease-surveillance system should document how to respond to each of these questions so that disease reporting is performed in a consistent manner for each disease.

Entry of Data into the Surveillance Information System

With the availability of microcomputers, many health departments enter morbidity reports into computerized data bases. Ideally, data are entered directly from the source documents. These data may have to be coded before they are entered into the data base. To minimize data transcription or coding errors, the data collection and entry processes should be separated from the coding of the data. Alternatively, the computerized information system could make reference file lookups available to assist with use of standard codes during data entry. The use of intermediate or temporary files during data entry allows the staff member to check and edit data before entering potential data errors in the master data base. Once reviewed for duplicates and errors, the temporary files can be merged into the master data base. Original data should be stored in the master data base; data transformations needed during analysis can be performed using an analysis file derived from the master data base.

Data-editing procedures should be clearly documented to allow staff to detect probable errors easily and to provide directions to aid in the resolution of such errors. It is critical that data be checked at several points throughout the data management process so that errors can be identified as early as possible. Each step in the data management process places the data further from the point of collection and decreases the likelihood that errors can be corrected.

Once public health surveillance data are entered into an electronic medium, every effort should be made to maintain those data electronically rather than to duplicate data entry efforts at various points within the public health system. Through the use of individual interface programs that reformat proprietary data, electronic transfer of information is already occurring between and within public health jurisdictions. Over time, use of EDI methodologies, e.g., HL7, which incorporate core data elements and data standards, should minimize the duplication of effort and paperwork and should increase the accuracy and timeliness of surveillance data.

Ideally, local and state health departments will agree on a public health surveillance and information model that can provide the foundation for the development of integrated health information systems and the redesign of categorical or stand-alone surveillance information systems. Such efforts should enhance public health-information management: This would minimize redundant data, maximize the effective use of limited resources, emphasize the development of interfaces between information systems to promote information sharing, and allow future changes in information content or surveillance protocols to be incorporated with minimal impact.

Surveillance information management in a public health jurisdiction requires input from a variety of stakeholders. However, at the level of a specific surveillance information system, it is essential that one person be responsible for man-

Table 5–2 Concerns of the Data-Base Manager

1. Who will enter the data? What credentials must this person have? Who is this person's back-up? Who will update records? Back-up the computer file?
2. Are staff adequately trained and supervised?
3. Will data be entered on an as-received basis or according to an established schedule?
4. Does the data-entry screen replicate the paper form from which data are to be entered? Does the data need to be coded prior to entry? If so, who will code the data?
5. Does the data-entry program allow for certain data items to be entered automatically on subsequent screens until the data recorder makes a change? (For example, the county initially entered will appear on each subsequent screen until the recorder types in a different county. This allows the recorder to batch records for more efficient entry.)
6. Does the data-entry program effectively validate the data being entered for completeness use of "must-enter" fields and "look-up" files?
7. Does the data-entry program have the ability to do range checking on values entered? If so, does the system allow for acceptable ranges to change, reflecting values entered in the data base over time? Is there a logic audit procedure in the system—to locate such errors as misspelled names or addresses, incorrectly coded race, gender, or code for disease?
8. At what level (state or local) will records be changed or deleted? Who owns the data records?
9. If the data base is distributed to other users as an electronic file or on diskette, are there safeguards to prevent overwriting another user's data? Safeguards against computer viruses?
10. Is the system able to respond quickly to new information requirements? Are the data-entry programs flexible enough to allow variables to be modified as prescribed by changes in state regulations and national recommendations?
11. Are production reports automatically generated for quality assurance of data entry?
12. How and with what frequency are data copied and stored for back-up purposes? Are paper copies maintained (in the event of computer failure)?
13. Are double-entry systems used for quality assurance?

agement of the surveillance data base (i.e., to be designated and to act as the data-base manager [DBM]) (*17*). A primary responsibility of the DBM is to maintain the integrity and completeness of the data base. Concerns of the DBM are summarized in Table 5–2.

Checklist for Data-Base Manager

With any surveillance information system, there is a need to establish procedures for maintenance and retention of paper disease-report forms (source documents). In general, the individual disease reports are filed by year of report (or onset), by disease, and in alphabetical order by the patient's last name. If not already specified by disease-reporting laws, retention periods should be designated for maintaining these files for reference purposes. Electronic reporting may obviate the need for redundant paper records (see also Chapter 11). Because the public health sector's information needs evolve, computerized surveillance information data bases should be organized to allow the timely expansion, updating, and retrieval of data and information for a variety of purposes. The extent to which surveillance data should be collected and maintained using paper forms or electronic data bases may vary both within and among public health departments.

Similarly, information systems vary. They range from highly centralized models with a central data base to widely distributed models with links to satellite clinics or health departments. Regardless of the information model or system design, the DBM should collaboratively develop and implement comprehensive, written policies on data management, quality control, access, release, and security.

Documentation and Training

Documentation is a critical step in the development of a surveillance information system—but one that is often neglected. A users' manual for a computerized system should provide both general and detailed descriptions of the system, including the following topics (*17*):

- general description of the entire system
- detailed procedures for installing the system
- detailed procedures for operating the system
- detailed procedures for maintaining the system

Both computerized and paper-based information systems need to document explicitly their policies and procedures. A description of the information content is required—whether for the data elements and formats to be included in the electronic record or for the printing specifications for a hard-copy data collection form. Similarly, protocols for data transmission and sharing are needed—whether conforming to EDI and data security standards or specifying how completed data collection forms should be transferred and stored securely within the health department.

The DBM should maintain contact with the chief programmer for the surveillance information system so that modifications to record formats and programs can be documented by the manager; the programmer should also maintain a file of all such changes. Thorough, clear documentation facilitates the addition of new programs and modifications in equipment or operations (*17*).

A formal training program should be established for persons involved in the daily operation of the surveillance system. These staff members must feel that they can participate in shaping the system, and their ideas and comments should be elicited as part of the training process (*17*). The DBM should schedule a series of training classes that include hands-on experience with the data-base software. Written operational procedures—including guidelines for interpreting information contained in the disease report forms—should be distributed and explained at this time. Software tutorial packages and videotapes (interactive or presentational) can also be useful tools for training. In addition, the computerized system should allow the user to easily navigate the system and should provide some form of user support, e.g., via the use of on-line HELP services.

Management personnel of the organization responsible for the surveillance system should also be oriented to the system in one or several briefing sessions. Comprehensive training for staff should include information on data security and confidentiality procedures.

ANALYSIS AND INFORMATION DISSEMINATION

Surveillance information is being used by an increasingly wide range of "consumers," i.e., people who are interested in disease prevention and control. Such people range from epidemiologists to community-based organizations and the general public. Surveillance information systems must therefore ensure that data maintained in the surveillance data base can be analyzed and disseminated in numerous formats for a varied audience.

An effective surveillance system must be designed to cover all the following areas in its reporting process:

- determining whether a condition is being reported more frequently than expected
- responding appropriately to reports of individual cases
- detecting clusters of cases
- notifying public health practitioners of the presence of specific conditions in their areas
- reinforcing the importance of reporting through facilitating effective control and prevention activities
- monitoring the quality of surveillance data

In order to ensure consistency, quality, and comparability of information, surveillance data must be aggregated and cross-checked at each level of the public health system before being used, fed back, or reported to a higher level. Validity checks during data entry can ensure the data type and format; more detailed logic checks can be programmed into the information system. Surveillance staff should determine what variable or combination of variables uniquely identifies a record so that duplicated data can be identified and resolved. Frequency distributions by each data variable can identify out-of-range values and the percentage of missing or unknown responses. Simple cross-tabulations of data can identify logical inconsistencies among related variables, e.g., the category "pregnant males."

The completeness and timeliness of case reports in the surveillance system should be assessed regularly (*18*). This assessment should include both the proportion of the reports with each variable, such as age of patient or date of onset of the condition, date completed, and time between onset of condition and receipt of report. At the local health department, this information can be analyzed by reporting source (e.g., by clinician, hospital, or diagnostic laboratory) or, at the state level by health jurisdiction. To support these analyses and other data-management activities, the information system should allow the user to scroll forward and backward through the data to generate line-lists, to sort data by selected variables, to search the data base by selected variables, and to subset the database by selected variables. These analyses should identify groups or institutions in need of additional information or training on disease reporting. Additionally, these analyses may allow staff to identify process improvements that will decrease the time to detect a health event or that will increase data completeness of core data elements.

Some prevention programs have developed so-called "surveillance indicators" to measure or quantify different surveillance and case investigation processes (19). The indicators range from process measures (Is the computerized surveillance information system installed and functioning? Has the program identified a surveillance coordinator?) to outcome measures (How many case reports are laboratory-confirmed and have complete information on laboratory test results? What is the lag time between date of specimen collection and receipt of the case report by the local health department?). Surveillance indicators should be updated routinely. Typically, the information is compared against some standard measure or management objective and can provide program management with information to act upon.

Most surveillance systems for infectious disease rely primarily on receipt of case reports from physicians, laboratories, and other health-care providers. To encourage reporting by these health professionals, many local health departments and most state health departments disseminate surveillance data and other public health information via printed newsletter, e-mail, or the Internet for contributors to the data base (4). Such information may include standard tabular reports of the occurrence of a reportable condition by week or month with a year-to-date summary. It may also include narrative reports about conditions of interest or about other topics relevant to public health. This feedback is important to demonstrate to those involved with the system that the data are being used, as well as to accomplish communications goals (see also Chapters 7 and 16).

Feedback is a critical component of the surveillance process. If decisions regarding disease interventions, program planning, and policy development are linked to the surveillance information system, the incentive to convert data into information will be encouraged. The information needs of management and operations personnel should be considered as programs are developed for standard reports from the data base. Standard reports should include information on time, place, and person, and should be produced in a form that can be easily interpreted by epidemiologists and management. The purpose of each report should dictate the appearance of the output (e.g., a table, map, or graph). Most types of reports should be produced on a regular basis and according to a set schedule, but others may be created only on an as-needed basis.

Each surveillance information system should allow various aspects of the surveillance system (e.g., representativeness, completeness, flexibility, timeliness) to be evaluated (see also Chapter 8) (18). However, each health outcome under surveillance may require different levels of each attribute; e.g., representativeness of *Chlamydia* case reports may be more important than completeness of each case report. Another example: improving the timeliness of a report of *Escherichia coli* O157:H7 infection in order to allow earlier implementation of control measures may be more important than increasing the flexibility of the computerized information system to allow the collection of additional risk-factor information.

DATA SHARING AND INTEGRATION

In some situations reports of disease case reports may be shared by various local or state health departments, particularly if the conditions reported require additional investigation or follow-up. For example, when a resident of one county or state is examined and given a particular diagnosis at a hospital in a neighboring county or state, health authorities need to be able to track the condition back to its source in order to respond appropriately.

Policies to share public health surveillance data should support the tenet that surveillance data and information should be available to those who will take public health action in response to this information. Occasionally, disease reports are sent directly to the state health department, bypassing the local health department. If that happens, the state should notify the local health department so that appropriate case management can be ensured, additional case finding can be performed, and the reports can be added to the disease reporting system at the local level. Additional data that the local or state health departments may collect should also be shared (electronically) across health department jurisdictions as needed and appropriate.

Staff of surveillance-information-system management and operations units must specify their policies for data release and data sharing. Such policies must be consistent with local and state laws that regulate the use and sharing of health information. Before releasing surveillance data to others (e.g., community planning groups), health departments may consider converting individual-specific data to a more general form (e.g., by aggregating or grouping data) in order to render them non-identifiable. Since surveillance data are being used by an increasingly wide variety of consumers, there is a critical need to develop and distribute data that describe the surveillance information system itself, the conditions under surveillance, the sources of reports, and any limitations in the data (i.e., the system's metadata), in order to facilitate the appropriate interpretation of those surveillance data.

In the context of a broad public health information model, the DBM should be aware of other sources of information that may need to be accessed and compared with or added to the data collected in his or her own system—laboratory results, epidemiologic information for specific conditions, population estimates, risk behaviors, socioeconomic data, and mortality records. Through careful planning and coordination on the part of managers of health information systems, core data elements and data classification and EDI standards can be adopted as data systems evolve. These actions facilitate the sharing and use of information.

Individual or categorical surveillance information systems will continue to be very useful and to provide a wide variety of information; however, integrating or linking data across a variety of data sources can provide more robust information for testing hypotheses or for assessing prevention and control activities. Integration of information systems does not imply a single information system. Rather, it implies the linkage of systems via the use of data and communications standards to allow information produced in any information system to be accessed and made available either directly or indirectly. Integrating surveillance information systems requires agreement on data access, data sharing, and confidentiality policies and procedures. Policies regarding ownership of data, resolution of data discrepancies, and synchronization of data bases must be documented. Integration of surveillance information can occur at the local, state, and federal level (20–22).

One form of information integration, data repositories or data warehouses—whether virtual (diverse health information databases maintained separately, but linked by common interfaces and EDI) or centralized (data bases consolidated in a central location via data mapping)—are being considered to enhance knowledge and to increase the cost-effectiveness of data management. Data warehouses may provide a new framework for the management and dissemination of information from public health surveillance systems. However, it is important to remember that the utility of these systems is directly dependent upon the quality and integrity of each individual data source.

SYSTEM MAINTENANCE AND SECURITY

Maintenance of a system should be directed a) toward reducing errors that are introduced through flaws in design and through changes in content (e.g., changes in the list of notifiable conditions) and b) toward improving the system's scope and services. Related activities can be categorized as routine maintenance, emergency maintenance, requests for special reports, and system improvements. Maintenance should not be performed on an informal or "first-come, first-served" basis. An effective maintenance program includes the following steps (17):

- Back up data and system files according to an established schedule, and maintain records in a secure environment.
- Require that requests for emergency maintenance be made in writing and entered into a log.
- Assign priorities to special requests on the basis of urgency of need and time and resources required.
- Institutionalize routine maintenance, such as procedures associated with changing to a new reporting year.
- Document maintenance as it is conducted.

In order to maintain the integrity of a computer system, only one person should have the authority to access the system and to assign and change passwords. The DBM should be the only staff member with authority to install or modify production software. This same rule should apply to access to the physical computer files. Authority to add or delete files from subdirectories or environments of computers should be delegated to only one individual, who is then held accountable for all modifications. A second computer should be available for testing changes to the system so that the computer used for the surveillance information system can be reserved for production only. The second computer could also serve as a backup computer should the primary machine fail.

The numerous risks to the security of a data base include mechanical failure, human carelessness, malicious damage, crime, and invasion of privacy. Therefore, back-up copies of the data base should be kept securely off site to ensure that the system cannot be deliberately or unintentionally destroyed. Updating of the off site copies should be done on a routine basis, and new diskettes or other storage media should be used to make back-up copies at least once each year.

A monthly, total-system back-up is recommended, if a valid copy of the current system is available. Data files that are changed during the day should be backed up at the end of the day.

Computer viruses have become a threat to data-base and computer-system security. These programs can be highly sophisticated and are capable of attaching themselves to software or data being loaded on the computer or data being sent from one computer to another. Software is available to scan entire systems or diskettes for virus infections and to remove the virus once detected; such software should be updated periodically because of the addition of new viruses. Data received via telecommunications channels or on diskettes from other sources should always be scanned before data files and programs are copied to the computer's disk. Software downloaded from the Web should be carefully examined before being incorporated into a system.

In the event of extended mechanical failure, a contingency plan should be in place for shifting the base of operations to another computer.

Notifiable disease surveillance data are generally received by a local health department, forwarded through a regional health center, and eventually directed to the state health department. The complete reporting form, which includes confidential information on patients, is usually shared by local and state health departments for purposes of follow up (if necessary) and for identifying and deleting any redundant (duplicate) reports. Morbidity report forms and other data-collection forms must be maintained securely by restricting access to only those staff persons who need access to the information and should be physically secured at all times; once computerized, additional safeguards, e.g., multi-level password controls and data encryption, should be implemented to ensure confidentiality and data security. Systems or procedures to track and audit access to and alteration of surveillance report forms and data should be established and monitored.

Persons who report disease should be familiar with the types of activities that may follow the receipt of a report. For example, for purposes of prevention or treatment, all cases of syphilis may be investigated to determine the source of the infection and the potential spread of the infection to others. Disease-reporting laws may specify who has access to the confidential portions of a disease report, and it is important to ensure that the confidentiality of the report is maintained (22). Failure to keep the reports confidential is likely to lead to an unwillingness to report on the part of physicians, laboratories, and other health-care providers. Reports and files that do not require personal identifiers should not contain them. In the United States, notifiable-disease reports received from states by the Centers for Disease Control and Prevention (CDC) do not include personal identifiers (such as name, address, and telephone number).

MODIFICATION OF REPORTING SYSTEMS

Increasingly, public health surveillance data are being using to improve public health practice and medical treatment. As new disease agents and syndromes of public health importance are recognized, surveillance activities and the information systems that support them must be flexible enough to allow them to be responsive to new information needs. The basic steps shown below are intended to ensure that a computer-based surveillance information system will meet current and future needs. A systems analyst, an epidemiologist, and the final users of information from the system should work together to produce a system that is user-friendly and functional (17). A primary objective of data base management is to ensure high-quality data. Good information system design, which balances system requirements and resources, creates the potential for obtaining good information.

1. Review current methods of processing disease information. Obtain copies of paper forms or computer-screen forms or reports. Determine whether suggested report forms or screens are available from state or national agencies. Often, ready-to-use surveillance software is available. Use of such systems facilitates standardization, quality control, and comparability of data.
2. Review with management and users any problems with the current method for processing data and any desired future enhancements. Establish clear lines of authority and responsibility for the data management system.
3. Document the current system and the proposed future system. Allow concerned parties to review and comment on their understanding of objectives for the system.
4. Document developmental specifications to meet the objectives above. In addition, document proposed testing schedules and methodology for implementing the system when it is completed.
5. Develop prototypic computer screens and paper report forms for management and end users to review, so that misunderstandings and problems can be identified and resolved during development.
6. Once all parties are in agreement, establish self-contained modules of development that can be completed, and proceed to the testing stage while other modules are being developed.
7. Begin development in a test environment separate from any current computer-based production system. Document any changes to developmental specifications that become necessary during actual development.
8. Produce processing manuals for users (to include not only the operation of the computerized system but also proper handling of paper forms, data quality assurance procedures, storage of electronic and paper data, data security procedures, and distribution of final reports). This documentation should be as thoroughly tested as the actual computer system.
9. Establish training sessions or develop tutorial manuals for users. If such manuals are to be effective, a development or test system for users must be in place during their training stage.

10. Finalize specification documents to include all current stages of the system, as well as all expected future enhancements. This documentation should include a schedule and methodology for maintaining and troubleshooting the system and for maintaining ongoing documentation of the system.
11. Establish and document proper back-up and data-recovery techniques. This step includes selecting a data-base manager (DBM).

SUMMARY

A surveillance information system of high quality and integrity can only be developed through careful planning, documentation, implementation, training, and long-term support. Because of the changing nature of disease reporting (e.g., new conditions being added or case definitions being modified), useful surveillance systems must be flexible enough to allow for such changes with a minimal amount of disruption.

Also important is the coordination of disease-reporting activities among local health departments, from local health departments to their appropriate state health departments, and among state health departments. The CSTE has played an important role in the state-to-state coordination of disease reporting, as well as in establishing reporting practices from states to CDC.

Although there are many complicated aspects of a public health surveillance system, it is important to remember the overall purpose: to prevent disease, disability, and death, thereby improving the public health. This makes all the effort worthwhile.

REFERENCES

1. Finney DJ. Numbers and data. *Biometrics* 1975;31:375–86.
2. Thacker SB, Stroup DF. Future directions for comprehensive public health surveillance and health information systems in the United States. *Am J Epidemiol* 1994; 140:383–97.
3. Roush SW, Birkhead GS, Koo D, Cobb AN, Fleming DW. Mandatory reporting of diseases and conditions by health-care professionals and laboratories. *JAMA* 1999; 282:164–70.
4. Uehler JW. Surveillance. In: Rothman KJ, Greenland S (eds.). Modern epidemiology. Philadelphia: Lippincott-Raven Publishers, 1998:435–57.
5. Harman J. Topics for our times: New health-care data—new horizons for public health. *AJPH* 1998;88:1019–21.
6. McDonald CJ, Overhage JM, Dexter P, Takesue BY, Dwyer DM. A framework for capturing clinical data sets from computerized sources. *Ann Intern Med* 1997;127: 675–82.
7. World Health Organization. The international statistical classification of diseases and related health problems. Tenth revision. Volumes 1, 2, 3. Geneva: World Health Organization, 1998.

8. Health Care Financing Administration. International classification of disease. Ninth revision. Clinical Modifications (ICD-9-CM). Rockville, Md.: Health Care Financing Administration, 1989. As of July 1999, additional information is available at http://www.mcis.duke.edu/standards/termcode/icd9cm.htm.

9. American Medical Association. Physicians' current procedural terminology (CPT95). Fourth edition. Chicago: American Medical Association, 1994. As of July 1999, additional information available at http://www.ama-assn.org/med-sci/cpt/cpt5.htm

10. Forrey AW, McDonald CJ, DeMoor G et al. Logical observation identifier names and codes (LOINC) data base: a public use set of codes and names for electronic reporting of clinical laboratory test results. *Clinical Chemistry* 1996;42:81–90. As of July 1999, additional information available at http://www.mcis.duke.edu/standards/termcode/loinclab/loinc.html.

11. College of American Pathologists. Systematized nomenclature of medicine (SNOMED). Version 3.4. As of July 1999, additional information available at http://www.snomed.org

12. American National Standards Institute. X.12N—Electronic data interchange (EDI) for health insurance. Gaithersburg, Md.: Washington Publishing Company, 1999. As of July 1999, additional information available at http://polaris.disa.org/x12/x12n or http://www.mcis.duke.edu/standards/X12N/x12.htm.

13. Health Level Seven, Inc. As of July 1999, additional information available at http://www.mcis.duke.edu/standards/HL7/h17.htm.

14. Aller RD. Software standards and the laboratory information system. *Am J Clin Pathol* 1996;105(Suppl):S48–S53.

15. Centers for Disease Control and Prevention (CDC), Council of State and Territorial Epidemiologists, Association of Public Health Laboratories. Electronic reporting of laboratory data for public health: meeting report and recommendations. Atlanta: U.S. Department of Health and Human Services, CDC, 1997.

16. Koo D, Wharton M, Birkhead G. Case definitions for infectious conditions under public health surveillance. *MMWR* 1997;46(RR-10):1–55.

17. Murdick, RG. MIS concepts and design. Englewood Cliffs, N.J: Prentice-Hall, 1980.

18. Klaucke DN, Buehler JW, Thacker SB, Parrish RG, Trowbridge FL, Berkelman RL et al. Guidelines for evaluating surveillance systems. *MMWR* 1988;37(S-5):1–18.

19. Centers for Disease Control and Prevention (CDC). Manual for the surveillance of vaccine-preventable diseases. Atlanta: U.S. Department of Health and Human Services, CDC, 1997:15.1–10.

20. Wei F, Wright K, Cook MA, Heaton TM. St. Louis integrated immunization information system. *J Public Health Management Practice* 1997;3:72–9.

21. Chapman KA, Moulton AD. The Georgia Information Network for Public Health Officials (INPHO): a demonstration of the CDC INPHO concept. *J Public Health Management Practice* 1995;1:39–43.

22. Centers for Disease Control and Prevention (CDC). Integrating public health information and surveillance systems. A report and recommendations from the CDC/ATSDR steering committee on public health information and surveillance system development. Atlanta: U.S. Department of Health and Human Services, CDC, 1995.

23. Gostin LO, Lassarini Z, Neslund VS, Osterholm MT. The public health information infrastructure: a national review of the law on health information privacy. *JAMA* 1996;275:1921–7.

6

Descriptive Epidemiology: Analyzing and Interpreting Surveillance Data

GAIL R. JANES
LORI HUTWAGNER
WILLARD CATES JR.
DONNA F. STROUP
G. DAVID WILLIAMSON

Where is the wisdom we have lost in knowledge? Where is the knowledge we have lost in information?

T. S. Eliot

Where is the information we have lost in data?
Editors

Historically, the core processes of public health surveillance have involved using appropriate methods to aggregate the units of data being collected—analysis—and also creative approaches to assess the emerging data patterns—interpretation (*1*).

The analysis and interpretation of surveillance data establish the foundation for many observational studies (*2*), placing surveillance at the forefront of the spectrum of descriptive epidemiology. Surveillance has a myriad of uses (*3,4*), each of which requires careful analysis and interpretation. Whether surveillance is used to detect epidemics, suggest hypotheses, characterize trends in disease or injury, evaluate prevention programs, or project future public health needs, data from a surveillance system must be analyzed carefully and interpreted prudently. In this chapter, we address practical and methodologically sound approaches to analyzing surveillance; discuss the presentation of surveillance data by time, place, and person—including the analysis of temporal and geographic patterns of disease occurrence; review the concept of rates and standardization of rates; go over approaches to exploratory data analysis; detail the use of graphics and maps; and, finally, discuss the systematic interpretation of surveillance data.

112

APPROACHES TO SURVEILLANCE ANALYSIS

A Practical Approach

The fundamental approach to analyzing surveillance data is relatively straight-forward. Data from surveillance systems are observational in nature; they do not come from a designed study or a randomized trial. Because of this, surveillance data cannot be used for formal hypothesis testing (5). Rather, the regular scrutiny of systematically collected information, distributed across a temporal and spatial continuum, allows epidemiologists to describe patterns of disease and injury in human populations, organized by a variety of submeasures. Moreover, the analysis (and subsequent interpretation) proceeds from the specific elements of the data themselves. Thus, surveillance analysis represents an inductive reasoning process in which the assembly of individual units eventually produces a more general picture of health-related conditions in a population.

Analyzing surveillance data should be of primary importance, although the time-consuming problems of collecting, managing, and storing surveillance data often supersede the analysis itself. If the analyses are implemented as part of a routine surveillance program, results can be monitored as the initial data are up-dated with subsequent reports. Approaches to analyzing surveillance data include the following steps:

1. Know the inherent idiosyncracies of the surveillance data set. It is tempting to begin immediately to examine trends over time. However, intimate knowledge of the day-to-day strengths and weaknesses of the data-collection methods and the reporting process can provide a "real world" sense of the trends that emerge.
2. Although surveillance data are increasingly reported at the individual level, it is still not uncommon to encounter aggregated surveillance data. If aggregated, the distribution of cases in the underlying population cannot be assessed directly. This problem is compounded by arbitrarily or politically defined areas of aggregation with frequently inconsistent case definitions. In addition, because surveillance data include both temporal and spatial components, aberrations may only become apparent when looking across time or across areas at a given point in time.
3. Proceed from the simplest to the most complex. Using the concepts of exploratory data analysis, discussed in this chapter, examine each condition separately. How many cases were reported each year? How many cases were reported in each age group each year? Perform subgroup analyses, to determine whether trends vary by factors such as race/ethnicity or sex. In addition to looking at each variable separately, also consider that the surveillance process is generally a multi-variate one (5). Multiple health events under surveillance may be observed at a given time and place, or the relationship may be delayed in time for the same or nearby areas if diagnosis is uncertain or confirmation is delayed. The multivariate nature of this process should be used to improve the ability of any method to detect aberrations from a baseline.

4. Realize when inaccuracies in the data preclude more sophisticated analyses. Erratically collected or incomplete data cannot be corrected by complex analytic techniques. Differential reporting by different regions or by different health facilities render the resulting surveillance data set liable to misinterpretation.

Methodologic Considerations

Reliability and Validity

Appropriate analysis of surveillance information depends on the accuracy of that information. Attempts to analyze data that are haphazardly collected or have varying case definitions waste valuable time and resources. The two key concepts that determine the accuracy of surveillance data are reliability and validity (5). *Reliability* refers to whether a particular condition is reported consistently by different observers, whereas *validity* refers to whether the condition as reported reflects the true condition as it occurs. Ideally, both reliability and validity can be achieved, but in practice, reliability (i.e., reproducibility) is easier than validity to assess. In situations involving conditions where biologic measures complement clinical case definitions, such as laboratory testing for infectious diseases, the accuracy of the data can be more completely assured. However, the accuracy of more subjective behavioral aspects, such as those associated with life-styles, is more difficult to confirm.

Statistical Testing

The application of standard statistical techniques to the analysis of surveillance data is dictated by the limitations of the data themselves. Because the essentials of sampling theory are not satisfied by the often incomplete surveillance data, it is not appropriate to apply many standard statistical techniques to this data. However, some other statistical and analytic methods, some of which are described in this chapter, can be applied to surveillance data. If, for example, surveillance data are viewed as samples over time, apparent clusters of health events can be evaluated for their statistical "significance." Applying 95% confidence limits to these samples over time can allow a determination of whether any differences might have occurred by chance alone, although this practice should not be used in lieu of descriptive statistical and epidemiological analyses.

Ecologic Analysis

Surveillance data are often aggregate data; because of this, surveillance analyses are often ecologic, i.e., they describe trends in groups of individuals. Thus, the use of surveillance data may be especially prone to the problem of the "ecological fallacy" (6,7). In brief, this type of bias may occur when health officials interpreting observations about groups (e.g., aggregated surveillance data) make causal inferences about individual phenomena (8). These population-level analyses may suffer from two separate problems (7): a) aggregation bias—arising from loss of information when individuals are grouped, and b) specification bias—

arising from the definition of the group itself (*8*). The chances of the ecological fallacy can be reduced by analyzing subsets of surveillance data to reveal trends in the individual characteristics. However, when describing bodies of surveillance data, public health officials usually summarize the populations trends, thus opening the possibility for fallacious interpretation.

Clustering of Health Events

One foundation of the science of epidemiology is the study of the departure of the observed patterns of disease from the expected (*9*). Variations in the usual incidence of health events in different geographic areas or different time periods may provide important clues to specific risk factors or even to the etiology of the problem. The expected numbers of reported health events involve human behavior and transmission of disease, and patterns of occurrence within human populations may lead to hypotheses about the determinants of the health problem (*10*).

The public health community continues to struggle with nomenclature for such variations. The term *cluster* is used here to describe a group of events occurring unusually close together in time or space, in both time and space, or within the same demographic group (e.g., persons in the same occupation) (*11*). *Cluster* is usually used to describe uncommon events (e.g., leukemia, suicide) and tends to evoke emotional response from members of the public or from the media.
A related term is *epidemic,* historically used to describe aggregation of infectious diseases: "an outbreak of a disease spreading rapidly from person to person" (*11*). More recently, the concept has been broadened to the following: "the occurrence in a community or region of cases of an illness, specific health-related behavior, or other health-related events clearly in excess of normal expectancy." The number of cases indicating the presence of an epidemic will vary according to agent, size and type of population exposed, previous experience or lack of exposure to the disease, and time and place of occurrence; thus, "epidemicity is relative to the usual frequency of the disease in the same area, among the specified population, at the same season of the year" (*12*).

The term *epidemic* can evoke emotional responses beyond these definitions. The term *outbreak* has less evocative connotations. With all such definitions, a critical concept is the comparison of an observed number with what is usual or normal. The distinction made here is that aberration will be used to denote changes in the occurrence of health events that are statistically significant when compared with usual or normal history. The definition of an epidemic may require the existence of an aberration; e.g., CDC declares that an epidemic of a specific strain of influenza is occurring only if the number of reported deaths exceeds a 95% confidence limit in the forecast for two or more consecutive periods (*13*). In some instances, use of the term *epidemic* may require conditions beyond statistical ones, e.g., verification of laboratory isolates.

In this chapter, we use *aberration* to describe statistical departures from a usual. Such departures do not necessarily signal the "onset of an epidemic" or the "presence of a cluster." Conversely, one can have an epidemic even in the absence of a statistical increase, such as when infant mortality is low, but still higher than expected. The methods developed here are intended for routine use by the public health analyst, in conjunction with epidemiologic investigations and close communication with the source of the surveillance reports.

Time, Place, and Person

Surveillance data allow public health officials to describe health problems in terms of the basic epidemiologic parameters of time, place, and person. In addition, surveillance data permit comparisons among these different parameters (e.g., the patterns of disease or injury at one time compared with another, in one place compared with another, or among one population compared with another). These are the comparisons that define aberrant variation in disease distribution, such as clusters. Comparison of the risks of disease or injury in terms of the parameters of time, place, and person may be facilitated by use of appropriate census data as denominators, in order to calculate rates. Moreover, use of these fundamental variables permits epidemics to be detected, long-term trends to be monitored, seasonal patterns to be assessed, and future occurrence of disease or injury to be projected, thus possibly facilitating a more timely public health response.

Time: General Concepts

Analysis of surveillance data by time can reveal trends in disease, injury, or exposure. For most health conditions, a measurable delay occurs between the exposure and the problem. In the case of disease, an interval exists between exposure and expression of symptoms, as well as an interval between *a*) onset of symptoms and diagnosis of the problem, and *b*) eventual reporting of the illness to public health authorities so that it can be included in the surveillance data set. For an infectious disease, the interval may represent days or weeks, and for chronic disease the initial interval may be measured in years. Thus, choosing the appropriate interval for analysis must involve a consideration of the health condition being assessed.

Analysis of surveillance data by time can be conducted in several different ways to detect changes in incidence of disease or injury. The easiest analysis is usually an examination of the number of case reports received during a particular interval (e.g., weeks or months) over a time period of sufficient length to permit meaningful comparison across intervals. Such data can be organized into a table or graph to assess whether an abrupt increase has occurred, whether the trends are stable, or whether a gradual rise or fall in the numbers occurs. Another simple method of analysis compares the number of cases for a current time period (e.g., a given month) with the number reported during the same interval for the past several years. Similarly, the cumulative number of cases reported in the representative year-to-date period can be compared with the appropriate cumulative number for previous years.

Analyzing long-term (secular) trends is facilitated by graphing surveillance data over time. The watershed events that influence secular trends—such as changes in the case definition used for surveillance, new diagnostic criteria, changes in reporting requirements or practices, publicity about a particular condition, or new intervention programs—can be indicated on the graph.

Changes in the surveillance system itself also influence long-term trends, particularly when the intensity of active case detection increases (e.g., screening programs in particular communities).

Finally, additional epidemiologic measures enhance the analysis of surveillance data by time. Using denominators to calculate rates becomes especially important if changes occur in the community, such as the immigration of a new population. As the size of a population changes over time, so will the expected number of cases of diseases and injuries. In addition, analysis by date of onset rather than date of report more clearly defines the condition. Because of delays between diagnosis and reporting, using "date of onset" when practical and possible provides a better representation of actual disease incidence, particularly when the delay is substantial. Statistical methods for adjusting for these delays in reporting have been successfully applied to certain diseases such as HIV and AIDS (*14*).

Aberrations in Time: Methodologies

Since the definition of surveillance includes ongoing collection of data, perhaps the most fundamental question suggested by the analysis of a surveillance system is this: When does the value of reported events signal a change in the process from past patterns? Although fundamental, the analysis required to address this question suggests additional questions: How are "past patterns" defined? If an outbreak occurred in the past, should this affect the definition of a change? Other than the disease or injury process itself, what other factors could cause a change? In this development, the term *baseline* denotes historical data used to define past patterns and *current report* denotes the most recent data on which the assessment of an aberration is based. Details of four techniques for assessing deviations from baseline follow; CDC supports Software for Statistics in Surveillance (SSS1), which provides functions for several of these techniques, and is downloadable from the Epidemiology Program Office Website (http://www.cdc.gov/epo/epi/software.htm).

Graph of Current and Past Experience

In the United States, state health departments report the numbers of cases of about 50 notifiable diseases each week to CDC's NNDSS. The list of health events is determined collaboratively by the Council of State and Territorial Epidemiologists and CDC (*15,16*). Each week, provisional reports are published in the *MMWR* and are made available to epidemiologists, clinicians, and other public health professionals in a timely manner. Although the tables of the *MMWR* continue to provide important information, the volume of data and the need for ease of interpretation encouraged the development of a graphic display to highlight unusually high or low numbers of reported cases.

An analytic and graphical method was adopted for this system to achieve the following objectives: *a*) to portray in a single comprehensible figure the weekly reports of data for multiple diseases and to compare those data with past results, and *b*) to highlight for further analysis the results most likely to reflect either long-term trends or epidemics. These objectives were formulated to reflect most recent behavior in as short a time period as possible for weekly publication, but a period long enough to assure stable results. To facilitate comprehension, the same method is used for all diseases portrayed.

The analytic method currently used for constructing Figure 1 in the *MMWR* (Figure 6–1), compares the number of reported cases in the current 4-week period for a given health event with historical data on the same condition from the preceding 5 years (*17,18*). Numbers of cases in the current month are listed to facilitate interpretation of instability caused by small numbers.

The choice of 4 weeks as the "current period" is based on evidence that weekly fluctuations in data from disease reports usually reflect irregular reporting practices rather than actual incidence of disease. The use of 5 years of history achieves the objective of using the same model for all conditions portrayed, since some health events were made notifiable more recently. Also, modeling of data from influenza mortality surveillance has shown that more accurate forecasts are based on more recent data (*18*). To increase the historical sample size and to account for any seasonal effect, the baseline is taken to be the average of the reported number of cases for the preceding 4-week period, the corresponding 4-week period, and the

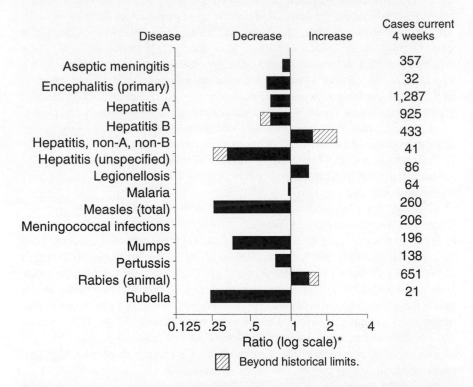

Figure 6–1 Deviation bar chart of notifiable-disease reports, comparison of 4-week totals ending May 23, 1992, with historical data—United States. *Ratio of current 4-week total to the mean 15 4-week totals (from previous, comparable, and subsequent 4-week periods for the past 5 years). The point where the hatched area begins is based on the mean and two standard deivations of these 4-week totals.

following 4-week period, for the previous 5 years. This yields 15 correlated observations, referred to as the historical observations, or baseline (Figure 6–2).

The deviation from unity of the ratio of the current 4-week total to the historical average indicates a departure from past patterns. This ratio is plotted on a logarithmic scale so that an n-fold increase projects to the right the same distance as an n-fold decrease projects to the left, and no change from past patterns (a ratio of 1:1) produces a bar of zero length (*19*). To distinguish the conditions that may require further epidemiologic investigation, the hatching on the bars begins at a point based on the mean and standard deviation of the historical observations. Historical limits of the ratio of current reports to the historical mean are calculated as 1 plus or minus 2 times the standard deviation divided by the mean, where the mean and the standard deviation are calculated from the 15 historical 4-week periods. An evaluation of this method shows that it has good statistical robustness and high sensitivity and predictive value positive for epidemiologically confirmed outbreaks (*20,21*).

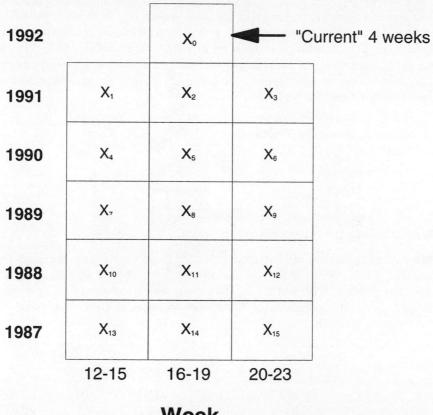

Figure 6–2 Example: Data used for report published during week 20 (May 23, 1992). For example, x_0 is the total number of cases reported for weeks 16–19, 1992.

Scan Statistic

The scan statistic (22) offers a relatively simple approach to determining whether the number of cases reported for a certain time period is excessive. The scan statistic is the maximum number of reported cases (i.e., events) in an interval of predetermined length over the time frame of interest. It is used to test the null hypothesis of uniformity of reporting against an alternative of temporal clustering. Consider the following setting: Surveillance data are reported over a time period T, containing k intervals of equal length:

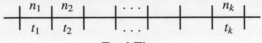

Total Time

where t_i, $i = 1, 2, \ldots, k$ are of equal length t
and $T = t_1 + t_2 + \ldots + t_k$.

The total number of events reported in the entire time period is called N and is the sum of the numbers of events in each of the intervals $n_1 + n_2 + \ldots + n_k$. Let $n = \max \{n_i\}$, $i = 1, 2, \ldots, k$, or the largest report in any of the intervals. The statistical question addressed by the scan statistic is: "What is the probability that the maximum number of cases in any interval of length t is equal to or exceeds n?" The calculation is based on $L = T/t$, or the number of intervals in the entire time period. For example, assume that the frequency of trisomies among karyotyped spontaneous abortions for a defined geographic area by calendar month of last menstrual period in 1992 is as follows:

Month	Number of Cases	Month	Number of Cases
January	1	July	2
February	3	August	4
March	2	September	4
April	2	October	2
May	4	November	3
June	3	December	10

What is the probability of 10 or more trisomies in December given there were a total of 40 in 1992? Using the notation defined above, $N = 40$, $T = 12$; $L = 12/1 = 12$; $n = 10$; and $t = 1$. Then from tabulated values (23) (partially printed below) the probability of 10 or more trisomies in December, given 40 for the year, is 0.083.

	L = 8		L = 12		L = 15	
N	n	p	n	p	n	p
35	14	0.002	11	0.007	10	0.007
40	13	0.040	10	**0.083**	9	0.082
40	14	0.012	11	0.024	10	0.021
40	15	0.003	12	0.006	11	0.005
45	14	0.042	11	0.064	10	0.053

If the results of the scan statistic are to be useful, the lengths of the entire time frame (T) and the scanning interval (t) must be determined *a priori*. The method is intended to detect relatively infrequent elevations in a series of relatively small numbers of events. The lack of extensive tabulated values and the computer-intensive calculations for series with large numbers of events limit the usefulness of the method. Approximations to the exact distribution can be helpful (*23,24*).

Time–Series Methods

Several methods have been used to determine cause-specific expected number of deaths; these have included the median number of deaths during a non-epidemic year (*25*) and regression modeling of incidence data (*26*). In 1979 CDC proposed a new method to estimate expected deaths using a group of methods called *time series;* the methodology of time series is appropriate for data available sequentially over time (*27*). The advantage of time-series models for surveillance over other modeling methods, such as regression, is that the estimation process accounts for period-to-period correlations and seasonality, as well as long-term secular trends. The process of model fitting consists of identification, estimation, and diagnostic validation. One then evaluates competing models on the basis of the fit of the models to the observed data and of the accuracy of the forecasts (*28*).

Most common methods of time-series analysis, such as the Auto Regressive Integrated Moving Average (ARIMA) models (*29*), are appropriate for relatively long series of data that exhibit certain regular properties over the entire series. Differencing, or forming a new series by subtracting adjacent observations, is generally used to create a series with a stationary mean, i.e., without trend. An additional property, stationarity of the variance, is generally required, so that the process does not become more or less variable over time. An autoregressive model includes terms that predict data at one point in time as a function of previous data. A moving-average term creates a series from averages of adjacent observations and is used to model cycles in the data.

Quality–Control Methods

Quality-control methods, traditionally used in manufacturing to detect the number of defective parts produced (*30,31*), have recently been adopted for disease surveillance, to assess whether the observed number of cases exceeds the expected, based on historical norms. The *Salmonella* Outbreak Detection Algorithm (SODA) examines data from the National *Salmonella* Surveillance System to detect outbreaks at the state, regional and national level using a quality control method commonly used in manufacturing (CUSUM) (*32*). SODA compares the count of *Salmonella* cases in the current week to data from the same week for the previous 5 years, to see if there has been a significant increase. A 1-week interval is used in SODA due to the seasonality of *Salmonella*. In addition, the specificity of CUSUM increases with increasing variation; this is a second reason why SODA uses an interval of 1 week rather than 1 month for comparison over the 5-year period. Previous outbreaks and other anomalies are not adjusted for in the data. The CDC has used SODA in its weekly surveillance summaries since 1995. An international outbreak of *Salmonella* serotype Stanley (Figure 6–3), traceable to alfalfa sprouts, was one of the first

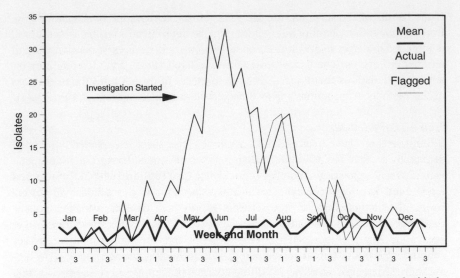

Figure 6–3 Number of *Salmonella* serotype Stanley isolates per week compared with the mean number of isolates reported in the previous 5 years—United States, January 1995–December 1995.

outbreaks identified by SODA (May 1995) (*33*). A recently described approach combines elements of time-series (ARIMA) and quality control methods (statistical process control), to detect changes in reported disease incidence (*34*).

Place: General Concepts

In addition to analysis of surveillance data by time, analysis by place is used. The location from which the condition was reported (such as a hospital) may not be the place where the exposure actually occurred (in the community). Similarly, for medical procedures, the place an operation took place may not be the place of residence of the client. For example, the District of Columbia has the highest rate of legal abortions in the United States, but more than 50% of the women reside outside the District (*35*).

Aberrations in Place: Methodologies

Locating the geographic area with the highest rates can facilitate efforts to identify causes and allow appropriate interventions to be applied. John Snow's removing the Broad Street pump handle remains the classic example of an intervention based on analysis by location (*36*). Even when the numbers of a particular problem are decreasing, focal areas with high levels of the condition may remain, and the identification of these areas allows prevention resources to be targeted effectively. The size of the unit for this type of geographic analysis is determined by the type of condition involved. For some rare conditions, large areas such as states may be appropriate, whereas for events that occur at relatively high frequency or for outbreak situations, areas defined by postal codes or other geographic boundaries may be the most desirable.

The availability of computers, as well as software for spatial mapping, allows more sophisticated analysis of surveillance data by place. Public health officials are now able to use surveillance data to follow the geographic course of a particular condition and assist their efforts to plan intervention strategies (see maps shown later in this chapter).

Geographic Information Systems (GIS) is an increasingly popular technology which helps temporally embellish a spot map by storing spatially referenced data in layers (37). This facilitates examination of spatial associations within the data, and supports the ability to view additional data which underly the map ("drill down"). Some GIS maps attempt to reflect the distribution of individual disease cases over a large geographical area. Other GIS maps aggregate the cases to area units such as census tracts or counties and present the relative risk for each unit; however, areas with small populations often present estimation problems. In these instances, smoothing methods are often used before mapping the relative risk (29). GIS maps can also be used for inferential analysis. Methods for inferential analysis, such as Kriging (37), account for the spatial correlation between data points. The application of other statistical methods such as multilevel modeling to control for hierarchical or neighborhood effects increases inference reliability (38). In summary, GIS methodology enables one to make more reliable inferences about the distribution and association of diseases.

Aberrations in Place and Time: Methodologies

When health events are reported from a specific geographic area over a defined time period, do they form a spatial–temporal cluster? Traditional approaches to the analysis of health-event aggregation in geographic areas have been based on randomization arguments (39,40). A representative discussion follows.

One proposed method divides the study area into subareas (e.g., counties or census tracts) and the study time period into intervals of constant length (e.g., months or years) (41). The cases of the health event for each time–space "cell" are then calculated. The maximum count within any time interval is summed across all subareas to obtain a test statistic.

This method assumes equal population density across all area cells, which may be a limitation in some applications. An alternative method (42) addresses this problem. All possible pairs of cases are examined, and each pair is classified according to whether the case-patients in the pair lived close together and had onset of the health problem (or report) close in time, resulting in a 2-by-2 table:

		Reports close in time?	
		Yes	No
Reports close	Yes	a	b
in space?	No	c	d

Under the hypothesis of no clustering, the expected number may be calculated in the usual way, with an adjustment in the significance test, since the statistic is based on pairs of cases (43). A brief example follows.

Consider cases of a disease with the following spatial and temporal relationships:

		Cases close in space?		
		Yes	No	All
	Yes	1		5
Cases close in time?	No			23
	All	6	22	28

The test statistic to be computed is X = number of pairs close in space and time, *1* in this example. We use row and column marginal totals to compute an expected value for this cell: $(6 \times 5) / 28 = 1.07$. Now use the Poisson distribution to compute the probability of seeing one (or more) cases close in space and time, given that we expect 1.07; this value is at least 0.63. Therefore, we conclude that these data provide no evidence for space or time clustering.

A criticism of this method is that the choice of the critical time and space distances is arbitrary. This problem was addressed for the question of spatial clustering (*44*), and the method does not require spatial boundaries or assessment of the entire population base. An alternative approach uses a sensitivity analysis of the time and space critical values (*45*).

A second criticism of this method is that it makes no allowance for edge effects that arise either from natural geographic boundaries (e.g., coastlines) or because unrecorded cases occur outside the designated study region. By altering the interpretation of expected pairs of close cases and replacing the simple count of close pairs by a weighted sum (*46*), this problem can be reduced. This method has been used to investigate Legionnaires' disease in Scotland (*47*).

Because of the diverse and complicated nature of clusters, there is no single test to use in all situations. The statistical sources referenced here are intended only to augment other epidemiologic methods in a systematic, integrated approach, coupled with flexibility in methods of analysis and interpretation of significance levels (*48*).

Person: General Concepts

Analyzing surveillance data by the characteristics of persons who have the condition provides further specification (*49*). The demographic variables most frequently used are age, gender, and race and ethnicity, when available. Surveillance data on race and ethnicity are critical for evaluating health status, health-care access, and the effectiveness of public health interventions, which target racial and ethnic subgroups. Most federally funded public health surveillance systems are required to collect data on race and ethnicity, and will be required to use the revised OMB Statistical Directive 15 for categorization of race (American Indian or Alaska Native, Asian, Black or African American, Native Hawaiian or Other Pacific Islander) and ethnicity ("Hispanic or Latino" and "Not Hispanic or Latino") by 2003 (*50*). Despite this, the completeness of most surveillance data for race and ethnicity is poor, at least partially due to sensitivity about collection of the data and concern about its accuracy (*51*). Other variables such as marital status, occupation, and levels of income and education may also be helpful, although most surveillance systems do not routinely collect such information.

Analysis of trends in disease or injury by age depends on the specific health condition of interest. For childhood diseases, relatively narrow age categories (e.g., by single years) can identify the age group associated with the peak incidence of a particular health condition. Conversely, for conditions that primarily affect older populations, broader 10-year-age intervals are frequently used. In general, the typical age distribution associated with the health condition provides the best guide to deciding which age categories to use, with several narrower categories for the ages associated with peak incidence and broader categories covering the remainder of the age spectrum.

Surveillance systems have also been used to analyze behavioral characteristics of populations; the BRFSS was recently used to describe the state-specific prevalence of adult tobacco usage (52). Such systems generally depend on self-reported behavior and may be based on repeated surveys of representative groups, trends in markers for specific types of behavior (e.g., sales of a particular product), or active surveillance of a particular behavioral characteristic or indicator in a defined group (e.g., testing urine for drugs in school or work settings).

If possible, the characteristics of persons included in any surveillance system should be related to denominators. Although assessing the number of cases alone can be sufficient, variable-specific rates are more helpful in allowing comparisons of the risk involved. Thus, even if the number of cases of a particular condition is higher in one part of a population, the rate may be lower if that group represents a large proportion of the population. In this way, comparing the rates within surveillance data of certain populations is analogous to calculating relative risks within observational cohort studies. Rates will be discussed in the next section.

Person: Confidentiality and Inadvertent Disclosure

Surveillance systems often collect personal data under a pledge of confidentiality. Therefore, the identity of those who participated in the surveillance system must be protected before data are disseminated. However, even if personal identifiers are not used, if the demographic data collected about a respondent are very detailed, if the prevalence of the health condition or some other identifying feature is low, or if the region in which the respondent lives is sparsely populated, it may be relatively easy to infer, with high probability of accuracy, the identity of the respondent. This is often referred to as the problem of small cell size or "inadvertent disclosure." Several approaches can minimize this problem. First, because precise data facilitate identification of individuals, disclosure prevention techniques have focused on limiting the nature and content of the data released, as well as limiting who gains access to the data. These techniques are often used in preparation of public use data sets and include collapsing continuous variables into categories, collapsing response categories for categorical variables, dropping variables that pose a large risk of disclosure, and adding random noise or error to selected variables. Second, in preparing tables or statistical analyses for publication, analyses or tables with cells with small numbers can be suppressed, ensuring that no characteristic of individuals will be identifiable by calculation from other tabulated data in the same or other public data sets. Third, care must be exercised with contextual data, which impart information about a geographic region, such as a county or a census tract. Contextual data might include population-based estimates of the percentage employed or foreign-born, and are thought often to be related to health behavior or status; however, release of contextual data increases the probability of inadvertent disclosure. The U.S. Bureau of Census and the National Center for Health Statistics have standards for the release of data containing contextual variables, as well as standards for the release of data from small cells (53).

Interactions among Time, Place, and Person

By proceeding from the simple (e.g., crude rates) to the more complex (e.g., variable-specific rates), meaningful trends may be revealed. This is because interactions among the time-place-person parameters of surveillance data can obscure important patterns of disease or injury in specific populations. For example, in the United States in the 1980s, the overall number of syphilis cases fell during the first two-thirds of the decade but rose beginning in 1987 (Figure 6–4, Panel A). When analyzed by gender (Figure 6–4, Panel B), the decline in syphilis occurred primarily among men; cases among women were low for the first 5 years, increased slightly in 1986, and rose more rapidly for the rest of the decade. Finally, when stratified by both gender and race (Figure 6–4, Panel C), the decrease in numbers of cases of syphilis was seen only among white males—presumably among men who have sex with other men and who had changed their sexual practices in response to HIV prevention activities (54). Conversely, the increase in syphilis occurred among black men and women, with both trends beginning in 1986, and being linked to unsafe sexual behavior associated with use of crack cocaine (55). If more specific analysis by person had not occurred, the offsetting trends in the mid-1980s of declines among white males might have delayed recognition by public health officials of the syphilis epidemic among minorities.

RATES AND RATE STANDARDIZATION

A rate measures the frequency of an event. It comprises a numerator (i.e., the upper portion of a fraction denoting the number of occurrences of an event during a specified time) and a denominator (i.e., the lower portion of a fraction denoting the size of the population in which the events occur). A crucial aspect of a rate is the specification of the time period under consideration. An optional component is a multiplier, a power of 10 that is used to convert awkward fractions to more workable numbers (56). The general form of a rate is shown below:

$$\text{rate} = \frac{\text{number of occurrences of event in specified time}}{\text{average or mid-interval population}} \times 10^n$$

where the denominator represents the size of the population during the specified period in which the events occur and the size of n usually ranges from 2 to 6

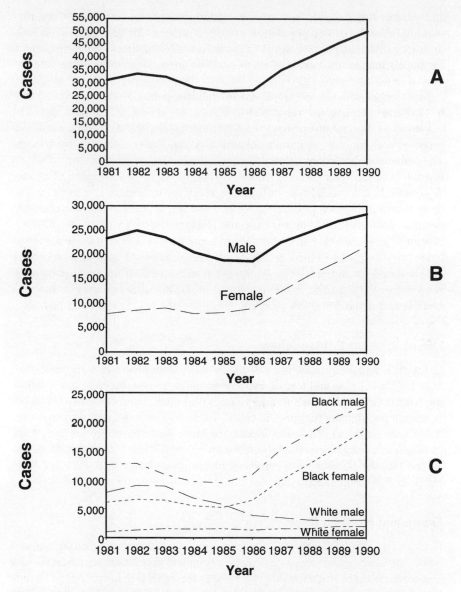

Figure 6–4 Crude gender-specific and gender-race-specific cases of primary and secondary syphilis—United States, 1981–1990. A comparison of differential trends.

(i.e., the number at risk varies between 100 and 1,000,000). The selection of n depends on the incidence or prevalence of the event.

Although surveillance often provides numerator data only, the use of raw numbers such as cases of a disease or injury has limitations. Raw numbers quantify occurrences of an event during a specified time without regard to population size and dynamics, or other demographic characteristics such as distribution by race and gender. Rates enable one to make more appropriate, informative comparisons of occurrences in a population over time, among different subpopulations, or among different populations at the same or different times, since the size of the population and the period of time specified are accounted for in the calculation of rates.

Many different rates are employed in standard public health practice (Table 6–1). These measures are calculated in numerous ways and may have different connotations. Special distinction should be made among the terms *rate, ratio,* and *proportion.* A *ratio* is any quotient obtained by dividing one quantity by another. The numerator and denominator are generally distinct quantities, neither of which is a subset of the other. No restrictions exist on the value or dimension of a ratio. A *proportion* is a special type of ratio for which the numerator is a subset of the denominator population, thus requiring the resulting quotient to be dimensionless, positive, and less than 1, or less than 100 if expressed as a percentage (*57*). Although all rates are ratios, in epidemiology a *rate* may be a proportion (e.g., prevalence rate) or may be limited in scope by further restrictions such as representing the number of occurrences of a health event in a specified time and population per unit time (e.g., hazard or incidence rate) (*58*). This latter definition is most restrictive and is the definition generally used for rates in chemistry and physics.

Use of Rates in Epidemiology

Calculation and analysis of rates is critical in epidemiologic investigations, not only for formulating and testing hypotheses about causes, but also for identifying risk factors for disease and injury. Rates also allow valid comparisons within or among populations for specific times. To determine rates, one must have reliable numerator and denominator data, the latter being generally more difficult to obtain in most epidemiologic investigations, particularly if the data to be analyzed (i.e, the number of occurrences of an event) have been collected from public health surveillance systems.

Crude and Specific Rates

Rates can be calculated either for the entire population or for certain subpopulations within the larger group. Rates describing a complete population are termed *crude.* The computation of crude rates is performed as the initial step in analysis since they are important in obtaining information about and contrasting entire populations. For example, the data in Figure 6–4, Panel A, could be divided by the total population each year to calculate the crude rate of primary and secondary syphilis.

Within a population, the rate at which a particular health event occurs may not be constant throughout the entire population. To examine the differences, the population is partitioned into relevant *specific* subpopulations, and a *specific* rate is calculated for each subset. For example, if one calculates death rates by age group (because death rate is not constant for all age categories), the resulting rates are termed *age-specific death rates.* In Figure 6–4, Panel B, dividing the sex-specific occurrences by the sex-specific populations yields the sex-specific rates.

Variation of rates among population subgroups results from several factors: natural history of the health problem, differential distribution of susceptibility or causes, and genetic differences among subpopulations. For example, mortality rates are higher among men than women and blacks than whites (*59*). The distribution of subgroups within the population may also be so disparate that a summary rate may not convey useful information. Therefore, the magnitude of a crude rate depends on the magnitude of the rates of the subpopulations as well as on the demographics of the entire population (*60*). These variations in rates across a population would remain unknown if only crude rates were calculated.

Standardized Rates

When rates are compared across different populations or for the same population over time, crude rates are appropriate only if the populations are similar with respect to factors associated with the health event being investigated (*61*). Such factors could include age, race, gender, socioeconomic status, or risk factors (e.g., number of cigarettes smoked). If the populations are dissimilar, variable-specific rates should be computed and compared. Alternatively, the rates can be adjusted for the effect of a confounding variable in order to obtain an undistorted view of the effect that other variables have on risk. This adjustment of rates when comparing populations is called *standardization* and yields "standardized" or "adjusted" rates. The two techniques of standardization are *direct* and *indirect*.

Direct Standardization

A directly standardized rate is obtained for a study population by averaging the specific rates for the population, using the distribution of a selected standard population as the averaging weights. This adjusted rate represents "what the crude rate would have been in the study population if that population had the same distribution as the standard population with respect to the variable(s) for which the adjustment or standardization was carried out" (*56*).

The rate is termed *directly standardized* because specific rates are used directly in the calculation. If data for the same standard population are used to calculate directly standardized rates for two or more study populations, those standardized rates can be appropriately compared. Any difference among the standardized rates cannot be attributed to differential population distributions of the standardized variable because the calculations have been adjusted for that variable (*62*). The following data must be available in order to use direct adjustment:

- specific rates for the study population
- distribution for the selected standard population across the same strata as those used in determining the specific rates

Indirect Standardization

An indirectly standardized rate is calculated for a study population by averaging the specific rates for a select standard population, using the distribution of the study population as weights. One should use indirect adjustment when any of the

Table 6–1 Rates and Quantities That Involve Rates Commonly Used in Epidemiology

Measure	Numerator	Denominator	Expressed per number at risk
Measures of morbidity			
Incidence rate	Number of new cases of specified condition/given time	Population at start of time interval	variable: 10^x where x = 2,3,4,5,6
Attack rate	Number of new cases of specified condition/epidemic period	Population at start of epidemic period	variable: 10^x where x = 2,3,4,5,6
Secondary attack rate	Number of new cases of specified condition among contacts of known patients	Size of contact population at risk	variable: 10^x where x = 2,3,4,5,6
Point prevalence	Number of current cases of specified condition at given time	Estimated population at same point in time	variable: 10^x where x = 2,3,4,5,6
Period prevalence	Number of old cases plus new cases of specified condition identified in given time interval	Estimated mid-interval population	variable: $10x$ where x = 2,3,4,5,6
Measures of mortality			
Crude death rate	Total number of deaths reported in given time interval	Estimated mid-interval population	1,000 or 100,000
Cause-specific death rate	Number of deaths from specific cause in given time interval	Estimated mid-interval population	100,000

Table 6-1 Rates and Quantities That Involve Rates Commonly Used in Epidemiology (Continued)

Measure	Numerator	Denominator	Expressed per number at risk
Proportionate mortality	Number of deaths from specific cause in given time interval	Total number of deaths from all causes in same interval	100 or 1,000
Death-to- case ratio (Case-fatality rate, case-fatality ratio)	Number of deaths from specific condition in given time interval	Number of new cases of that condition in same time interval	100
Neonatal mortality rate	Number of deaths (<28 days of age) in given time interval	Number of live births in same time interval	1,000
Infant mortality rate	Number of deaths (<1 year of age) in given time interval	Number of live births in same time interval	1,000
Maternal mortality rate	Number of deaths from pregnancy-related causes in given time interval	Number of live births in same time interval	100,000
Measures of natality			
Crude birth rate	Number of live births reported in given time interval	Estimated total mid-interval population	1,000
Crude fertility rate	Number of live births reported in given time interval	Estimated number of women ages 15–44 years at mid-interval	1,000
Crude rate of natural increase	Number of live births minus number of deaths in given time interval	Estimated total mid-interval population	1,000
Low birth weight ratio	Number of live births (<2,500 grams) in given time interval	Number of live births reported in same time interval	100

specific rates in the study population are unavailable or when such small numbers exist in the categories of strata that the data are unreliable (i.e., the resulting rates are unstable). This commonly occurs in occupational mortality or in small geographic areas. For these reasons, indirect standardization is used more often than direct standardization. Indirectly standardized rates for two or more populations of interest can be appropriately compared if the same standard population is used in the computations. The following data are required to make an indirect adjustment to a rate:

- specific rates for the selected standard population
- distribution for the study population across the same strata as those used in calculating the specific rates
- crude rate for the study population
- crude rate for the standard population

A special application of the indirect standardized rate, when the health event of interest is death, is the standardized mortality ratio (SMR). It is the number of deaths occurring in a study population or subpopulation, expressed as a percentage of the number of deaths expected to occur if the given population and the selected standard population had the same specific rates (63). Explicitly, the SMR is an indirect, age-adjusted ratio calculated as the indirect standardized mortality rate for the study population, divided by the crude mortality rate for the standard population. Additional information is available on the use of the SMR, as well as on computation of variance and confidence intervals for direct and indirect measures (62).

Choice of Standard Population

If crude rates are to be adjusted, an appropriate standardized population needs to be chosen. In extreme cases, the choice of different standardized populations can lead to different results. For example, use of one standardized population may yield an adjusted rate higher for population A than for population B, while choice of another standard population may yield a higher rate for population B (62). Two factors should be considered when choosing a standard population:

- Select a population that is representative of the study populations being compared.
- Understand how choice of a standard population affects directly standardized rates (e.g., if the age-specific rates for population A are greater than for population B at young ages and the opposite is true at older ages, a standard population with distribution skewed to younger ages will yield a higher directly standardized rate for population A than for population B).

Generally, the choice of standard population makes little difference in comparing adjusted rates. Although magnitudes of the adjusted rates depend upon choice of standard population, no meaning is attached to those magnitudes; only relative differences in the adjusted rates can be assessed.

Various choices are available for a standard population. Customary selections include the combined or pooled population of the overall population to be studied, the population of one of the study groups, a large population, or a hypothetical population. Calculating standardized rates using different standard populations allows comparisons of different distributions (64).

In 1998, the DHHS announced its decision to adopt the projected population for the year 2000, produced by the Bureau of the Census, as its uniform population standard for age-adjusting death rates (65). This will effectively standardize mortality data provided by the DHHS, and eliminate the multiplicity of mortality rates that have resulted from disparate population standards.

To Standardize or Not To Standardize

The decision to standardize is not always straightforward. Several factors, most of which are data-driven, must be considered in the decision process. Reasons to present standardized rates include the following (61):

- Standardization adjusts for confounding variables to yield a more realistic view of the effect of other variables on risk.
- A summary measure for a population is easier to compare with similar summary measures than are sets of specific rates.
- A standardized rate has a smaller standard error than any of the specific rates (this is important when comparing subpopulations or geographic areas).
- Specific rates may be imprecise or unstable because of sparse data in the strata.
- Specific rates may be unavailable for certain groups of interest (e.g., small populations or those designated by specific geographic areas).

The major disadvantage of standardization is evident when the specific rates vary differently across strata, such as when they move in different directions or at different magnitudes, in individual age groups. In this case the trend in the standardized rate is a weighted average of the trends in the specific rates, where the weights depend on the standard population selected. When this occurs, the standardized rate tends to mask the differences, and no single summary measure will reveal these differences.

Another unfavorable characteristic of standardized rates is that their magnitude is arbitrary and depends entirely on the standard population. Although generally not the case, relative rankings of summary measures from different study populations may change if a different standard population is selected.

Regardless of the decision made regarding standardization, the variable-specific rates must be evaluated to characterize accurately and to understand more fully the variation among study populations. Standardized rates should never be used as a substitute for specific rates, nor should they be the basis of inferences when specific rates can be computed. A compromise to the use of a summary measure versus a set of specific measures is to use the specific rates but to eliminate or combine categories to minimize the number of rates required for comparison. Additional discussion is available on advantages and disadvantages of standardization and on analyzing crude and specific rates (66).

Table 6–2 Crude Death Rates—Dade and Pinellas Counties, Florida, 1980

	Population	Deaths	Crude Death Rate (per 1,000 population)
Dade County	1,706,097	16,859	9.9
Pinellas County	732,685	11,531	15.7

Sources: Bureau of the Census, 1983.
    National Center for Health Statistics, Centers for Disease Control and Prevention.

Rate Standardization: Practical Example

To demonstrate how crude, specific, and standardized rates are obtained, we compare death rates in two Florida counties. This example shows how standardized rates can be misleading if they are not properly scrutinized. We will use population and death totals for Pinellas and Dade counties in Florida for 1980 (Table 6–2). The crude death rate for Pinellas County is about 60% higher than for Dade County. When the age distributions of each county are used, the resulting age-specific death rates are generally slightly higher in Dade County (Table 6–3), even though the crude death rate is substantially higher for Pinellas County. This seeming anomaly in the data results from the different age distributions of each county. Specifically, the population in Pinellas is older than the population in Dade. Directly standardizing the rates for Pinellas and Dade counties to the 1980 U.S. population corrects for the differences in population (Table 6–4). Once differences in age-related distributions in the two counties have been taken into account, the adjusted death rate for Pinellas County is lower than that for Dade County (7.7 and 7.9, respectively).

Table 6–3 Age-Specific Death Rates—Dade and Pinellas Counties, Florida, 1980

Age Group (years)	Dade			Pinellas		
	Population	Deaths	Rate (per 1,000 pop.)	Population	Deaths	Rate (per 1,000 pop.)
0–4	97,870	383	3.9	31,005	101	3.3
5–14	221,452	75	0.3	77,991	20	0.3
15–24	284,956	440	1.5	95,456	80	0.8
25–34	265,885	529	2.0	90,435	129	1.4
35–44	207,564	538	2.6	65,519	168	2.6
45–54	193,505	1,107	5.7	69,572	460	6.6
55–64	175,579	2,164	12.3	98,132	1,198	12.2
65–74	152,172	3,789	24.9	114,686	2,746	23.9
>75	107,114	7,834*	73.1	89,889	6,629*	73.7
Total	1,706,097	16,859	9.9	732,685	11,531	15.7

Sources: Bureau of the Census, 1983.
    National Center for Health Statistics, Centers for Disease Control and Prevention.
*Deaths >75 include six persons of unknown age for Dade County and one of unknown age for Pinellas County.

Table 6–4 Directly Standardized Death Rates—Dade and Pinellas Counties, Florida, 1980*

Age Group (years)	A: 1980 U.S. Population (percentage distribution)	B: Age-Specific Death Rates (per 1,000 pop.)		C: Expected Deaths in 1980 U.S. Population Using County Age-Specific Rates[†]	
		Dade	Pinellas	Dade	Pinellas
0–4	7.2	3.9	3.3	28	24
5–14	15.3	0.3	0.3	5	5
15–24	18.7	1.5	0.8	28	15
25–34	16.5	2.0	1.4	33	23
35–44	11.4	2.6	2.6	30	30
45–54	10.0	5.7	6.6	57	66
55–64	9.6	12.3	12.2	118	117
65–74	6.9	24.9	23.9	172	165
>75	4.4	73.1	73.7	322	324
Totals	100.0	9.9	15.7	793	769
Directly adjusted death rates (per 1,000 pop.)¶				7.9	7.7

*U.S. population, 1980, used as standard.
[†]$C_{ij} = A_i \times B_{ij}$ where $i = 1,...,9$ age groups and $j = 1,2$ counties.
$\sum_i C_{ij} /100.$

The indirect method of adjustment increases the relative difference between death rates for the two counties (Table 6–5). The adjusting factor is computed as the 1980 death rate for the total U.S. population divided by the expected death rate. Then, adjusted death rate is calculated as the adjusting factor multiplied by the crude death rate. In this example, indirect adjustment reinforces and accen-tuates the results of direct adjustment by yielding rates of 7.5 and 7.8 deaths per 1,000 population for Pinellas and Dade counties, respectively.

This example illustrates the importance of being thoroughly familiar with the data. Comparison of crude death rates alone can be misleading. However, calculating age-specific and adjusted rates permits an accurate understanding of death rates in these counties and shows that the high crude rate in Pinellas County reflects its older population. The example also illustrates how the magnitude of adjusted rates depends on the choice of standard population.

Analysis of Rates

When numerator and denominator data are available, analysis of rates should always begin with calculation of crude rates and proceed to subsequent computation of relevant specific rates. If appropriate, a standard population can be chosen to determine standardized rates. Tables and especially maps are important

Table 6–5 Indirectly Standardized Death Rates—Dade and Pinellas Counties, Florida, 1980*

Age Group (years)	A: Death Rates (per 1,000 pop.) U.S. 1980	B: 1980 Population		C: Expected Number of Deaths in County Based on U.S.-Specific Rates†	
		Dade	Pinellas	Dade	Pinellas
0–4	3.3	97,870	31,005	323	102
5–14	0.3	221,452	77,991	66	23
15–24	1.2	284,956	95,456	342	115
25–34	1.3	265,885	90,435	346	118
35–44	2.3	207,564	65,519	477	151
45–54	5.9	193,505	69,572	1,142	410
55–64	13.4	175,579	98,132	2,353	1,315
65–74	29.8	152,172	114,686	4,535	3,418
>75	87.2¶	107,114	89,889	9,340	7,838
Totals	8.8	1,706,097	732,685	18,924	13,490
Expected death rates (per 1,000 pop.)§				11.1	18.4
Adjusting factors**				0.79	0.48
Crude death rates (per 1,000 pop.)				9.9	15.7
Indirectly adjusted death rates (per 1,000 pop.)††				7.8	7.5

*U.S. age-specific death rates, 1980, used as standard.
†$C_{ij} = A_i \times B_{ij}$ where i = 1,...,9 age groups and j = 1,2 counties.
¶Deaths >75 include 568 of unknown age for United States.
§$\sum_i C_{ij} / B_{ij}$ for j = 1,2.
**U.S. total death rate/expected death rate.
††Crude death rate × adjusting factor.

means of presenting rates at different times or locations (see various tables, graphs, and maps in this chapter).

Several statistical procedures are available to analyze data. Inference on a single proportion is performed using a z test, and assessing the difference between two proportions can be accomplished with a z or χ^2 test (note that Fleiss does not distinguish between rates and proportions or the analysis of them) (61). Use of Poisson parameters is helpful in comparing two rates (67). A series of χ^2 tests can be used to compare proportions from several independent samples (60), and Poisson regression is frequently used for comparing several rates (68). Other modeling procedures that can be used to analyze rates include smoothing, Box-Jenkins, and Kalman filter approaches, as well as the full-range of non-parametric approaches, including Bayes smooths (29).

EXPLORATORY DATA ANALYSIS

Exploratory data analysis (EDA) is enumerative, numeric, or graphic detective work (63). It is the application of a set of techniques to a body of data to make the data more understandable.

A philosophy that minimizes assumptions, EDA allows the data to motivate the analysis, and combines ease of description with quantitative knowledge. It leads the analyst to uncover characteristics often hidden within the data.

Practice of EDA involves four fundamental steps (69,70).

1. Use visual displays to convey the structure of the data and analyses.
2. Transform the data mathematically to simplify their distribution and to clarify their analysis.
3. Investigate the influence that unusual observations (outliers) have on the results of analysis.
4. Examine the residuals (the difference between the observed data and a fitted model) to provide additional insight into the data.

The initial step in any analysis is EDA. It allows the investigator to become familiar with the data and forms the foundation for further analysis. Although most public health surveillance systems are established for specific topics, proper EDA of the data can provide insight into demographic, temporal, and spatial patterns otherwise overlooked in the collection of numbers. Additionally, EDA may contribute to more timely detection of unusual observations, which may in turn facilitate a quicker public health response to factors that cause increased morbidity or mortality.

Data Displays

A first step in any analysis of data is a visual examination of the data. A few of the techniques that should be used initially are described below for application to a single set of numbers, for exploration of relationships between two factors, and for comparisons among several populations.

Data Plots

A dot plot is a one-dimensional plot (Figure 6–5) of the individual values of a set of numbers. The x axis represents one or more categories of a noncontinuous variable, and the y axis represents the range of values displayed by the observations. Observations with identical values are plotted side by side on the same horizontal plane.

Stem-and-Leaf Displays

A stem-and-leaf display is a graphic (Figure 6–6) that allows the digits of the observation values to sort the numbers into numerical order for display. This is a variation of the conventional histogram. The basic principle used in constructing a stem-and-leaf display is the splitting of each data value between a suitable pair of adjacent digits to form a set of leading digits and a set of trailing digits. The set of leading digits forms the stems, and the set of the first trailing digit from the data forms the leaves. Remaining trailing digits are ignored for the purpose of the graphic. Variations to the stem-and-leaf display are possible (69).

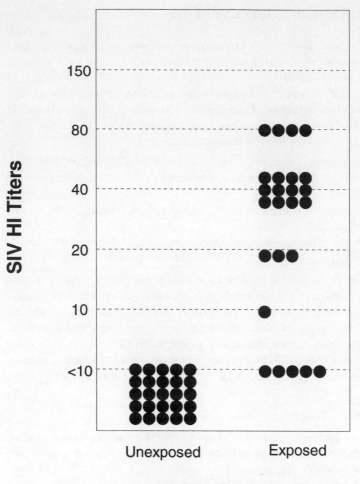

Swine Exhibitors

Figure 6–5 Dot plot of results of swine influenza virus (SIV) hemagglutination-inhibition (HI) antibody testing among exposed and unexposed swine exhibitors—Wisconsin, 1988.

Although many investigators begin an evaluation of data with a histogram, the stem-and-leaf display has several advantages over it. Because every observation is plotted in the stem-and-leaf display, it contains more detail than the histogram and allows computation of percentages. Moreover, transformations can be applied directly to stem-and-leaf data.

Scatter Plots

The scatter plot or scatter diagram is a plot (Figure 6–7) that reveals the relationship between two variables. Each observation comprises a pair of values, one for each variable. The observation is plotted by measuring the value of one variable on the horizontal axis and the value of the other on the vertical axis.

1987: 226, 307, 350, 236, 222, 258, 197, 167, 138, 108, 191, 190, 201
1988: 216, 238, 331, 270, 265, 156, 164, 142, 112, 111, 153, 138, 159
1989: 145, 306, 314, 264, 222, 195, 155, 149, 102, 117, 174, 158, 159

Stem	Leaf
	0
34	1
32	674
30	
28	450
26	8
24	22668
22	16
20	157
18	474
16	259356899
14	88
12	28127
10	

Figure 6–6 Ordered data series and stem-and-leaf display of 39 4-week totals of reported cases of meningococcal infections—United States, 1987–89.

Data Summaries

A data set can be summarized by calculating a few numbers that are relatively easy to interpret. For example, measures of central tendency and variability are frequently used to describe data. In particular, two types of summary displays have proven useful in characterizing data, i.e., the 5-number summary and the box plot.

Five-Number Summaries

The 5-number summary of a data set is a simple display (Table 6–6) involving the median, hinge, and extreme values. The median is a measure of the central tendency of the data that splits an ordered data set in half. The hinges are a measure of the variability of the data and are the values in the middle of each half. Therefore, the hinges are the data values that are approximately one-quarter and three-quarters from the beginning of the ordered data set. They are determined by formulas (70) and are similar to quartiles that are defined so that one-quarter of the observations lie below the lower quartile and one-quarter lie above the upper quartile. The extremes also reflect the variability of the data and are the smallest and largest values in the data.

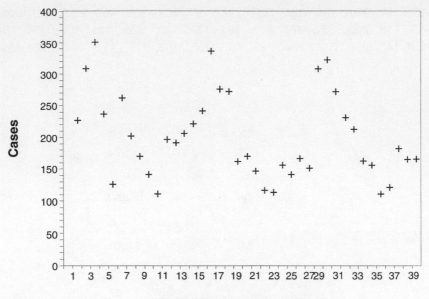

1987-1989 (4-week periods)

Figure 6–7 Scatter plot of 39 4-week totals of reported cases of meningococcal infections—United States, 1987–89.

Box Plots

The box plot is a graphic representation (Figure 6–8) of the 5-number summary with the two ends of the box representing the hinges and the line through the box representing the median. A line runs from each end of the box (i.e., from each hinge) to the corresponding lower and upper extreme values. This plot al-

Table 6–6 Common Power Transformations $(y \rightarrow y^p)$

p	Transformation	Name	Notes
•			
•			Higher powers
•			
2	y^2	Square	
1	y	Raw	No transformation
$^1/_2$	$\sqrt{y}$	Square root	Appropriate for count data
0	$\log(y)$	Logarithm	Generally logarithm to base 10; widely used
$-^1/_2$	$-1/\sqrt{y}$	Reciprocal root	Minus sign preserves order
-1	$-1/y$	Reciprocal	
-2	$-1/y^2$	Reciprocal square	
•			
•			Lower powers
•			

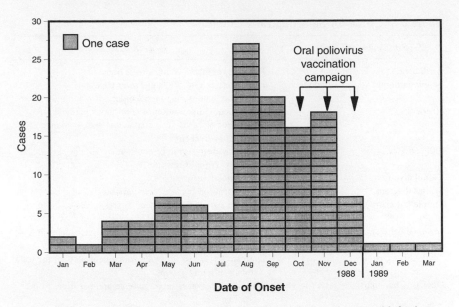

Figure 6–8 Box plot of 39 4-week totals of reported cases of meningococal infections— United States, 1987–89.

lows the reader to see quickly the median level, the variability, and the symmetry of the data. Variations of the box plot, including identification of outlier values, are possible (*21*).

Transformations

Transformation or re-expression of data is a powerful tool that facilitates understanding their implications. If numbers are collected in a manner that renders them hard to grasp, the data analyst should use a transformation method, while preserving as much of the original information as can be used. When used appropriately, transformed data can be readily analyzed and interpreted.

Raw data are transformed for a number of reasons, including the achievement of symmetry, to produce a straight-line relationship, to allow use of an additive model, to reduce variability, and to attain normally distributed data. Symmetry is highly desirable when analyzing a single data set, since it ensures that a "typical" value (such as the mean or median) more nearly summarizes the data. When analyzing pairs of data, a straight-line relationship is important because linear associations are simple, both in form and in interpretation. One or both variables can be transformed to achieve linearity. A desirable feature of additive models is that data in complex tables can be typically decomposed into additive effects and analyzed accordingly. Reduced variability of the data is crucial when comparing several data sets. If the data spread varies with the data set, then "typical" values are obtained more accurately in the data with smaller spread. Finally, normally distributed data are needed so that normal theory statistics can be applied to test hypotheses and to draw inferences.

Table 6–7 Guide for Selecting Data Graphics

Type of Graph or Chart	When to Use
Arithmetic-scale line graph	Trends in numbers or rates over time
Semilogarithmic-scale line graph	1. Emphasize rate of change over time
	2. Display values ranging >2 orders of magnitude
Histogram	1. Frequency distribution of continuous variable
	2. Number of cases during epidemic (i.e., epidemic curve) or over time
Frequency polygon	Frequency distribution of continuous variable, especially to show components
Cumulative frequency	Cumulative frequency
Scatter diagram	Plot association between two variables
Simple bar chart	Compare size or frequency of different categories of single variable
Grouped bar chart	Compare size or frequency of different categories of 2–4 series of data
Stacked bar chart	Compare totals and illustrate component parts of the total among different groups
Deviation bar chart	Illustrate differences, both positive and negative, from baseline
Pie chart	Show components of a whole
Spot map	Show location of cases or events
Chloropleth map	Display events or rates geographically
Box plot	Visualize statistical characteristics (e.g., median, range, skewness) of variable

Not all data sets can be transformed. The ratio of the largest to smallest value in the original data set is a simple indicator of whether a group of numbers will be affected substantially by transforming. If the ratio is near 1:1, a transformation will not severely alter the appearance of the data. Since transformations affect larger and smaller values differently, the further the ratio is from *1*, the greater the need is for transformation to display and understand the data most simply.

Transformations are generally accomplished by raising each value of the data set to some power p. Different values of p yield different effects on a data set, but those effects are ordered if the values of p are ordered. Some transformations are especially effective in certain instances (Table 6–7). For example, the square root transformation is particularly capable of reducing variability in count data. Guidelines are available to assist in selecting appropriate transformations (*69,70*).

Smoothing

Smoothing refers to EDA techniques that summarize consecutive, overlapping segments of a series of data to produce a smoother curve. Its goal is to represent patterns in the data more clearly without becoming encumbered with any detailed peaks and valleys. Variations in the data set caused by irregular components are smoothed so that the overall trend can be determined more readily. Thus, smoothing allows investigators to search for patterns that may otherwise be masked.

Smoothing is used on data series to explore the relationship between two variables. The values along the *x* axis should be equally spaced. The *y* values are called a *time series* if they are collected over successive time intervals, although these values need not be defined by time (e.g., in a data sequence of birth rates by mother's age). As long as the x axis defines an order and the order is not too irregular, the y sequence can be called a time series, and smoothing techniques can be applied. In time-series analysis, models are frequently developed on the smoothed data because these data are generally easier to model.

Numerous smoothing approaches exist, each having its own assets and liabilities. The simplest example of smoothing is a moving average of three intervals in which observation y_i in the data sequence is replaced with the mean of y_{i-1}, y_i, and y_{i+1}. Discussions of smoothing functions, including suggestions on how to overcome the problem of obtaining end points for the smoothed series, appear elsewhere (*29,70,71*).

SELECTION OF ANALYTIC METHODS

Once EDA has been completed, and the investigator has gained a sense of the characteristics of the data, the next step entails a more probing analysis. No single method can be used to detect all epidemics or all types of aberrations. Several questions provide a framework for choosing an analytic method. We will use the "Figure 1" methodology from the *MMWR* to illustrate these concepts.

- *What is the purpose of the surveillance system?* The analyses in Figure 1 reveal aggregated national patterns in selected health conditions, thereby facilitating prevention and intervention efforts. Since the data are reported weekly by state health departments, CDC is able to collate this information for national trends. Additionally, the data are maintained historically for the archival purposes of measuring trends and assessing the effects of interventions.
- *What is the purpose of the analytic method?* Since a single method cannot be expected to distinguish between a change in historical trend and a one-time outbreak with unsustained increases, the analyst must identify the purpose of the analysis before choosing an analytic method. If the nature of the data is determined and the questions are well defined, the results of the analytic method can be used to augment other sources of information.

  The purpose of Figure 1 is to facilitate the routine analysis of surveillance data and to supplement other sources of information. The method is most useful for conditions without long-term historical trends. When the data have complex patterns, it may be helpful to remove (simplify) some of this pattern by modeling. The classical methods of time-series analysis are appropriate for this situation, but these may not be accessible to the practicing public health official.
- *Which conditions should be monitored?* Routine analyses should be used for conditions for which public health interventions exist. The Figure 1 methodology is used for national surveillance of notifiable conditions to facilitate prevention and intervention efforts. It is most useful for conditions that occur often enough so that a single case or two does not constitute a significant flag. The Figure 1 method may be limited if the sur-

veillance data are not already analyzed for trend and period effects, if the variance of the numerator (present cases) cannot be assumed to have the same variance as the observations in the denominator (baseline data), or if the series exhibits considerable correlation for first-order (adjacent) observations. For rare conditions, the instability caused by small numbers of reported cases may make the results unsuitable for repeated use.

- *What is the (person, place, or time) unit of analysis?* We chose national data for presentation of Figure 1. The objective was to use as short and recent a time period as possible for weekly publication, thus making the results useful for timely intervention. However, variability in weekly reports reflecting factors other than the disease process—e.g., reports delayed because of outbreaks—may make the results unstable. We chose a 4-week window to address this problem.

   Because of the interest in analytic techniques for the analysis of aberrations in surveillance data at the state level, six state health departments evaluated the usefulness of Figure 1 (*21*). During the 4-month period of study, a total of 210 episodes were observed, of which 27 episodes were flagged as exceeding historical limits; one state had no episodes of unusual reporting. Overall, 14 episodes (52%) represented epidemiologically confirmed outbreaks. Many were small, and none were detected when aggregated with other state data for the national analyses. Each disease exceeded historical limits at least twice during the study period, and for all but meningococcal disease, at least one incident represented an outbreak. Although the numbers are clearly small, the proportion of episodes that represented outbreaks varies. This is expected for conditions with different epidemiology.

   The five outbreaks that the health department knew about but that were not detected by the Figure 1 method highlight some of its limitations. In three outbreaks, cases were not reported nationally as current reports; thus, they were not included with the data used for the calculation. The other two outbreaks were not detected because of concurrent increases in the corresponding baseline.

- *What provision is there for updating or correcting the data using later reports?* In the NNDSS, cases are reported as early as possible and then later confirmed or modified. The methodology of Figure 1 is applied to the provisional (earliest reported) data. In our study of six states, two of the five outbreaks that were not detected reflected late reports not included in the current reporting period.

- *How is the baseline determined?* The choice of 5 years as a baseline period was based on a consideration of appropriate sample size balanced by a desire to use the same method for all conditions. Although a longer baseline might be used for some conditions with a long reporting history, epidemics or changes in trend in the baseline will increase the variance of the baseline and thus offset any benefit of additional data. An additional source of variation may be increases in reporting due to intensive investigation. In these cases, the analyst may choose to omit or adjust the increased baseline data.

- *How are outbreaks in the baseline handled?* As presented here, Figure 1 does not adjust for epidemics in the baseline. The result of this is a progressive decline in sensitivity—when an outbreak moves in and then out of the baseline window. To address this point, one could use a median of the baseline reports (rather than a mean). This replacement may require altering the technique used to compute the point for signaling aberrations, and the alternative methods for calculating this are not as accessible to the practicing epidemiologist as the Figure 1 methodology.
- *What are the sensitivity and predictive value positive of the method?* The application of Figure 1 by states showed a sensitivity of 74% and a positive predictive value of 52%. We investigated the predictive value positive of Figure 1 from six state health departments by asking each department to follow up on aberrations detected by this system (*21*). In addition, we asked that outbreaks that came to their attention through other sources, but had not been identified by Figure 1, be noted.
- *What are the mechanics of operation?* For any analytic method to be useful, it must be easily implemented in the routine work of the practicing epidemiologist. In evaluating the states' use of Figure 1, an epidemiologist at CDC routinely evaluated each aberration, analyzed state distributions, and conveyed results to each CDC program responsible for the control of the condition. Additional information was provided by epidemiologists in state health departments. Investigation was based on this evidence in addition to that obtained through other analysis. Software is being developed so that health departments can generate Figure 1 locally.

DATA GRAPHICS

Visual tools also play a critical role in public health surveillance; some simple data graphics have already been introduced in the discussion of EDA. Data graphics visually display measured quantities using points, lines, a coordinate system, numbers, symbols, words, shading, and color (*72*). Graphics allow researchers to mesh presentation and analysis. Data graphics are essential to organizing, summarizing, and displaying information clearly and effectively. The design and quality of such graphics largely determine how effectively scientists can present their information.

Many visual tools are available to assist in analysis and presentation of results. The data to be presented and the purpose for the presentation are the key factors in deciding which visual tools should be used (Table 6–7). Further discussion and guidance in producing effective, high-quality data graphics are available from several sources (*72–77*).

Tables

A table arranges data in rows and columns and is used to demonstrate data patterns and relationships among variables and to serve as a source of information for other types of data graphics (*73*). Table entries can be counts, means, rates, or other analytic measures.

A table should be simple; two or three small tables are simpler to understand than one large one. A table should be self-explanatory so that if taken out of context readers can still understand the data. The guidelines below should be used to increase effectiveness of a table and to ensure that it is self-explanatory (74).

- Describe what, when, and where in a clear, concise table title.
- Label each row and column clearly and concisely.
- Provide units of measure for the data.
- Provide row and column totals.
- Define abbreviations and symbols.
- Note data exclusions.
- If the data are not original, reference the source.

Single-Variable Tables

One of the most basic tables is a frequency distribution by category for a single variable. For example, the first column of the table contains the categories of the factor of interest, and the second column lists the number of persons or events that appear in each category and gives the total count. Often a third column contains percentages of total events in each category (Table 6–8).

Multi-Variable Tables

Most phenomena monitored by public health surveillance systems are complex and require analysis of the interrelationships of several factors. When data are available on more than one variable, multivariable cross-classified tables can elucidate associations. These tables are also called *contingency tables* when all the primary table entries (e.g., frequencies, persons, or events) are classified by each of the variables in the table (Table 6–9).

The most frequently used type of table in epidemiologic analysis is the two-by-two contingency table, which is appropriate when two variables, each having

Table 6–8 Primary and Secondary Morbidity from Syphilis, by Age Category—United States, 1989

Age Group (years)	Cases	
	Number	Percentage*
≤14	230	0.5
15–19	4,378	10.0
20–24	10,405	23.6
25–29	9,610	21.8
30–34	8,648	19.6
35–44	6,901	15.7
45–54	2,631	6.0
>55	1,278	2.9
Total	44,081	100.0

*Percentages do not add to 100.0 due to rounding.

Table 6–9 Primary and Secondary Morbidity from Syphilis, by Age Category, Race, And Gender—United States, 1989

Age (years)	White			Black			Other			Total		
	Male	Female	Total	Male	Female	Total	Male	Female	Total	Male	Female	Total
<15	2	14	16	31	165	196	7	11	18	40	190	230
15–19	88	253	341	1,412	2,257	3,669	210	158	368	1,710	2,668	4,378
20–24	407	475	883	4,059	4,503	8,562	654	307	961	5,120	5,285	10,405
25–29	550	433	983	4,121	3,590	7,711	633	283	916	5,304	4,306	9,610
30–34	564	316	880	4,453	2,628	7,081	520	167	687	5,537	3,111	8,648
35–44	654	243	897	3,858	1,505	5,363	492	149	641	5,004	1,897	6,901
45–54	323	55	378	1,619	392	2,011	202	40	242	2,144	487	2,631
>55	216	24	240	823	92	915	108	15	123	1,147	131	1,278
Total	2,804	1,813	4,617	20,376	15,132	35,508	2,826	1,130	3,956	26,006	18,075	44,081

two categories, are studied. This special case is particularly suited for analyzing case-control and cohort studies for which the categories of the variables are "case" and "control" (or "ill" and "well") and "exposed" and "unexposed."

Graphs

A graph is a visual display of quantitative information involving a system of co-ordinates. Two-dimensional graphs are generally depicted along an x axis (horizontal orientation) and y axis (vertical orientation) coordinate system. Graphs are primary analytic tools used to assist the reader to visualize patterns, trends, aberrations, similarities, and differences in data.

Simplicity is the key to designing graphs. Simple, uncluttered graphs are more likely than complicated presentations to convey information effectively. Several specific principles should be observed when constructing graphs (74):

- Ensure that a graph is self-explanatory by clear, concise labeling of title, source, axes, scales, and legends.
- Clearly differentiate variables by legends or keys.
- Minimize the number of coordinate lines.
- Portray frequency on the vertical scale, starting at zero, and the method of classification on the horizontal scale.
- Assure that scales for each axis are appropriate for the data.
- Clearly indicate scale division, any scale breaks, and units of measure.
- Define abbreviations and symbols.
- Note data exclusions.
- If the data are not original, reference the source.

Several commonly used types of graphs are described below. The scatter plot, an extremely helpful graph for detecting the relationship between two variables, has already been described (See "Data Displays" earlier in this chapter).

Arithmetic-Scale Line Graphs

An arithmetic-scale line graph is one in which equal distances along the x and y axes represent equal quantities along that axis. This type of graph is typically used to demonstrate an overall trend over time rather than focus on particular observation values. It is most helpful for examining long series of data or for comparing several data sets.

The scale of the x axis is usually presented in the same increments as the data are collected (e.g., weekly or monthly). Several factors should be considered when selecting a scale for the y axis (68).

- Choose a length for the y axis that is suitably proportional to that of the x axis. (A common recommendation is a 5:3 ratio for the ratio of x axis to y axis.)
- Identify the maximum y axis value and round the value up slightly.
- Select an interval size that provides enough detail for the purpose of the graph.

Scale breaks can be used for either or both axes if the range of the data is excessive. However, care should be taken to avoid misrepresentation and misinterpretation of the data when scale breaks are used.

Semilogarithmic-Scale Line Graphs

A semilogarithmic-scale line graph or semilog graph is characterized by one axis being measured on an arithmetic scale (usually the x axis) and the other being measured on a logarithmic scale. A logarithm is the exponent expressing the power to which a base number is raised (e.g., log 100 = log 10^2 = 2 for base 10). The axis portraying the logarithmic scale on semilog graph paper is divided into several cycles, with each cycle representing an order of magnitude and values 10 times greater than the preceding cycle (e.g., a 3-cycle semilog graph could represent 1 to 10 in the first cycle, 10 to 100 in the second cycle, and 100 to 1,000 in the third cycle).

A semilogarithmic-scale line graph is particularly valuable when examining the rate of change in surveillance data, because a straight line represents a constant rate of change. For absolute changes, an arithmetic-scale line graph would be more appropriate. The semilog scale is also useful when large differences in magnitude or outliers occur because this type of graph allows the plotting of wide ranges of values. With semilog graphs, the slope of the line indicates the rate of increase or decrease; thus a horizontal line indicates no change in rate. Also, parallel lines for two conditions demonstrate identical rates of change *(74)*.

Histograms

A histogram is a graph in which a frequency distribution is represented by adjoining vertical bars. The area represented by each bar is proportional to the frequency for that interval (i.e., the height multiplied by the width of each bar yields the number of events for that interval). Thus, scale breaks should never be used in histograms because they misrepresent the data.

Histograms can be constructed with equal- and unequal-class intervals. Equal-class intervals occur when the height of each bar is proportional to the frequency of the events in that interval. We do not recommend using histograms with unequal class intervals because they are difficult to construct and interpret correctly.

The epidemic curve is a special type of histogram in which time is the variable plotted on the x axis. The epidemic curve represents the occurrence of cases of a health problem by date of onset during an epidemic, (e.g., an outbreak of paralytic poliomyelitis in Oman) (Figure 6–9). Usually the class intervals on the x axis should be less than one-fourth of the incubation period of the disease, and the intervals should begin before the first reported case during the epidemic in order to portray any identified background cases of the condition being graphed.

Cumulative Frequency and Survival Curves

A cumulative frequency curve is used for both continuous and categorical data. It plots the cumulative frequency on the y axis and the value of the variable on the x axis. Cumulative frequencies can be expressed either as the number of cases or as a percentage of total cases. For categorical data, the cumulative frequency

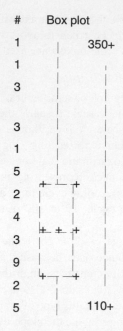

Figure 6–9 Reported cases of paralytic poliomyelitis*—Oman, January 1988–March 1989. The histogram displays the epidemic curve of the outbreak.

is plotted at the right-most end of each class interval (rather than at the midpoint) to depict more realistically the number or percentage of cases above and below the x axis value (Figure 6–10). When percentages are graphed, the cumulative frequency curve allows easy identification of medians, quartiles, and other percentiles of interest.

A survival curve (Figure 6–11) is useful in a follow-up study for graphing the percentage of subjects remaining until an event occurs in the study. The x axis represents time, and the y axis is percentage surviving. A difference in orientation exists between cumulative frequency and survival curves (Figures 6–10 and 6–11).

Frequency Polygons

A frequency polygon is constructed from a histogram by connecting the midpoints of the class intervals with a straight line. A frequency polygon is useful for comparing frequency distributions from different data sets (Figure 6–12). Detailed instructions for constructing frequency polygons are presented elsewhere (*73,74*).

Charts

Charts are useful graphics for illustrating statistical information. Many types of charts can be used (*73–75*). They are most suited and helpful for comparing magnitudes of events in categories of a variable. In the paragraphs below, we describe several of the most frequently used types of charts.

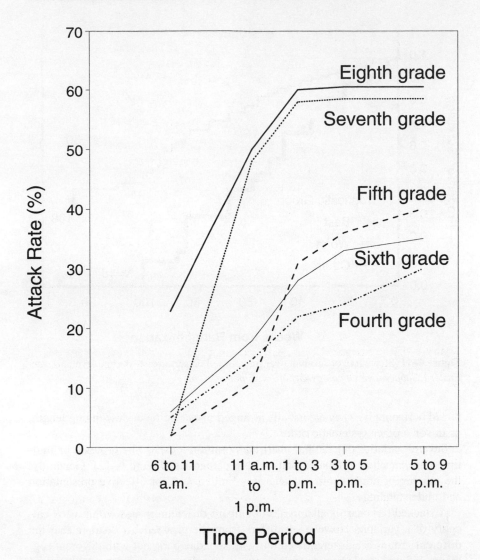

Figure 6–10 Sample cumulative attack rate, by grade in school and time of onset—North Carolina, 1985.

Bar Charts

A bar chart is one of the simplest and most effective ways to present comparative data. A bar chart uses bars of the same width to represent different categories of a factor. Comparison of the categories is based on linear values since the length of a bar is proportional to the frequency of the event in that category. Therefore, scale breaks could cause the data to be misinterpreted and should not be used in bar charts. Bars from different categories are separated by spaces (unlike the bars in a histogram). Although most bars are vertical, they may be de-

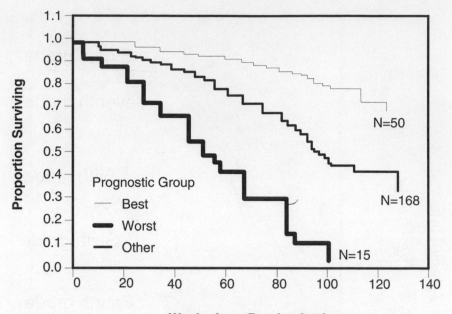

Figure 6–11 Step curve of survival over time, based on serum testosterone level. *Source: Eastern Cooperative Oncology Group, with permission.*

picted horizontally. They are usually arranged in ascending or descending length, or in some other systematic order.

Several variations of the bar chart are commonly used. The grouped or multiple-unit bar chart compares units within categories (Figure 6–13). Generally, the number of units within a category is limited to 3 for effective presentation and understanding.

A stacked bar chart is also used to compare different groups within each category of a variable. However, it differs from the grouped bar chart in that the different groups are differentiated not with separate bars, but with different segments within a single bar for each category. The distinct segments are illustrated by different types of shading, hatching, or coloring, which are defined in a legend (Figure 6–14).

The deviation bar chart illustrates differences in either direction from a baseline. This type of chart is especially useful for demonstrating positive–negative and profit–loss data or comparisons of data at different times (Figure 6–1). The incorporation of a confidence interval-like portion in the bars provides additional useful information.

Pie Charts

A pie chart represents the different percentages of categories of a variable by proportionally sized pieces of pie (Figure 6–15). The pieces are usually denoted

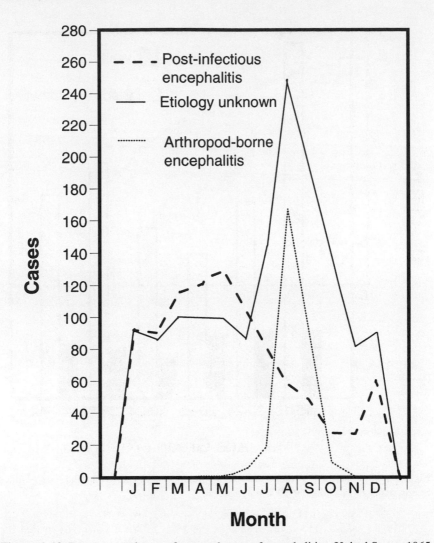

Figure 6–12 Frequency polygon of reported cases of encephalitis—United States, 1965.

with different colors or shading, and the percentages are written inside or outside the pieces to allow the reader to make accurate comparisons.

Maps

Maps are the graphic representation of data using location and geographic coordinates (78). A map generally provides a clear, quick method for grasping data and is particularly effective for readers who are familiar with the physical area being portrayed. A few popular types of maps that depict incidence or distribution of health conditions are described below.

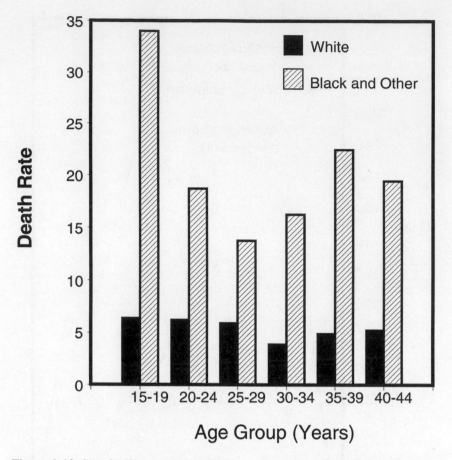

Figure 6–13 Case-fatality rates from ectopic pregnancy, by age group and race—United States, 1970–87. Deaths per 1000 pregnancies.

Spot Maps

A spot map is produced by placing a dot or other symbol on the map where the health condition occurred or exists (Figure 6–16). Different symbols can be used for multiple events at a single location. Although a spot map is beneficial for displaying geographic distribution of an event, it does not provide a measure of risk since population size is not taken into account.

Chloropleth Maps

A chloropleth map, also called a shaded or area map, is a frequently used statistical map involving different types of shading, hatching, or coloring to portray range-graded values (Figure 6–17). Chloropleth maps are useful for depicting rates of a health condition in specific areas.

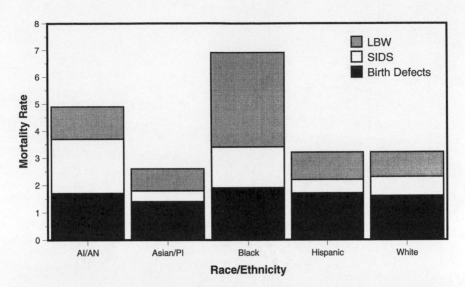

Figure 6–14 Infant mortality rate, by underlying cause and race/ethnicity—United States, 1996. Deaths per 1000 live births. LBW = low birth weight, prematurity, respiratory distress syndrom; SIDS = sudden infant death syndrome; AI/AN = American Indian/Alaskan native; Asian/PI = Asian/Pacific islander.

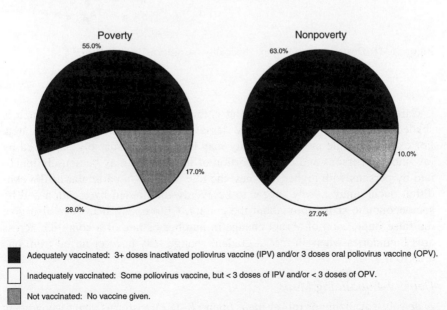

Figure 6–15 Poliomyelitis vaccination status of children ages 1–4 years in cities with populations >250,000, by financial status—United States, 1969.

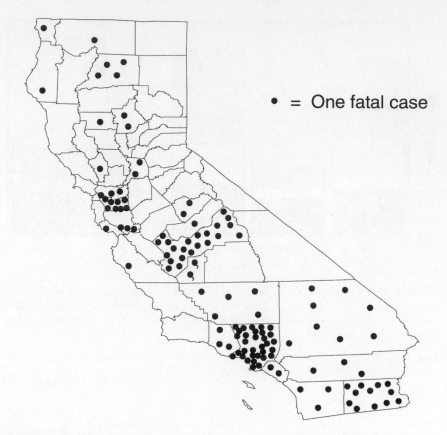

• = One fatal case

Figure 6–16 Deaths from smallpox, by county—California, 1915–1924.

Care must be taken in interpreting chloropleth maps because each area is shaded uniformly regardless of any demographic differences within an area. For example, while most of a county may be relatively sparsely populated by low-income persons and a small portion of that county may be densely inhabited by persons with higher incomes, the rate at which a particular health condition occurs may falsely appear to be evenly distributed by location and by socioeconomic status throughout the county. Chloropleth maps can also give the false impression of abrupt change in number or rate of a condition across area boundaries when, in fact, a gradual change may have occurred from one area to the next.

Density–Equalizing Maps

A density-equalizing or rubber map (Figure 6–18) transforms actual geographic coordinates to produce an artificial figure in which area or population density is equal throughout the map (*77,79*). Density-equalizing maps correct for the con-

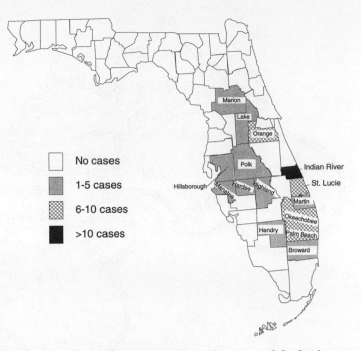

Figure 6–17 Chloropleth map of confirmed and presumptive cases of St. Louis encephalitis, by county—Florida, 1990. Reported October 17, 1990.

founding effect of population density and thus are particularly useful in analyzing geographic clusters of public health events.

Several algorithms exist to transform coordinates of maps. Any transformation routine should define a continuous transformation over the map domain, solve for the unique solution that minimizes map distortion, accept optional constraints, and avoid overlapping of transformed areas (80).

ADDITIONAL ANALYTIC METHODS

In addition to the more traditional analytic methods that have been mentioned, other less frequently used approaches also offer valuable opportunities for surveillance practice. For example, in the analysis of surveillance data, a group of Bayesian methods (81) offers a mechanism to include in the analysis information beyond the data, such as expert knowledge of a change in a surveillance case definition that may influence reporting (82). The empirical Bayes procedure for increasing the stability of observed rates is very useful for surveillance of areas with small populations (83). This methodology has been used to produce maps of injury-related mortality in the United States in recent years.

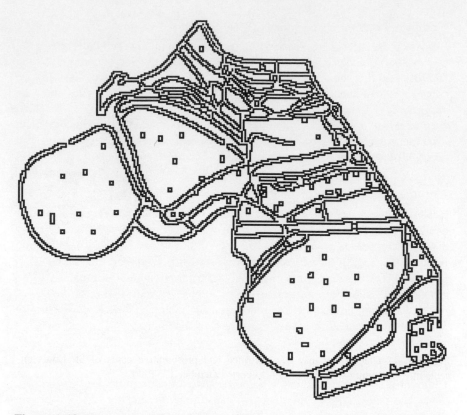

Figure 6–18 Density-equalizing map of California (based upon population density), depicting deaths from smallpox, 1915–1924.

INTERPRETATION OF SURVEILLANCE DATA

The real art of conducting surveillance lies in interpreting what the data say. Data need to be interpreted in the context of our understanding of the etiology, epidemiology, and natural history of the disease or injury. The interpretation should focus on aspects that might lead to improved control of the condition. By proceeding from the simple to the complex, investigators can use surveillance as a basis for taking appropriate public health action. Epidemics can be recognized, preventive strategies applied, and the effect of such actions can be assessed. The key to interpretation lies in knowing the limitations of the data and being meticulous in describing them. One axiom to be always kept in mind is that, because of the descriptive nature of surveillance data, correlation does not equal causation.

Limitations in Data

Although no surveillance system is perfect, most can be useful. Several problems inherent in data obtained through surveillance must be recognized if the data are to be interpreted correctly.

Under–Reporting

Because most surveillance systems are based on conditions reported by health-care providers, under-reporting is inevitable. Depending on the condition, 5% to 80% of cases that actually occur will be reported (*84–87*). However, the need for completeness of reporting—particularly for common health problems—may be exaggerated. Disease trends by time, place, and person can frequently be detected even with incomplete data. So long as the under-reporting is relatively consistent, incomplete data can still be applied to derive useful inferences. For problems that occur infrequently, the need for completeness becomes more important.

Unrepresentativeness of Reported Cases

Health conditions are not reported randomly. For example, illnesses dealt with in a public health facility are reported disproportionately more frequently than those diagnosed by private practitioners. A health problem that leads to hospitalization is more likely to be reported than problems dealt with on an outpatient basis. Thus, reporting biases can distort interpretation. When it is possible, adjusting for skewed reporting will allow investigators to obtain a more accurate picture of the occurrence of a health problem. Collecting data from multiple sources may help provide ways to improve the representativeness of the information.

Inconsistent Case Definitions

Different practitioners frequently use different case definitions for health problems. The more complex the diagnostic syndrome, the greater the difficulty in reaching consensus on a case definition. Moreover, with newly emerging problems, as understanding of their natural history progresses, we frequently adjust the case definition to allow greater accuracy of diagnosis. Persons who interpret surveillance data must be aware of any changes in case definitions and must adjust their interpretations accordingly.

Approach to Interpretation

Creative interpretation of surveillance data requires more common sense than sophisticated reasoning. The data can speak for themselves. Brainstorm and test, if possible, all potential explanations for an observed pattern. Has the nature of reporting changed? Have providers or new geographic areas entered the surveillance system? Has the case definition changed? Has a new intervention, such as screening or therapy, been introduced?

Consistency among different surveillance systems is probably the most crucial factor affecting interpretation. If different surveillance data sets from different locations show similar trends, the likelihood that the effect is real increases. Examine trends in different age groups. Finally, choose the surveillance system you think represents the highest-quality local information. If the trends of the health problem are evident there, you can be more confident about your interpretations.

INTERPRETIVE USES FOR SURVEILLANCE DATA

Identifying Epidemics

An important use of surveillance data is in determining whether increases in numbers of cases of a health condition at the local or national level represent outbreak (i.e., epidemic) situations that require immediate investigation and intervention. Thus, a surveillance system can function as an early–warning signal for public health officials. Some of the methodological issues involved in defining an epidemic have already been discussed.

A few examples of outbreaks and the responses they triggered include the documented increases in numbers of cases of hepatitis B among military recruits that provided the stimulus to intervene with drug-prevention programs (*88*). CDC's Birth Defects Monitoring System identified increases in renal agenesis (*89*) during the 1970s and 1980s, which prompted an investigation. Monitoring of regional trends in rubella and congenital rubella identified outbreaks among the Amish in 1989–1990 (*90*). A national registry of anti-abortion-associated violence clearly documented an "epidemic" of attacks in the mid-1980s, which have varied depending on the level of prosecution allowed (*91*). Documentation of the number of fatal car trunk entrapments involving children over the past decade has resulted in evaluation of design changes to auto trunk locks, allowing lock release from within the trunk (*92*).

The utility of surveillance data in detecting epidemics is highest in situations in which cases of the health condition occur over a wide geographic area or gradually over time. In such situations, the time–place–person links among cases probably would not be recognized by individual practitioners (*3*). Typical examples occur with infectious diseases when laboratory monitoring of unusual serotypes or antibiotic-resistance patterns identify outbreaks of specific microorganisms that might otherwise have gone unnoticed. Nationwide epidemics of *Salmonella newport* (*93*), *S. enteritidis* (*94*), and *Shigella sonnei* (*95*) have been detected through surveillance.

Identifying New Syndromes

The most dramatic use of surveillance data occurs when a "new" syndrome emerges from an ongoing monitoring system. Legionnaires' disease was detected and subsequently characterized as the result of an outbreak of non-influenza pneumonia within a specific place and population (*96*). AIDS was recognized both because of rapid increases in requests for CDC's pentamidine supply and because it occurred in a specific time (early 1981), in two specific places (California, New York), and among specific persons (men having sex with men) (*97*). Finally, the national scope of the epidemic of eosinophilia myalgia syndrome (EMS) was noticed because its unique features were like those of toxic oil syndrome (*98*).

Monitoring Trends

Even if specific outbreaks or new syndromes cannot be identified by tracking surveillance data, the baseline level of the health condition being monitored reflects any variation in its occurrence over time. This purpose is especially relevant to assessing events associated with reproductive health (e.g., ectopic pregnancy or neonatal mortality), chronic disease, or infections with a long latency. The downward trend in pregnancy rates among adolescents during 1992–1995, after 5 years of steady increase during 1985–1990, reflects this monitoring function (*99*).

Evaluating Public Policy

Surveillance data can assess the health impact—pro or con—of specific interventions or of public policy. The rapid fall in numbers of cases of poliomyelitis and measles after national vaccination campaigns were instituted is a classic example of the usefulness of surveillance data (*100,101*). More recently, the Florida Youth Tobacco Survey was used to test the effectiveness of the Florida Pilot Program on Tobacco Control, a youth-oriented, countermarketing media campaign developed to reduce the allure of smoking (*102*). Following implementation of the program, evidence of a significant decline in tobacco use among middle and high school students has spurred adoption of similar programs in other states. Creative interpretation of surveillance data has also been applied to other noninfectious conditions; however, the impact in such situations is somewhat more difficult to assess. For example, in Washington, D.C. the adoption of a gun-licensing law coincided with an abrupt decline in firearm-related homicides and suicides (*103*). No similar reductions occurred in the number of homicides or suicides committed by other means, nor did states adjacent to the District experience any reductions in their rates of firearm-related homicides or suicides. Also, surveillance of legal abortions and of deaths associated with illegal abortion has helped trace the public health impact of this controversial health problem (*8,104,105*). After legal abortions became widely available, deaths from illegal abortions decreased markedly; however, restriction of federal funds for abortions had a negligible effect on health parameters (*106*).

Though it is tempting to use trends in disease and injury to monitor the impact of community interventions, such evaluation becomes increasingly suspect when several factors contribute to the occurrence of the disease or health condition being monitored. In addition, if only a portion of the population accepts an intervention, analysis and interpretation of surveillance data are made even more difficult. Frequently, surveillance of process measures or other health problems can act as proxies for the intended outcome. For example, decreases in unsafe sexual behaviors or other sexually transmitted diseases after HIV campaigns have been used as surrogates for trends in HIV incidence. Moreover, finding comparability in data from several populations that have attempted similar public health programs strengthens evidence that the interpretation is correct. For example, to evaluate the effectiveness of allowing people to exchange used hypodermic needles for new ones as a means of preventing AIDS, epidemiologists could simultaneously examine trends in numbers of needles distributed, surveys of needle use, and incidence of higher-prevalence infections such as hepatitis B.

Projecting Future Needs

Mathematical models based on surveillance data can be used to project future trends. This tool helps health officials determine the eventual need for preventive and curative services. Recently such modeling assisted in estimating the impact of AIDS on the U.S. health-care system in the 1990s (*107*). Such projections addressed not only the demand for AZT by HIV-infected persons with low CD-4 lymphocyte counts, but also the requirements for hospital care for persons with life-threatening superinfections later in the course of HIV-related disease. In addition, models based on surveillance data can predict the decline of morbidity and mortality when there are changes in risk factors among the population at risk. Examples of this application include projecting the decline in cardiovascular disease on the basis of decreased smoking of cigarettes (*108*), the decline in cirrhosis-related mortality in the presence of lower levels of alcohol use (*109*), and decreased rates of mortality from cervical cancer associated with an increase in the prevalence of hysterectomy (*110*).

REFERENCES

1. Thacker SB, Berkelman RL. Public health surveillance in the United States. *Epidemiol Rev* 1988;10:164–90.
2. Doll R. Surveillance and monitoring. *Int J Epidemiol* 1974;3:305–13.
3. Berkelman RL, Buehler JW. Surveillance. In: Holland WW, Detels R, Knox G (eds.). Oxford textbook of public health. Second edition, Volume 2. Methods of public health. Oxford: Oxford University Press, 1991:161–76.
4. Buehler JW. Surveillance. In: Rothman KJ, Greenland S (eds.). Modern epidemiology. Second edition. Philadelphia: Lippencott-Raven, 1998:435–57.
5. Thacker SB, Berkelman RL, Stroup DF. The science of public health surveillance. *J Pub Health Pol* 1989;10:187–203.
6. Morgenstern H. Uses of ecologic analysis in epidemiologic research. *Am J Public Health* 1982;72:1336–44.
7. Piantadosi S, Byar DP, Green SB. The ecological fallacy. *Am J Epidemiol* 1988;127:893–904.
8. Robinson WS. Ecological correlations and the behavior of individuals. Am Sociol Rev 1950;15:351–7.
9. Lilienfeld AE, Lilienfeld DE. Foundations of epidemiology. Second edition. Oxford: Oxford University Press, 1980.
10. Macmahon B, Pugh TF. Epidemiology: principles and methods. Boston: Little, Brown and Co., 1970.
11. Baker AD, Margerison FM. New medical dictionary. London: Northcliff, 1935.
12. Last JM. A dictionary of epidemiology. Second edition. Oxford: Oxford University Press, 1988.

13. Centers for Disease Control and Prevention. Update: Influenza activity—United States and worldwide, 1998–99 season and composition of the 1999–2000 influenza vaccine. *MMWR* 1999; 48:374–8.
14. Brookmeyer R, Gail MH. AIDS epidemiology: a quantitative approach. Oxford: Oxford University Press, 1994.
15. Thacker SB. The surveillance of infectious diseases. *JAMA* 1983;249:1181–5.
16. Centers for Disease Control and Prevention. Summary of notifiable diseases—United States, 1997. *MMWR* 1998;46(54).
17. Stroup DF, Williamson GD, Herndon JL, Karon JM. Detection of aberrations in the occurrence of notifiable diseases surveillance data. *Stat Med* 1989;8:323–32.
18. Centers for Disease Control. Proposed changes in format for presentation of notifiable disease report data. *MMWR* 1989;38(47):805–9.
19. Morgenstern H, Greenland S. Graphing ratio measures of effect. *J Clin Epidemiol* 1990;43:539–42.
20. Stroup DF, Wharton M, Kafadar K, Dean AG. An evaluation of a method for detecting aberrations in public health surveillance data. *Am J Epidemiol* 1993;137: 373–80.
21. Wharton M, Price W, Hoesly F et al. Evaluation of a method for outbreak detection in six states. *Am J Prev Med* 1993;9:45–9.
22. Wallenstein S. A test for detection of clustering over time. *Am J Epidemiol* 1980; 111:367–72.
23. Naus JI. Approximations for distributions of scan statistics. *J Amer Stat Assn* 1982;77:177–83.
24. Glaz J. Approximations and bounds for the distribution of the scan statistic. *J Amer Stat Assn* 1989;84:560–6.
25. Collins SD. Excess mortality from causes other than influenza and pneumonia during influenza epidemics. *Publ Health Rep* 1932;47:2159–80.
26. Serfling RE. Methods for current statistical analysis of excess pneumonia-influenza deaths. *Public Health Rep* 1963;78:494–505.
27. Choi K, Thacker SB. An evaluation of influenza mortality surveillance, 1962–1979. I. Time series forecasts of expected pneumonia and influenza deaths. *Amer J Epidemiol* 192;113:215–26.
28. Kafadar K, Andrews JS Jr. Investigating health effects and hazards in the community. In: Statistics in public health. Stroup DF, Teutsch SM (eds.). Oxford: Oxford University Press, 1998:93–122.
29. Devine O, Parrish RG. Monitoring the health of a population. In: Statistics in public health. Stroup DF and Teutsch SM (eds.). Oxford: Oxford University Press, 1998: 59–91.
30. Banks J. Principles of quality control. New York: John Wiley and Sons, 1989.
31. Montgomery DC. Introduction to statistical quality control. New York: John Wiley and Sons, 1985.
32. Hutwagner LC, Maloney EK, Bean NH, Slutsker L, Martin SM. Using laboratory-based surveillance data for prevention: an algorithm for detecting *Salmonella* outbreaks. *Emerging Infectious Diseases* 1997;3:395–400.
33. Mahon B, Ponka A, Hall W, Komatsu K, Dietrich S, Siitonen A *et al*. An international outbreak of *Salmonella* infections caused by alfalfa sprouts grown from contaminated seed. *J Infect Dis* 1997;175:876–82.
34. Williamson GD, Hudson GW. A monitoring system for detecting aberrations in public health surveillance reports. *Statistics in Medicine* (in press).

35. Koonin LM, Kochanek KD, Smith JC, Ramick M. Abortion surveillance, United States, 1988. In: CDC surveillance summaries, July 1991. *MMWR* 1991;40(No. SS-2):15–42.
36. Snow J. Snow on cholera. New York: Hafner Press, 1965.
37. Cressie NAC . Statistics for spatial data. New York: John Wiley and Sons, 1993.
38. Langford IH, Leyland AH, Rasbash J, Goldstein H. Multilevel modelling of the geographical distributions of diseases. *Applied Statistics* 1999;48(Pt2):253–68.
39. Mantel N. The detection of disease clustering and a generalized regression approach. *Cancer Res* 1967;27:209–20.
40. Aldrich TE, Wilson CC, Warner SS, Easterly CE. Studying case clusters: a primer for disease surveillance. *Am J Epidemiol* 1989;120:223–30.
41. Ederer F, Myers MH, Mantel N. A statistical problem in space and time: do leukaemia cases come in clusters? *Biometrics* 1964;20:626–39.
42. Knox EG. The detection of space-time interaction. *Appl Statist* 1964;13:25–9.
43. David FN, Barton DE. Two space-time interaction tests for epidemicity. *Brit J Prev Soc Med* 1966;20:44–8.
44. Cuzick J, Edwards R. Spatial clustering for inhomogeneous populations. *J R Statist Soc* 1990;652:73–104.
45. Williams EH, Smith PG, Day NE *et al.* Space-time clustering of Burkitt's lymphoma in the west Nile district of Uganda: 1961–1975. *Brit J Cancer* 1978;37:109–22.
46. Diggle PJ, Chetwynd AG, Haggkvist R. Second order analysis of space-time clustering. Department of Mathematics technical report. Lancaster, Penn.: Lancaster University, 1991.
47. Bhopal RS, Diggle PJ, Rowlingson B. Pinpointing clusters of apparently sporadic cases of Legionnaire's disease. *BMJ* 1992;304:1022–7.
48. Centers for Disease Control. Guidelines for investigating clusters of health events. *MMWR* 1990;39(No. RR-11).
49. Firebaugh G. A rule for inferring individual relationships from aggregate data. *Am Sociol Rev* 1978;43:557–72.
50. Executive Office of the President, Office of Management and Budget. Revisions to the standards for the classification of federal data on race and ethnicity. *Federal Register* 1997;62:58782–90.
51. Centers for Disease Control and Prevention. Reporting race and ethnicity data—National Electronic Telecommunications System for Surveillance, 1994–1997. *MMWR* 1999;48:305–12.
52. Centers for Disease Control and Prevention. State-specific prevalence among adults of current cigarette smoking and smokeless tobacco use and per capita tax-paid sales of cigarettes—United States, 1997. *MMWR* 1998;47:922–6.
53. Statistical Policy Office, Office of Information and Regulatory Affairs, Office of Management and Budget. Report on statistical disclosure limitation methodology. Statistical policy working paper 22, 1994. This report can be accessed at http://www.bts.gov/NTL/DOCS/wp22.html.
54. Rolfs RT, Nakashima AK. Epidemiology of primary and secondary syphilis in the United States, 1981–1989. *JAMA* 1990;254:1432–7.
55. Marx R, Aral SO, Rolfs RT, Sterk CE, Kahn JG. Crack, sex, and STD. *Sex Transm Dis* 1991;18:92–101.
56. Last JM (ed.). A dictionary of epidemiology. Second edition. New York: Oxford University Press, 1988.
57. Kleinman JC (updated by Kiely JL). Infant mortality. National Center for Health Statistics. *Healthy People 2000 Statistical Notes* 1(2), 1991.

58. Briss PA, Sacks JJ, Adiss DG, Kresnow M-J, O'Neill J. Injuries from falls on playgrounds: Effects of day care regulation and enforcement. *Arch Pediatr Adolesc Med* 1995; 149(8):906–11.
59. National Center for Health Statistics. Health, United States, 1998, with socioeconomic status and health chartbook. Hyattsville, Md.: 1998.
60. Ahlbom A, Norell S. Introduction to modern epidemiology. Chestnut Hill, Mass.: Epidemiology Resources, 1984.
61. Fleiss JL. Statistical methods for rates and proportions. Second edition. New York: John Wiley & Sons, 1981.
62. Kahn HA, Sempos CT. Statistical methods in epidemiology. Volume 12. MacMahon B (ed.). Monographs in epidemiology and biostatistics. New York: Oxford University Press, 1989.
63. Lilienfeld AM, Lilienfeld DE. Foundations of epidemiology. Second edition. New York: Oxford University Press, 1980.
64. Peavy JV. Adjusted rates. DHHS Publ No (PHS) 00–1833. Atlanta: Centers for Disease Control, 1988.
65. Anderson R, Rosenberg HM (eds.). Proceedings of the second workshop on age adjustment. National Center for Health Statistics. *Vital and Health Statistics* (in press).
66. Mausner JS, Bahn AK. Epidemiology: an introductory text. Philadelphia: W.B. Saunders, 1974.
67. Haight F. Handbook of the Poisson distribution. New York: John Wiley & Sons, 1967.
68. Kleinbaum DG, Kupper LL, Muller KE, Nizam A. Applied regression analysis and multivariable methods. Third edition. Boston: Duxbury Press, 1988.
69. Tukey JW. Exploratory data analysis. Reading, Mass.: Addison-Wesley Publishing Company, 1977.
70. Velleman PF, Hoaglin DC. Applications, basics, and computing of exploratory data analysis. Boston: Duxbury Press, 1981.
71. McNeil DR. Interactive data analysis. New York: John Wiley & Sons, 1977.
72. Tufte ER. The visual display of quantitative information. Cheshire, Conn.: Graphics Press, 1987.
73. Principles of epidemiology. Second edition (developmental). Washington, D.C.; American Public Health Association, 1992.
74. Peavy JV, Dyal WW, Eddins DL. Descriptive statistics: tables, graphs, and charts. DHHS Publ No (PHS) 00–1834. Atlanta: Centers for Disease Control, 1986.
75. Schmid CF. Statistical graphics design principles and practices. New York: John Wiley & Sons, 1983.
76. Chambers JM, Cleveland WS, Kleiner B, Tukey PA. Graphical methods for data analysis. Boston: Duxbury Press, 1983.
77. Tufte ER. Envisioning information. Cheshire, Conn.: Graphics Press, 1990.
78. Haggett P, Cliff AD, Frey A. Locational analysis in human geography. Second edition. Bristol, England: J.W. Arrowsmith, 1977.
79. Gillihan AF. Population maps. *Am J Public Health* 1927;17:316–9.
80. Merrill DW, Selvin S, Mohr MS. Analyzing geographic clustered response. In: American Statistical Association 1991 Proceedings of the Section on Statistics and the Environment. Alexandria, Va.: American Statistical Association, 1993.
81. Harrison PJ, Stevens CF. Bayesian forecasting (with discussion). *J Royal Stat Soc* 1976;38:205–47B.
82. Stroup DF, Thacker SB. A Bayesian approach to the detection of aberrations in public health surveillance data. *Epidemiol* 1993;4(5):435–43.

83. Devine OJ. A modified empirical Bayes approach for stabilizing mortality rates in areas with small populations. Proceedings of the National Meeting of the American Statistical Association, Atlanta, August 1991.
84. Eylenbosch WJ, Noah ND. Surveillance in health and disease. Oxford: Oxford University Press, 1988.
85. Vogt RL, LaRue D, Klaucke DN, Jillson DA. Comparison of active and passive surveillance systems of primary care providers for hepatitis, measles, rubella, and salmonellosis in Vermont. *Am J Public Health* 1983;73:795–7.
86. Levy BS, Mature J, Washburn JW. Intensive hepatitis surveillance in Minnesota: methods and results. *Am J Epidemiol* 1977;105:127–34.
87. Marier R. The reporting of communicable diseases. *Am J Epidemiol* 1977;105:587–90.
88. Cowan DN, Prier RE. Changes in hepatitis morbidity in the United States Army, Europe. *Milit Med* 1984;149:260–5.
89. Edmonds LD, James LM. Temporal trends in the prevalence of congenital malformations at birth based on the Birth Defects Monitoring Program, United States, 1979–1987. In: CDC surveillance summaries, December 1990. *MMWR* 1990;39(No. SS-4):19–23.
90. Centers for Disease Control. Outbreak of rubella among the Amish—United States, 1991. *MMWR* 1991;40:264.
91. Grimes DA, Forrest JD, Kirkman AL, Radford B. An epidemic of anti-abortion violence in the United States. *Am J Obstet Gynecol* 1991;165:1263–8.
92. Centers for Disease Control. Fatal car entrapment involving children—United States, 1987–1998. *MMWR* 1998;47:1019–22.
93. Holmberg SD, Osterholm MT, Senger KA, Cohen ML. Drug-resistant *Salmonella* from animals fed antimicrobials. *N Engl J Med* 1984;311:617–22.
94. St Louis ME Morse DL, Potter ME *et al.* The emergence of grade A eggs as a major source of *Salmonella enteritidis* infections: new implications for the control of salmonellosis. *JAMA* 1988;259:2103–7.
95. Centers for Disease Control. Nationwide dissemination of multi-resistant *Shigella sonnei* following a common-source outbreak. *MMWR* 1987;36:633–4.
96. Fraser DW, Tsai TR, Orenstein W *et al.* Legionnaires' disease: description of an epidemic of pneumonia. *N Engl J Med* 1977;297:1189–97.
97. Centers for Disease Control. Pneumocystic pneumonia—Los Angeles. *MMWR* 1981; 30:250–2.
98. Swygert LA, Maes EF, Sewell LE, Miller L, Falk H, Kilbourne EM. Eosinophilia-myalgia syndrome: results of national surveillance. *JAMA* 1990;264:1698–703.
99. Centers for Disease Control and Prevention. State-specific pregnancy rates among adolescents—United States, 1992–1995. *MMWR* 1998; 47:497–504.
100. Centers for Disease Control. Measles prevention: recommendations of the Immuniza-tion Practices Advisory Committee (ACIP). *MMWR* 1989;38(No. S-9):1–18.
101. Centers for Disease Control. Progress toward eradicating poliomyelitis from the Americas. *MMWR* 1989;38:532–5.
102. Centers for Disease Control and Prevention. Tobacco use among middle and high school students—Florida, 1998 and 1999. *MMWR* 1999; 48:248–53.
103. Loftin C, McDowall D, Wiersema B, Cottey TJ. Effects of restrictive licensing of handguns on homicide and suicide in the District of Columbia. *N Engl J Med* 1991; 325:1615–20.
104. Cates W Jr, Rochat RW, Grimes DA, Tyler CW Jr. Legalized abortion: effect on national trends of maternal and abortion-related mortality (1940–1976). *Am J Obstet Gynecol* 1978;132:211–4.

105. Cates W Jr. Legal abortion: the public health record. *Science* 1982;215:1586–90.
106. Cates W Jr. The Hyde amendment in action: how did the restriction of federal funds for abortion affect low-income women? *JAMA* 1981;246:1109–12.
107. Centers for Disease Control. HIV prevalence estimates and AIDS case projections for the United States: report based upon a workshop. *MMWR* 1990;39(No. RR-16).
108. Kullback S, Cornfield J. An information theoretic contingency table analysis of the Dorn study of smoking and mortality. *Comput Biomed Res* 1976;9:409–37.
109. Skog O. The risk function for liver cirrhosis from lifetime alcohol consumption. *J Stud Alcohol* 1984;45:199–208.
110. Centers for Disease Control. Hysterectomy prevalence and death rates for cervical cancer—United States, 1965–1988. *MMWR* 1992;41:17–20.

7

Communicating Information for Action within the Public Health System

RICHARD A. GOODMAN
PATRICK L. REMINGTON
ROBERT J. HOWARD

All I know is just what I read in the papers.
Will Rogers

Standard definitions for public health surveillance specify the requirement for the timely dissemination of findings to those who have contributed and others who need to know (*1–3*). In the United States, surveillance findings have been disseminated through the *MMWR* series of publications, public health bulletins in states, and special reports in peer-reviewed journals. Even though new technologies and epidemiologic methodologies have dramatically improved the collection and analysis of surveillance data, however, public health programs have lagged in developing effective approaches to the dissemination of surveillance findings—and to the ultimately successful communication of those findings (see also Chapter 16).

As recently as the 1970s, public health surveillance in the United States focused almost exclusively on the detection and monitoring of cases of specific communicable diseases, and surveillance data were disseminated primarily in a basic tabular format. However, surveillance efforts have expanded rapidly and now include chronic diseases, injuries, occupationally acquired conditions, and other problems. In addition, surveillance encompasses problems as diverse as personal behavior (e.g., cigarette smoking and seat-belt use); environmental insults (e.g., hazardous materials incidents); and preventive practices (e.g., Pap smears and mammographic screening).

Because of the fundamental changes in public health programs and priorities, programs at all levels require innovative approaches to convey surveillance findings to new and more diverse constituencies. This chapter provides a practical framework for optimizing dissemination and communication of information developed through public health surveillance efforts.

BASIC CONCEPTS FOR DISSEMINATING AND COMMUNICATING SURVEILLANCE INFORMATION

Surveillance has been characterized as a process that provides "information for action." This concept is inherently consistent with the definition of communications as "...a process, which is a series of actions or operations, always in motion, directed toward a particular goal" (*3*). On the basis of this definition, then, public health programs must ensure more than the mere transmission or dissemination of surveillance results to others; rather, surveillance data should be presented in a manner that facilitates their use for public health actions. One fundamental concept is that the terms *dissemination* and *communication* cannot be used interchangeably. Dissemination is a one-way process through which information is conveyed from one point to another. In comparison, communications is a loop—involving at least a sender and a recipient—a collaborative process. The communicator's job is completed when the targeted recipient of the information acknowledges receipt and comprehension of that information.

A basic framework for disseminating the results of public health surveillance with the intent of communicating can be adapted from fundamental models for communications. One such model—which emphasizes the effect of communications—includes the sender, the message, the receiver, the channel, and the impact (*3*). The sender is the person responsible for surveillance of each health condition being monitored. For applications in public health practice, this model can be modified (See Table 7–1).

Each of these steps is discussed in greater detail in the paragraphs below. They should all be read with the understanding that one should never disseminate more information than s/he can evaluate and revise, as needed, during the communications process.

Establish the Message

The primary message or communications objective for the findings of any public health surveillance effort should reflect the basic purposes of the surveillance system. In this textbook, the purposes of surveillance systems have been described (see Chapters 1 and 2). For each of these categories, the findings and interpretation of surveillance data may necessitate a different type of public health response. In addition to disseminating data to those who may have contributed, the com-

Table 7–1 Controlling and Directing Information Dissemination

Steps	*Questions To Be Answered*
Establish communications message	What should be said?
Define the audience	To whom should it be?
Select the channel	Through what communication medium?
Market the message	How should the message be stated?
Evaluate the impact	What effect did the message create?

munications objectives should also dictate the delivery of the information to the relevant target groups and the stimulation of appropriate public health action.

To Detect and Control Outbreaks

When the purpose of a surveillance system is to detect outbreaks or other occurrences of disease in excess of predicted levels, the primary communications objective should be to inform two groups: *a*) the population at risk of exposure or disease, and *b*) persons and organizations responsible for immediate control measures and other interventions. For example, when surveillance efforts detect influenza activity in a specific locality, public health agencies can promptly disseminate this information to health-care providers, who may in turn intensify efforts to vaccinate or provide amantadine chemoprophylaxis to persons at high risk of complications from influenza. The release and timing of such messages should be carefully considered and coordinated with appropriate agencies.

In the context of this example, the impact of releasing a message recommending the use of amantadine or influenza vaccine may be enhanced if the release has been coordinated with public health units, local pharmaceutical suppliers, and medical organizations.

To Determine the Etiology and Natural History of Disease

Public health surveillance for newly recognized or detected problems may be initiated to assist in determining the epidemiology, etiology, and natural history of such conditions. In such circumstances, the communications objective may simply be to provide information which is sufficient to initiate surveillance.

For example, when EMS was recognized in the United States in October 1989, a case definition was developed and disseminated to the public health community to enable the immediate implementation of national surveillance for EMS (*4*). Surveillance efforts were critical in characterizing the epidemiology and natural history of EMS, as well as in assisting in the development of hypotheses regarding its cause.

To Evaluate Control Measures

For many public health conditions, surveillance is the principal means for assessing the impact of control measures. Epidemiologic trends and patterns that are based on surveillance findings must be conveyed to persons involved in control efforts in order to refine control activities and guide the allocation of resources in support of those activities.

Following a period of relative quiescence, as of the mid-1980s the incidence of measles in the United States surged. When surveillance indicated that vaccination coverage had declined substantially in some groups (e.g., children residing in inner-city locations), key findings were conveyed to and used by public health programs and primary care providers in targeting measles vaccination efforts.

To Detect Changes in Disease Agents

In addition to monitoring trends in the occurrence of public health problems, surveillance systems may be fundamental to the process of detecting changes in disease agents and the impact of these changes on public health. For example, in the late 1980s in the United States, surveillance documented an increase in the incidence of tuberculosis—an increase substantially in excess of predicted levels. In addition to this overall trend, transmission of multi-drug-resistant tuberculosis (MDR-TB) was detected in health-care and prison settings (5). The public health implications of these findings are similar to the basic considerations outlined above for detecting and controlling outbreaks: specifically, there is need for timely and effective notification of populations at risk and of organizations responsible for control and prevention measures. Therefore, in the case of MDR-TB, the communications objectives would include immediate notification of the public health community about the problem with the intent of facilitating implementation of proper diagnostic, therapeutic, and preventive measures.

To Detect Changes in Health Practices

Some surveillance systems monitor changes in health practices and behaviors in the population rather than changes in patterns of disease (6). This "life-style" information is particularly important for problems such as chronic disease, for which trends in risk behavior often precede changes in health outcome by years or even decades. The communications objective in this context is often to increase awareness regarding the role of behavior in causing disease or injury. In addition, this information may be used to identify high-risk groups in the population.

For example, surveillance data regarding trends in cigarette smoking indicate that smoking rates have not declined among persons with lower educational attainment. Accordingly, surveillance data which characterize risk factors (such as smoking), outcomes, health services, and other related factors may guide public health programs and decision makers in the implementation of targeted community-wide or state-wide intervention strategies (7).

To Facilitate Planning of Health Policies

For some conditions, the most appropriate control measure is promulgation of a public health policy. In this context, surveillance information about the public health impact of different conditions and problems must be effectively conveyed to legislators and makers of public health policy.

For example, in California surveillance information about smoking-attributable mortality, morbidity, and economic costs helped in enacting Proposition 99. This legislation provided for a 25-cent increase in the state cigarette tax, which in turn funded state-wide initiatives to prevent and control the use of tobacco. Subsequently, surveillance data regarding trends in the prevalence of smoking and the impact of this initiative assisted in ensuring the application of state funds to control tobacco use. Similarly, data for the United States have confirmed that increases in cigarette taxes have helped in reducing cigarette smoking (8).

Define the Audience

Identification of target groups is an essential part of the process of developing strategies for communicating surveillance results. Typically, public health surveillance information and reports have been disseminated in a standard format with only limited consideration of the target audiences and, more importantly, of the techniques to communicate effectively to these groups. Key target groups include public health practitioners, health-care providers, professional and voluntary organizations, and policy makers (e.g., from the executive and legislative branches of government).

In some instances, surveillance information should be disseminated widely, in which case communication strategies should be tailored to subgroups of greater interest. For example, information regarding trends in injecting drug-use-related risks for HIV is often communicated to the general public through the newspapers, however, this strategy may be inadequate for reaching the groups at highest risk, who use alternative media such as radio and television (9).

Select the Channel

Specification of the messages and audiences for surveillance results enable selection of the most suitable channels of communication for this information. Traditionally, surveillance information has been disseminated through published surveillance reports. However, in addition to conventional means for communicating with traditional audiences, the advent of new methods and technologies have made possible improved communications with both old and new audiences. This spectrum of communications options includes professional and trade publications, electronic channels, broadcast media, print media, and public forums:

- publications: government public health bulletins and surveillance reports, peer-reviewed public health and biomedical journals, newsletters
- electronic: telecommunications systems, faxes and batch faxes, audioconferences, videoconferences
- media: news releases, news conferences, fact sheets, video releases
- public forums: briefings, hearings and testimony, conferences, and other planned meetings

Market the Information

Once the message has been defined and the target audience and channel selected, it is critical to ensure that the information is communicated and marketed—not merely disseminated—to those who need to know. Today enormous quantities of information concerning public health are communicated through professional channels, as well as print and electronic media. Because of the volume of essential information, as well as time constraints, surveillance information must be carefully tailored for presentation to each targeted audience, including public health and health-care professionals, policy makers, and the public.

To ensure that surveillance information is readily communicated to target audiences, public health agencies should use those techniques that are most effective for marketing information. First, as a general principal, graphic formats and other visual displays are likely to be more effective in conveying information than conventional tabular presentations. Such formats include maps, bar graphs, histograms, diagrams, or other ways of visually depicting data which may not be readily comprehended through tabular presentation. For example, in December 1989 the CDC introduced a graphic format for displaying NNDSS data in the *MMWR* (*10*). This bar graph (Figure 6–1), which replaced a standard table, was designed both to facilitate interpretation of routine notifiable disease data and to enable timely public health responses to changes in disease patterns.

Second, the principal components of the message can be focused by selecting the most important point, then stating that point as a simple declarative sentence. This message, termed the *single overriding communications objective* (SOCO), should consider three questions:

- What is new?
- Who is affected?
- What works best?

For example, chronic disease surveillance information data indicate that compared with younger women, older women are less likely to have received a Pap test in the past, are more likely to have cervical cancer diagnosed at a late stage, and have higher mortality rates due to cervical cancer. Traditionally, this information might be disseminated to health-care and public health providers through vital statistics reports and other published accounts about cervical cancer. However, if these findings are to be used as a basis for action, they first must be synthesized, then effectively communicated. Thus, in addition to presenting these findings in detailed reports, they also may be expressed through a single message, the SOCO: "Older women need to get regular Pap tests."

Third, techniques must be used which present (or "package") the surveillance information in a manner which captures an audience's interest and focuses attention on a specific issue. Examples of these techniques are the use of introductory terms such as: "A new study . . ."; "Recent findings . . ."; and "Information recently released. . . ." These terms are likely to appeal more to a target audience than a presentation which begins with a conventional preface, such as "Based on recent surveillance findings. . . ."

Fourth, the method and forum of release of surveillance information may be critical—particularly when a timely release is required, or when the target audiences include the media, the public, or policymakers. Under such circumstances, news conferences or other news releases may be considered, and should be held when they are likely to be attended. Foremost, the presenter should involve reporters in the public health surveillance process by "walking them through it," and should recognize opportunities to articulate the SOCO on camera or in print. Important adjuncts for presenting the information include readily available handouts and effective, but simple, visuals.

Evaluate the Impact

Because public health surveillance is, by definition, oriented toward action, evaluation efforts should address two considerations: *a*) whether surveillance information has been communicated to those who need to know; and *b*) whether the information has had a beneficial effect upon the public health problem or condition of interest.

Assessment of whether surveillance information has been communicated to those who need to know may be accomplished through a process evaluation, such as by monitoring the distribution of the information or a user survey. In particular, the effectiveness of communication through newspapers can be evaluated by using clipping services which determine the number of published reports, the geographic distribution of the reports, and the proportion of the total audience to which the reports have been circulated. In addition, process evaluation efforts should include a review of the content of articles to assess both the accuracy and appropriateness of the communicated message.

The second consideration—the impact of the communications effort on the public health problem—requires an evaluation of outcomes (e.g., knowledge or practices) within specific target audiences.

Under ideal circumstances, this type of evaluation requires surveys of the target audiences both before and after the surveillance information has been communicated to detect changes in levels of outcomes. The potential for such evaluation is constrained, however, by technical and methodologic challenges, as well as substantial resource requirements.

SUMMARY

Effective communication of public health surveillance results represents the critical link in the translation of science into action. Recognition of the key components in this process—including the medium, the message, the audience, the response, and the evaluation of the process—is the first step in completing the communications loop. Without this loop, we are left with one-way information dissemination.

REFERENCES

1. Langmuir AD. The surveillance of communicable diseases of national importance. *N Engl J Med* 1963;288:182–92;
2. Thacker SB, Berkelman RL. Public health surveillance in the United States. *Epidemiologic Rev* 1988;10:164–90.
3. Hiebert RE, Ungurait DE, Bohn TW. The process of communication. In: Mass media: an introduction to modern communication III. New York: Longman, 1982:15–29.
4. Centers for Disease Control. Eosinophilia-myalgia syndrome—New Mexico. *MMWR* 1989;38:765–7.
5. Centers for Disease Control. Nosocomial transmission of multidrug-resistant tuberculosis among HIV-infected persons—Florida and New York, 1988–1991. *MMWR* 1991;40:585–91.
6. Remington PL, Smith MY, Williamson DF, Anda RF, Gentry EM, Hogelin GC. Design, characteristics, and usefulness of state-based risk factor surveillance 1981–1986. *Public Health Rep* 1988;103(4):366–75.

7. Boss LP, Suarez L. Uses of data to plan cancer prevention and control programs. *Public Health Rep* 1990;105:354–60.
8. Peterson DE, Zeger SL, Remington PL, Anderson HA. The effect of state cigarette tax increases on cigarette sales, 1955 to 1988. *Am J Public Health* 1992;82:94–6.
9. Centers for Disease Control. HIV-prevention messages for injecting drug users: sources of information and use of mass media—Baltimore, 1989. *MMWR* 1991;40: 465–9.
10. Centers for Disease Control. Proposed changes in format for presentation of notifiable disease report data. *MMWR* 1989;38:805–9.

8

EVALUATING PUBLIC HEALTH SURVEILLANCE

RAUL A. ROMAGUERA
ROBERT R. GERMAN
DOUGLAS N. KLAUCKE

The best way to escape from a problem is to solve it.
Brandon Francis

The highest-priority public health events should be monitored, and surveillance systems should meet their objectives as efficiently as possible. Thus, the overall purpose of evaluating public health surveillance is to obtain feedback about the overall operation of the system and to promote the most effective use of health resources.

Evaluation is the systematic investigation of the merit, worth, or significance of an object (*1*). When planning a surveillance system (see also Chapter 2), we need to ask the question, What do we want to know? Furthermore, when evaluating a surveillance system, it is necessary to determine whether the purposes of the surveillance system were met. The performance of the system can be assessed using specific criteria and standards of performance (*1*).

The evaluation of an operating surveillance system for a high-priority health event aims to increase the system's utility and efficiency. It may also compare two or more systems that involve the same health event. But most important, it will determine whether the system is meeting its objectives, serving a useful public health function, and operating as efficiently as possible. The evaluation of a surveillance system should include at least the following steps:

- an explicit statement of the purposes and objectives of the system
- a description of its operation
- documentation of how the surveillance system has been useful
- an assessment of the different attributes
- estimates of the cost of the system

ADAPTING THE EVALUATION

Determining the most efficient approach to surveillance for a given health event is an art. There is room for creativity and the opportunity to combine scientific rigor with practical realities. The methods discussed in this chapter should be used as a guide to the types of questions that need to be answered about the system. Each evaluation should be individually tailored. Few evaluations address fully all of the methods outlined in this chapter, and many profitably focus on only one or two major attributes, such as sensitivity and timeliness (2–10). Some of the elements of evaluation may also be useful for evaluating other health-information systems or evaluating the value of secondary data sources for surveillance (11).

Each of the listed aspects of a surveillance evaluation are covered in the section below under the following topics: public health importance, objectives and usefulness, operation of the system, system attributes (simplicity, flexibility, acceptability, sensitivity, predictive value positive, representativeness, and timeliness), and cost. This chapter also reviews the process through which public health surveillance systems are evaluated (12,13).

PUBLIC HEALTH IMPORTANCE

The first step in evaluating a surveillance system is to answer the question, Should this health event be under surveillance? This question should be answered from a perspective external to the surveillance system itself (see also Chapter 2). It should also be asked when deciding whether to start a new system or before conducting a detailed evaluation of an existing one. This is done primarily to assess the public health importance of a health event and how to determine its importance when compared with that of other health events. Once a health event is identified as being of high priority, it is important to consider both the options, feasibility, and cost of conducting surveillance for that event. If this assessment leads to a decision to discontinue or not to start a surveillance system, a detailed evaluation of that system becomes superfluous.

The public health importance of a health event and the need for surveillance of that health event can be described in a variety of ways. Health events that affect many people or require large expenditures of resources are clearly important in a public health context. However, health events that affect relatively few persons may also be important, especially if the events cluster in time and place— e.g., a limited outbreak of a severe disease. At other times, public concerns may focus attention on a particular health event, creating or heightening the sense of importance associated with it. Health problems that are now rare because of successful control measures may be perceived as unimportant, but their level of importance should be assessed on the basis of their potential to reemerge. Finally, the public health importance of a health event is influenced by its preventability and the ability of public health action to influence it.

Measures of the importance of a health event include the following:

- morbidity: total number of cases, incidence and prevalence, physician visits, hospital days
- severity: mortality rate and case-fatality ratio
- premature mortality: years of potential life lost (YPLL)
- economic cost: costs of medical care, lost productivity interventions
- preventability: [preventable] fraction

Measures of importance used should take into account the effect of previously implemented prevention strategies on the incidence or prevalence of the health event. For example, the number of cases of vaccine-preventable illness has declined following the implementation of school immunization laws, and the public health importance of diseases in this category is underestimated by case counts alone. In such instances, it may be possible to estimate the number of cases that would be expected in the absence of control programs (*14*).

Preventability can be defined at several levels—from preventing the occurrence of disease (primary prevention), through early detection and treatment (secondary prevention), to minimizing the effects of the health problem among those already ill (tertiary prevention). From the perspective of surveillance, preventability reflects the potential for effective interventions at any of these levels.

The need for surveillance may also be affected by factors other than those mentioned above. Political and public pressure may affect whether surveillance is undertaken—or, at the other extreme, forbidden—for a specific health event. Regulations, laws, and public health programs may be implemented on the basis of considerations other than those listed above. However, it is still important to make the scientific criteria for evaluation as clear and explicit at possible. Even when using quantitative measures, judgment is necessary to decide which criteria are most relevant for assessing the importance of each condition. It is important to make these judgments as explicit—and as early—as possible.

Attempts have been made to quantify the public health importance of health conditions and to prioritize public health interventions. Dean described an approach that involved using a score that accommodated for age-specific mortality and morbidity rates and health-care costs (*15*). The CDC conducted an evaluation of 19 prevention strategies to provide economic guidance for making prevention decisions and allocating public health resources. This evaluation was based on the health impact of the related disease, injury or disability on U.S. society; the effectiveness of the prevention strategy; the costs of the disease, injury or disability; and the cost-effectiveness of the strategy (*16*). The Canadian Laboratory Centre for Disease Control has used explicit criteria in setting national surveillance priorities for communicable diseases. Their criteria include the parameters listed above, plus several others such as interest on the part of the WHO or the Canadian Department of Agriculture, potential for outbreaks, public perception of risk, and necessity for immediate public health response. Their ratings for 60 communicable diseases can be useful in setting priorities for initiating a surveillance system (*17,18*).

OBJECTIVES AND USEFULNESS

The most important steps in evaluating a surveillance system are *a*) describing (or defining) the health event(s) under surveillance, *b*) stating explicitly the objectives of the system, and *c*) describing how the system has actually been used to help prevent and control disease or injury. These three steps alone often sufficiently indicate how the system can be improved.

The description of a health event under surveillance (also known as the *case definition* if the event is a disease or injury) should include symptoms, signs, laboratory results, and epidemiologic information; a scale of severity; and the extent to which the event meets the definition using terms such as *suspected, probable,* or *confirmed.* Definitions for nationally notifiable diseases have been published for Canada and the United States (*19,20*). Table 8–1 outlines a definition for measles developed by CDC and CSTE.

The possible objectives of surveillance systems and the uses of surveillance information are very similar and have been reviewed in Chapter 1. For example,

Table 8–1 Sample Case Definition Developed by CDC and CSTE

Measles (revised September 1996)

Clinical case definition
An illness characterized by all the following:
- a generalized rash lasting greater than or equal to 3 days
- a temperature greater than or equal to 101.0°F (greater than or equal to 38.3°C)
- cough, coryza, or conjunctivitis

Laboratory criteria for diagnosis
- positive serologic test for measles immunoglobulin M antibody, or
- significant rise in measles antibody level by any standard serologic assay, or
- isolation of measles virus from a clinical specimen

Case classification
suspected: any febrile illness accompanied by rash
probable: a case that meets the clinical case definition, has noncontributory or no serologic or virologic testing, and is not epidemiologically linked to a confirmed case
confirmed: a case that is laboratory confirmed or that meets the clinical case definition and is epidemiologically linked to a confirmed case. A laboratory-confirmed case does not need to meet the clinical case definition

Comment
Confirmed cases should be reported to NNDSS.
An *imported* case has its source outside the country or state. Rash onset occurs within 18 days after entering the jurisdiction, and illness cannot be linked to local transmission.
International: Imported cases should be classified as a case that is imported from another country.
Out-of-State: A case that is imported from another state in the United States. The possibility that a patient was exposed within his or her state of residence should be excluded; therefore, the patient either must have been out of state continuously for the entire period of possible exposure (at least 7–18 days before onset of rash) or have had one of the following types of exposure while out of state: a) face-to-face contact with a person who had either a probable or confirmed case or b) attendance in the same institution as a person who had a case of measles (e.g., in a school, classroom, or day-care center).
An *indigenous* case is defined as a case of measles that is not imported. Cases that are linked to imported cases should be classified as indigenous if the exposure to the imported case occurred in the reporting state. Any case that cannot be proved to be imported should be classified as indigenous.

---

the objective of a surveillance system might be to meet a statutory requirement resulting from political necessity or public pressure or to identify cases for additional studies. There may also be objectives, such as meeting the reporting requirements of the WHO, that might not be of immediate or direct benefit to the agency operating the surveillance system.

The usefulness of a system should be described specifically, including the public health interventions that have been taken as a result of the data and analysis from the surveillance system, and who used the data to make decisions and take actions. Other anticipated uses of the data should be noted and their feasibility determined.

A surveillance system should contribute to the control and prevention of adverse health events. This process may include an improved understanding of the public health consequences of the events. A surveillance system can also be useful if it determines that an adverse health event previously thought to have public health importance actually does not.

An assessment of the usefulness of a surveillance system begins with a review of the objectives of the system and should consider the dependence of policy decisions and control measures on the surveillance system. Depending on the objectives of a particular surveillance system, the system may be considered useful if it satisfactorily addresses one or more of the following questions. Does the system

- detect trends signaling changes in the occurrence of the health problem in question?
- detect epidemics?
- provide estimates of the magnitude of morbidity and mortality related to the health problem being monitored?
- stimulate epidemiologic research likely to lead to control or prevention?
- identify high-risk groups?
- identify risk factors involved in the occurrence of the health problem?
- permit assessment of the effects of control measures?
- lead to improved clinical practice by the health-care providers who are the constituents of the surveillance system?

Usefulness may be affected by all the attributes of surveillance described below. Increased sensitivity may afford a greater opportunity for identifying epidemics and understanding the natural course of an adverse health event in a community. More rapid reporting allows more timely control and prevention activities. Increased specificity enables public health officials to focus on productive activities. A representative surveillance system will characterize more accurately the epidemiologic features of a health event in the population.

OPERATION OF THE SYSTEM

To evaluate a surveillance system, one must know how it operates (see also Chapter 5). The system description should include the following:

- the people and organizations involved (see also Chapters 4, 5, and 11)
- the flow of information (up and down) (see also Chapters 2, 7, and 16)

- tools used for data collection, analysis, and dissemination (see also Chapters 6, 7, and 16)
- mechanisms of information transfer (see also Chapters 7 and 11)
- frequency of reporting and feedback (see also Chapter 5)
- quality control (See also Chapter 5)

The evaluation should address the following questions:

What is the population being monitored?

Who is responsible for reporting a case, and to which public health agency?

What data is collected on each case, and who is responsible for collecting it?

How is data collected and entered into the surveillance system?

Are data elements coded in a standard manner? If there are multiple administrative levels represented in the system, how are the data transferred from one level to another?

Are privacy and confidentiality guidelines in place?

How is information stored?

What format is used to store the information?

What type of data quality checks are done?

What type of system documentation is available?

How is the system maintained or upgraded?

Who is responsible for system maintenance?

What type of help or troubleshooting is available?

Who analyzes the data?

How are data analyzed, and how often?

Are there preliminary and final tabulations, analyses, and reports?

How often are reports disseminated and to whom?

What mechanisms or media are used to distribute reports and communicate relevant findings?

Are there any automatic responses to case reports (e.g., follow-up of individual cases of rabies, botulism, or poliomyelitis)?

A diagram is often useful to summarize the relationship between the various components of a system (Figure 8–1).

ATTRIBUTES OF THE SYSTEM

Each surveillance system has characteristics or attributes (e.g., simplicity, flexibility, acceptability, sensitivity, predictive value positive, representativeness, and timeliness) that contribute directly to its ability to meet its specific objectives. The combination of these attributes determines the strengths and weaknesses of the system. The attributes must be balanced against each other; for instance, high sensitivity may only be possible with a complex reporting system from a wide array of providers.

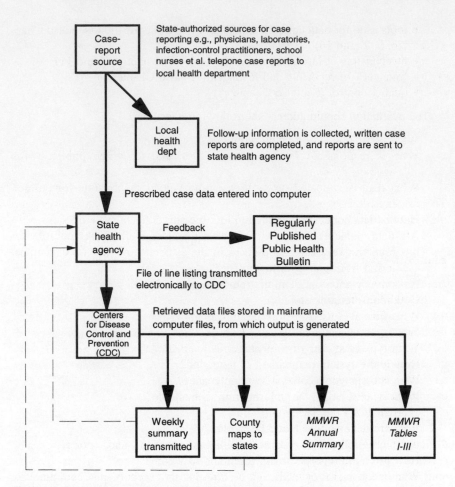

Figure 8–1 Components of a public health surveillance system.

Simplicity

Simplicity of a surveillance system refers both to its structure and to its ease of operation. Surveillance systems should be as simple as possible while still meeting their objectives. It may be useful to think of the simplicity of a surveillance system from two perspectives: the design of the system and the size of the system. An example of a system that is simple in design is one whose case definition is easy to apply and in which the person identifying the case will also be the one analyzing and using the information. A more complex system might involve special laboratory tests to confirm the case, telephone contact or a home visit by a public health nurse to collect additional data, multiple levels of reporting (e.g., case reports that start with doctors who make the diagnosis and then pass through local and state health departments before going to the federal government), and/or multiple sources of data.

The following measures might be considered in evaluating the simplicity of a system:

- amount and type of information necessary to establish a diagnosis
- number and type of data sources
- methods of transmitting case information and data
- staff training requirements
- type and extent of data analysis
- amount of computerization
- methods of distributing reports
- amount of time spent operating the system

The cost estimates for a system are also an indirect indicator of simplicity. Simple systems usually cost less than complex ones.

Flexibility

Another consideration is the ability of the system to adapt to changing needs such as the addition of new conditions or data-collection elements—a characteristic termed *flexibility*. Flexibility is probably best judged retrospectively, by observing how a system responded to a new demand. For example, when AIDS emerged in 1981, the existing notifiable-disease reporting system of state health departments was used to report cases. AIDS surveillance has since adapted to rapidly advancing knowledge about the disease, its diagnosis, and its risk factors. Another example is the capacity of the gonorrhea surveillance system to accommodate special surveillance for penicillianase-producing *Neisseria gonorrhoeae*.

Unless efforts have been made to adapt a system to another disease, it may be difficult to assess the flexibility of that system. In the absence of practical experience, one can look at the design and size of a system. Generally, simpler systems will tend to be more flexible, i.e., fewer components will need to be modified when adapting the system for use with another disease.

Acceptability

Acceptability reflects the willingness of individuals and organizations to participate in the surveillance system. This attribute refers to the acceptability of the system to health department staff, and at least equally importantly, to persons outside the sponsoring agency (e.g., physicians or laboratory staff) who are asked to report cases of certain kinds of health problems. To assess acceptability, one must consider the points of interaction between the system and its participants, including subjects (persons grouped under "cases") and reporters. Indicators of acceptability include: *a*) subject or agency participation rates; *b*) interview completion rates and question refusal rates, if the system involves case interviews; *c*) completeness of report forms; *d*) physician, laboratory, or hospital or facility reporting rates; and *e*) timeliness of reporting. Some of these indicators may be obtained from a review of surveillance report forms, while others would require special studies or surveys.

Sensitivity

The sensitivity of a surveillance system can be considered on two levels. First, the completeness of case reporting—the proportion of cases of a disease or health condition that are detected by the surveillance system (e.g., $A / (A + C)$ in Table 8–2)—can be evaluated. Second, the system can be evaluated for its ability to detect epidemics (21).

The sensitivity of a surveillance system is affected by the likelihood that

- persons with certain health conditions seek medical care
- the condition is correctly diagnosed, which reflects the skill of care providers and the accuracy of diagnostic tests
- the case is reported to the system once it has been diagnosed

These factors also apply to surveillance systems that do not fit the traditional model of passive reporting by health-care providers. For example, the sensitivity of a telephone-based surveillance system of morbidity or risk factors would be affected by

- the number of people who have telephones, who are at home when the surveyor calls, and who agree to participate
- the ability of persons to understand and correctly answer the questions
- the willingness of respondents to report their status

The extent to which these questions are explored depends on the system and on the resources available for the evaluation. The measurement of sensitivity in a surveillance system requires the validation of information collected through the system, so as to distinguish accurate from inaccurate case reports, and the collection of information external to the system, so as to determine the frequency of the condition in a community (i.e., a "gold standard") (22). From a practical standpoint, the primary emphasis in assessing sensitivity—assuming that most reported cases are correctly classified—is estimating what proportion of the to-

Table 8–2 The Detection of Health Conditions Using a Surveillance System*

		Condition present		
		Yes	No	
	Yes	True positive A	False positive B	A + B
Detected by surveillance				
	No	False positive C	True negative D	C + D
		A + C	B + D	Total

*Sensitivity = A / (A + C)
A / (A + C).
*Specificity = D / (B + D)
D / B(B + D)
*PVP = A / (A + B)

tal number of cases in the community are being detected by the system. If this proportion is estimated using methods that compare two or more surveillance systems, none of which is a gold standard, then this proportion should be called an estimate of "completeness of coverage" rather than of sensitivity. For surveillance systems that collect data from multiple sources, the sensitivity of each source can be examined by using the unduplicated multiple-source data base as the gold standard.

A surveillance system that does not have high sensitivity can still be useful in monitoring trends, as long as the sensitivity and predictive value positive (PVP) (discused below) remain reasonably constant. Questions concerning sensitivity in surveillance systems most commonly arise when changes in patterns of occurrence of the health problem are noted. Changes in sensitivity can be precipitated by heightened awareness of a health problem, introduction of new diagnostic tests, or changes in the method of conducting surveillance. A search for such surveillance "artifacts" is often an initial step in investigating an outbreak.

Several evaluations have looked at the sensitivity or completeness of coverage of surveillance systems (5–9,23–26).

Predictive Value Positive (PVP)

The PVP is defined as the proportion of persons identified as case-patients who actually have the condition being monitored (21). In Table 8–2 this is represented by $A / (A + B)$.

In assessing PVP, primary emphasis is placed on the confirmation of cases reported through the surveillance system. Its effect on the use of public health resources can be considered on two levels. At the level of an individual case, PVP affects the amount of resources required for investigation of cases. For example, where every reported case of hepatitis A is promptly investigated by a public health nurse, and family members at risk are referred for a prophylactic immune globulin injection, each reported case generates a requirement for follow-up. A surveillance system with low PVP, and therefore frequent false-positive case reports, would lead to resources being wasted on cases that do not in fact exist.

The other level is that of detection of epidemics. A high rate of erroneous case reports over the short term might trigger an inappropriate outbreak investigation, and conversely, a constant high level of false-positive reports might mask a true outbreak. In assessing this attribute, we want to know what proportion of epidemics identified by the surveillance system are true epidemics.

Calculating the PVP requires confirmation of all cases. Interventions initiated on the basis of information obtained from the surveillance system should be documented and kept on file. Personnel activity reports, travel records, and telephone logbooks may all be useful in estimating the impact of the PVP on the detection of epidemics. For surveillance systems that collect data from multiple sources, the PVP of each source can be examined by using the unduplicated multiple-source data base as the gold standard.

A low PVP means that a) non-cases are being investigated, and b) there may be mistaken reports of epidemics. False-positive reports to surveillance systems lead to unnecessary interventions, and falsely detected "epidemics" lead to costly investigations. A surveillance system with high PVP will lead to "less unnecessary and inappropriate expenditure of resources"(27).

The PVP for a health event may be enhanced by clear and specific case definitions. Good communications between the persons who report cases and the staff who operate the surveillance system can also improve PVP. The sensitivity and specificity of the case definition, as well as the prevalence of the condition in the population, contribute to the PVP (Table 8–2); the PVP increases with increasing specificity and prevalence.

Sensitivity and PVP are inversely related. The balance between assuring that all (or almost all) cases are identified (high sensitivity) and few false positives are identified (high PVP) must be based on the level of importance accorded to identifying all cases (e.g., for rabies or meningococcal meningitis), and the ability to use an indicator of the disease in the community (e.g., use of *Salmonella* laboratory isolates).

Several evaluations have examined the PVP of surveillance systems (5,7,9,23,25).

Representativeness

A truly representative surveillance system accurately describes the occurrence of a health event over time and its distribution in the population by place and person.

Representativeness is assessed by comparing the characteristics of reported events with those of all such events that occurred. Although this information is not generally available in specific detail, some judgment of the representativeness of surveillance data is possible, on the basis of knowledge of the following factors:

- characteristics of the population—e.g., age, socioeconomic status, geographic location (28)
- natural history of the condition—e.g., latency period, fatal outcome, prevailing medical practices—e.g., sites that perform diagnostic tests, physician-referral patterns (29,30)
- multiple sources of data—e.g., mortality rates for comparison with data on incidence and laboratory reports for comparison with physician reports

Representativeness can also be examined through special studies of a representative sample of the population (27).

The points at which bias can enter a surveillance system and decrease representativeness are illustrated in Figure 8–2.

Case Ascertainment Bias

This might also be called "sampling bias" and is the differential identification and reporting of cases from different populations or over time.

In order to generalize findings from surveillance data to the population at large, the data from a surveillance system should reflect the population characteristics that are important to the goals and objectives of that system. These characteris-

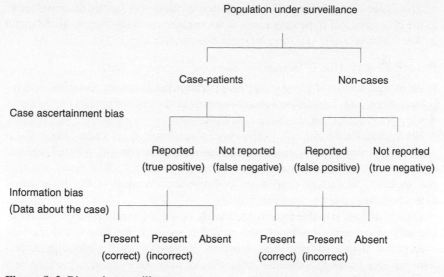

Figure 8–2 Biases in surveillance.

tics generally relate to time, place, and person. An important result of evaluating the representativeness of a surveillance system is the identification of subgroups in the population that may be systematically excluded from the reporting system. This will enable appropriate modification of data-collection practices and more accurate projections of incidence of the health event in the target population.

Changes in reporting practices over time can introduce bias into the system and make it difficult to follow long-term trends or to establish baseline rates to be used for the recognition of outbreaks. For example, switching from a passive to an active system or changing reporting sources may change the sensitivity of the system. Publicity can also increase rates of reporting in passive systems (*31*). While more complete reporting is desirable in principle, it is difficult to predict how a change in reporting practices or in publicity associated with the reportable condition will change the proportion of cases reported.

Differences in reporting practices by geographic location can bias the representativeness of the system. For example, the NNDSS aggregates data collected independently by the 50 states, the District of Columbia, and several territories. For some infectious diseases, some states collect data only from laboratories, whereas other states also accept cases reported by health practitioners (*32*). Also, despite efforts to achieve consistency, case definitions can be inconsistent across state and territorial boundaries (*20*).

Differential reporting rates of cases may occur in association with different characteristics of the person, so that cases among certain subpopulations may be less likely to be reported than those among other groups. For example, an evaluation of reporting on viral hepatitis in a county in Washington State suggested that cases of hepatitis B were under-reported among homosexual men and that cases of hepatitis non-A and non-B were under-reported among persons who had received blood transfusions. The importance of these risk factors as contributors to the occurrence of these diseases was apparently under-estimated, as indicated by the selective under-reporting of certain hepatitis cases (*33*).

Bias in Descriptive Information about a Reported Case

Even though a case of a reportable health condition has been identified and reported, there may be information bias (errors in the collection and recording of descriptive information about the case).

Most surveillance systems collect more than simple case counts. Information commonly collected includes the demographic characteristics of affected persons, details about the health event, and the presence or absence of defined potential risk factors. The quality, usefulness, and representativeness of this information depends on its completeness and validity.

Quality of data is influenced by the clarity of the information forms, the training and supervision of persons who complete surveillance forms, and the care exercised in management of data. A review of these facets of a surveillance system provides an indirect measure of quality of data. An examination of the percentage of "unknown" or "blank" responses to items on surveillance forms or questionnaires is straightforward. Assessing the validity of responses requires special studies, such as chart reviews or re-interviews of respondents.

Errors and bias can make their way into a surveillance system at any stage in the reporting and assessment process. Because surveillance data are used to identify high-risk groups, to target interventions, and to evaluate interventions, it is important to be aware of the strengths and limitations of the information in the system.

So far, the discussion of attributes has been aimed at the information collected for cases, but many surveillance systems also involve calculating morbidity and mortality rates. The denominators for these rate calculations are often obtained from a separate data system maintained by another agency, such as the Bureau of the Census or the NCHS of CDC. Although these data are regularly evaluated, thought should be given to the comparability of categories (e.g., race, age, or residence) used in the numerator and denominator of rate calculations.

Several studies have looked at quality-assurance problems associated with surveillance data. A sample of NEISS records was compared with emergency-room records to assess the quality of data recorded in the surveillance system (*34*). A study of the quality of national malaria surveillance reports was carried out in the United Kingdom (*35*). The quality of BRFSS data, which are obtained through monthly telephone surveys for behavioral risks associated with cardiovascular problems, has been examined in California (*36*). The CDC examined the completeness of race-ethnicity reporting in the NETSS (*37*).

Timeliness

Timeliness reflects the delay between any two (or more) steps in a surveillance system. The timeliness of the system can best be assessed by the ability of the system to take appropriate public health action based on the urgency of the prob-

lem and the nature of the public health response. Four points in time in the surveillance process are most often considered when measuring timeliness: *a*) time
of onset of disease or occurrence of an injury, *b*) time of diagnosis, *c*) time of
receipt of the report of case by public health agency responsible for control activities, and *d*) time of implementation of control activities. Usually one of the
first two, *a* or *b,* is used as the starting point, and one of the last two, *c* or *d,* is
used as an end point.

Another aspect of timeliness is the time required for the identification of trends,
outbreaks, or the effect of control measures. With infectious diseases, the onset
of symptoms can be measured. Sometimes the date of exposure is used. With
chronic diseases and other non-infectious health events, it may be more useful
to look at elapsed time from diagnosis rather than to estimate an onset date.

Timeliness is usually measured in days or weeks, but in hospital settings it
might be measured in hours or minutes; for diseases that do not necessitate an
immediate response, it might be measured in months or even years.

Evaluations of the timeliness with which shigellosis is reported in two different surveillance systems in the U.S. found median delays of 11 and 12.5 days
from time of onset of illness to receipt of report by the public health agency responsible for control measures. This delay did not allow public health officials
to intervene in a timely manner to prevent the occurrence of secondary or tertiary cases. However, such a time frame might still allow for effective intervention in settings, such as day-care facilities, in which outbreaks may persist for
weeks or months (*38*). Another study of timeliness in the reporting of salmonellosis, shigellosis, hepatitis A, and bacterial meningitis looked at the reporting delay between date of onset and date of report to CDC (*4*). Median reporting delays ranged from 20 days for bacterial meningitis to 33 days for hepatitis A. Wide
variations in reporting delays were found between states as well. A study in Australia showed that reports of infectious diseases from laboratories were received
by the Medical Officer of Health in a substantially shorter time than those received from medical practitioners (*39*).

In contrast, if there is a long latency between exposure and appearance of disease, the rapid identification of cases of illness may not be as important as the
rapid availability of data to interrupt and prevent exposures that lead to disease.

The need for rapid reporting to a surveillance system depends on the nature
of the public health problem under surveillance and the objectives of the system.
Recently, computer technology has been integrated into surveillance systems and
may promote timeliness of reporting (*40,41*).

COST

The final descriptive element is cost estimation of the resources used to operate
the system. The estimates generally are limited to direct costs and include the
costs of operating the system, e.g., personnel and resources required for collecting, processing, and analyzing surveillance data, as well as for the dissemination
of information resulting from the system.

Personnel costs may be determined from an estimate of the time it takes to operate the system for different personnel. While this can be expressed as person-time expended per year of operation, it is preferable to convert the estimate to dollar costs by multiplying the person-time by appropriate salary and benefit figures. Other costs may include those associated with travel, training, supplies, equipment, and services such as mail, telephone, rent, and computer time. The resources required at all relevant levels of the public health system—from the local health-care provider to municipal, county, state, and federal health agencies—should be included.

The approach to resources described here includes only those personnel and material resources required for the direct operation of surveillance. A more comprehensive evaluation of costs should examine consequential or indirect costs, such as follow-up laboratory testing or treatment, case investigations or outbreak control resulting from surveillance, costs of secondary data sources (e.g., vital statistics or survey data), costs incurred in processing and analyzing data, and costs averted (benefits) by surveillance.

Costs are judged relative to benefits, but few evaluations of surveillance systems have included a formal cost–benefit analysis, and such analyses are beyond the scope of this chapter. Estimating benefits, such as savings resulting from morbidity prevented through surveillance, may be possible in some instances, although this approach does not take into account the less tangible benefits that may result from surveillance systems. More realistically and in most instances, costs should be judged with respect to the objectives and usefulness of a specific surveillance system. Morris developed a framework for evaluating the cost-effectiveness of surveillance activities and conducted a detailed cost analysis for HIV/AIDS surveillance in England and Wales. This analysis demonstrated that the surveillance system would have to prevent 9.5 HIV infections per year to be cost-effective (*41*).

RECOMMENDATIONS

On the basis of the evaluation, an assessment of how well the surveillance system is meeting its current objectives should be made. Modifications to the system to enhance its usefulness and improve its attributes should be considered. A regular review of each surveillance system should assure that systems remain responsive to contemporary public health needs.

CONCLUSION

Evaluation of surveillance systems should be done on a regular basis and should be closely integrated into the operation of the systems. When time and resources are scarce, a rapid assessment of the importance of the problem, the current purpose of the system, and the usefulness of the system should be done. Based on that assessment, a more detailed evaluation may be in order. Careful evaluations have led to major revisions in surveillance systems, such as the improved and uniform reporting of gunshot wounds from multiple sources, and the change from a sentinel system to a school-based system for the surveillance of influenza-like illnesses (25,42). Regular evaluations should assure that surveillance systems operate efficiently and continue to meet contemporary public health needs.

The evaluation guidelines discussed in this chapter can also be used to evaluate information and administrative systems that may provide data for the development of integrated surveillance systems. Because some of these data bases were created to support administrative functions and not for public health surveillance, they should be validated and evaluated independently. Once the validation and evaluation of these systems is completed, these data bases can be combined into a larger data base to form an integrated surveillance system, or they could remain separate for easy electronic access. The evaluation of these integrated systems will require new approaches to assess the operation of the system, system attributes (simplicity, flexibility, acceptability, sensitivity, predictive value positive, representativeness, timeliness), and cost. In addition, the evaluation approach discussed in this chapter can be helpful in planning new surveillance systems.

REFERENCES

1. Centers for Disease Control and Prevention. Recommended framework for program evaluation in public health practice. *MMWR* 1999;48:RR11.
2. Harkess JR, Gildon BA, Archer PW, Istre GR. Is passive surveillance always insensitive? An evaluation of shigellosis surveillance in Oklahoma. *Am J Epidemiol* 1988;128:878–81.
3. Modesitt SK, Hulman S, Fleming D. Evaluation of active versus passive AIDS surveillance in Oregon. *Am J Public Health* 1990;80:463–4.
4. Birkhead G, Chorba TL, Root S, Klaucke DN, Gibbs NJ. Timeliness of national reporting of communicable diseases: the experience of the National Electronic Telecommunications System for Surveillance. *Am J Public Health* 1991;81:1313–5.
5. Thurman DJ *et al.* Surveillance of spinal cord injuries in Utah, USA. *Paraplegia* 1994;32(10):665–69.
6. Wendt RD *et al.* Evaluating the sensitivity of hazardous substances emergency events surveillance: a comparison of three surveillance systems. *J Environ Health* 1996; 58(9):13–7.
7. Archer PJ, Mallonee S, Schmidt AC, Ikeda RM. Oklahoma firearm-related injury surveillance. *Am J Prev Med* 1998;15(3S):83–91.
8. Barber CW *et al.* Massachusetts weapon-related injury surveillance system. *Am J Prev Med* 1998;15(3S):57–66.
9. Fox J, Stahlsmith L, Remington P, Tymus T, Hargarten S. The Wisconsin firearm-related injury surveillance system. *Am J Prev Med* 1998;15(3S):101–8.
10. Wilt SA, Gabrel CS. A weapon-related injury surveillance system in New York. *Am J Prev Med* 1998;15(3S):75–82.
11. Annest, JL, Mercy JA. Use of national data systems for firearm-related injury surveillance. *Am J Prev Med* 1998;15(3S):17–30.
12. Klaucke DN, Buehler JW, Thacker SB *et al.* Guidelines for evaluating surveillance systems. *MMWR* 1988;37(SS-5):1–18.

13. Thacker SB, Parrish RG, Trowbridge FL. A method for evaluating systems of epidemiological surveillance. *World Health Statistics Quarterly* 1988;41:11–8.
14. Hinman AR, Koplan JP. Pertussis and pertussis vaccine: reanalysis of benefits, risks, and costs. *JAMA* 1984;251:3109–13.
15. Dean AG, West DJ, Weir WM. Measuring loss of life, health, and income due to disease and injury. *Public Health Rep* 1982;97:38–47.
16. Messonier ML, Corso PS, Teutsch SM, Haddix AC, Harris JR. An ounce of prevention . . . what are the returns? *Am J Prev Med* 1999;16(3):248–63.
17. Laboratory Centre for Disease Control. Establishing goals, techniques and priorities for national communicable disease surveillance. *Canada Diseases Weekly Report* 1991;17:79–84.
18. Carter A. Setting priorities: the Canadian experience in communicable disease surveillance. In: Proceedings of the 1992 International Symposium on Public Health Surveillance. *MMWR* 1992;41(Suppl):79–84.
19. Laboratory Centre for Disease Control. Canadian communicable disease surveillance system. Disease-specific case definitions and surveillance methods. *Canada Diseases Weekly Report* 1991;17(Suppl 3):1–35.
20. Centers for Disease Control and Prevention. Case definitions for infectious conditions under public health surveillance. *MMWR* 1997;46(No. RR-10).
21. Weinstein MC, Fineberg HV. Clinical decision analysis. Philadelphia: W.B. Saunders Co., 1980.
22. Chandra Sekar C, Deming WE. On a method of estimating birth and death rates and the extent of registration. *J Am Stat Assoc* 1949;44:101–15.
23. Hedegaard H, Wake M, Hoffman R. Firearm-related injury surveillance in Colorado. *Am J Prev Med* 1998;15(3S):38–45.
24. Kim AN, Trent RB. Firearm-related injury surveillance in California. *Am J Prev Med* 1998;15(3S):31–7.
25. LeMier M, Cummings P, Keck D, Stehr-Green J, Ikeda R, Saltzman, L. Washington state gunshot-wound surveillance system. *Am J Prev Med* 1998;15(3S): 92–100.
26. Van Tuinen M, Crosby A. Missouri firearm-related injury surveillance system. *Am J Prev Med* 1998;15(3S):67–74.
27. Barker WH, Feldt KS, Feibel J *et al.* Assessment of hospital admission surveillance of stroke in a metropolitan community. *Am J Chron Dis* 1984;37:609–15.
28. Kimball AM, Thacker SB, Levy ME. *Shigella* surveillance in a large metropolitan area: assessment of a passive reporting system. *Am J Public Health* 1980;70:164–6.
29. Vogt RL, Larue D, Klaucke DN, Jillson DA. Comparison of active and passive surveillance systems of primary care providers for hepatitis, measles, rubella, and salmonellosis in Vermont. *Am J Public Health* 1983;73:795–7.
30. Thacker SB, Redmond S, Rothenberg R *et al.* A controlled trial of disease surveillance strategies. *Am J Prev Med* 1986;2:345–50.
31. Davis JP, Vergeront JM. The effect of publicity on the reporting of toxic-shock syndrome in Wisconsin. *J Infect Dis* 1982;145:449–57.
32. Sacks JJ. Utilization of case definitions and laboratory reporting in the surveillance of notifiable communicable diseases in the United States. *Am J Public Health* 1985; 75:1420–2.
33. Alter MJ, Mares A, Hadler SC *et al.* The effect of under-reporting on the apparent incidence and epidemiology of acute viral hepatitis. *Am J Epidemiol* 1987;125:133–9.
34. Hopkins RS. Consumer product-related injuries in Athens, Ohio, 1980–85: assessment of emergency-room-based surveillance. *Am J Prev Med* 1989;5(2):104–12.

35. Phillips-Howard PA, Mitchell J, Bradley DJ. Validation of malaria surveillance case reports: implications for studies of malaria risk. *J Epidemiol Community Health* 1990;44(2):155–61.
36. Jackson C, Jatulis DE, Fortmann SP. The behavioral risk factor survey and the Stanford five-city project survey: a comparison of cardiovascular risk behavior estimates. *Am J Public Health* 1991;82:412–6.
37. Centers for Disease Control and Prevention. Reporting race and ethnicity data—National Electronic Telecommunications System for Surveillance, 1994–1997. *MMWR* 1999;48:305–6.
38. Rosenberg ML. *Shigella* surveillance in the United States, 1975. *J Infect Dis* 1977; 136:458–9.
39. Murphy DJ, Seltzer BL, Yesalis CE. Comparison of two methodologies to measure agricultural occupational fatalities. *Am J Public Health* 1990;80:198–200.
40. Buehler JW. Surveillance. In: Rothman KJ, Greenland S (eds.). Modern epidemiology. Second edition. Philadelphia: Lippencott-Raven, 1998.
41. Morris S, Gray A, Noone A, Wiseman M, Jathanna S. The costs and effectiveness of surveillance of communicable disease: a case study of HIV and AIDS in England and Wales. *J Public Health Medicine* 1996;18(4):415–22.
42. Koo D, Wetterhall SF. History and current status of the National Notifiable Diseases Surveillance System. *J Public Health Management Practice* 1996;2(4):4–10.

9

Ethical Issues

DIXIE E. SNIDER
DONNA F. STROUP

*Epidemiology exudes an air of objectivity and many of its practitioners seem
loathe to accept that it is far from being value free either in its theory and methods or in its application. Indeed, even in its compilation and presentation of
data . . . , epidemiology involves value judgements and ethical choices.*

Mooney and Leeder

The above quotation helps to explain the primary reason for a chapter on ethics
in a book on surveillance. Effective public health activities, including public
health surveillance, depend on a trusting relationship between public health practitioners and the society they are trying to assist (*1*). This trust is placed at risk
when questions of ethics are raised about the appropriateness of certain public
health surveillance activities. Such situations have occurred, for example, in association with human immunodeficiency virus (HIV) serosurveys (*2*), screening
for genetic diseases (*3–5*), and some classification and labeling schemes used by
epidemiologists (*6,7*).

Second, surveillance activities have been authorized because society (through
its elected legislators and public health officials) has judged that the benefits
greatly outweigh the risks to individuals. Furthermore, surveillance usually is not
considered to be research (*8*). It should be noted, however, that some activities
classified initially as surveillance by public health officials and other epidemiologists may actually extend beyond surveillance and meet the definition of research. In that case, the activities are covered by federal regulations for protection of human subjects (*9*), in accordance with the Belmont Report (*10*), to ensure
patients' rights to relevant disclosure about potential risks and benefits of data
collection, and to ensure that benefits of the activity outweigh any harms. An example of such an activity is provided by the Behavioral Risk Factor Surveillance
System (BRFSS), which meets the definition of surveillance, but is also a research project (*11*).

A third reason to discuss ethics in a book on surveillance is that professional
societies of epidemiologists and statisticians have ethical guidelines, and the content of these guidelines applies to surveillance activities. Finally, public health
surveillance is inherently a social enterprise, usually funded by tax dollars, which

can directly and indirectly affect society (*12*). Therefore, the public has an interest in ensuring that surveillance activities are conducted in an ethical manner.

This chapter presents elements of the field of ethics that apply to epidemiology and public health surveillance. We begin with a discussion of underlying frameworks for ethics, summarize examples of professional standards of conduct for public health practitioners, delineate obligations of epidemiologists, present some legal issues related to ethical issues in surveillance, discuss the role of clinicians in surveillance activities, and provide several applications of these frameworks in surveillance practice. Because of the extension of surveillance into the research arena, we also give a brief overview of selected aspects of ethical issues in research. From reading this material, epidemiologists should gain awareness of the ethical issues underlying their discipline in practice and be able to respond to ethical issues that arise in the usual practice of their profession.

ETHICAL FRAMEWORKS

Last (*13*) defines *ethics* as "... the branch of philosophy that deals with the distinction between right and wrong, with the moral consequences of human actions" (*13*). Webster's definition says that ethics is the discipline that deals with "good and bad, or right and wrong, or with moral duty and obligation." It is often claimed that the basis for public health is social justice (*14–16*). However, adherence to this single principle (even if a uniform definition were accepted) is not adequate for the ethical practice of public health; for example, economic and social inequities of the contemporary world require different frameworks (*17,18*). Among the frameworks that are useful in public health are utilitarian theory, Kantian (deontological) theory, virtue theory, casuistry, rights-based theories, communitarianism, and principlism.

Utilitarianism is a consequence-based theory that holds that an action or practice is right if it leads to the greatest possible balance of good consequences or to the least possible balance of bad consequences for the greatest number of people (*19*). Kantianism is a duty-based (or deontological) theory espoused by Immanuel Kant (1734–1804), who held that an action has moral worth only when performed by a person who adheres to a categorical imperative of universal moral law (*1*); that is, a duty. For example, if a researcher discloses risk to a study participant only because she or he fears a lawsuit, and not because of a belief in the value of truth, the researcher is acting correctly but deserves no moral credit.

Virtue ethics, sometimes referred to as "character ethics," holds that the character of the person—not his/her duties or the consequence of actions—is the primary consideration in judging something as ethical (*20*). When the principle of virtue ethics is applied to epidemiology, examples of virtues of particular importance are honesty, self-effacement, integrity, fidelity, excellence, and prudence. A casuist analyzes an ethical problem by finding analogues in paradigm cases or precedents and then, in identifying salient similarities, arrives at the best decision (*1*).

Rights-based theories as applied to public health can be illustrated by the statement that public health can achieve its goals most effectively when it respects and promotes human rights. Violations of the rights of one individual or community (e.g., privacy) are permitted only when the violation is minor and in no other way affects the rights of other individuals or communities (21).

Communitarianism views everything fundamental in morality as deriving from communal values, the common good, social goals, traditional practices, and cooperative virtues (22). A key aspect of this approach is that issues traditionally outside the sphere of public health (e.g., housing, employment, and safety) should be considered when addressing health problems (23). Another implication of this approach is greater involvement of members of communities in decisions about public health activities (24,25).

Principlism, specifically the "four principles approach" to bioethics, is probably the most widely known tool for addressing ethical issues in health (15). The four principles are respect for autonomy or self-determination, beneficence (providing benefits and balancing these against risks and costs), nonmaleficence (avoiding causing harm), and justice (fairness in the distribution of benefits, risk, and costs). This framework has proven to be especially useful when evaluating the ethics of research proposals (26).

At times, ethical dimensions of public health and surveillance problems might best be determined in consultation with professionally trained ethicists, especially when confronting extremely difficult and controversial issues. At a minimum, a public health worker should be able to identify and address the major ethical issues associated with any given activity (e.g., development of a new surveillance system) by becoming familiar with and following professional ethical guidelines and federal, state, and local laws and regulations relevant to the activity (27).

Each of the ethical frameworks above has something to contribute to the development of guidelines for professional conduct. We propose the following questions based on all frameworks that the surveillance practitioner may want to address:

- Do my reasons for undertaking this activity reflect self-interest or a desire to benefit the community?
- What are the potential benefits and harms from the surveillance activity that is being considered?
- Who will benefit, who will be harmed and who will bear the costs?
- Am I maximizing the benefits and minimizing the harms to the population involved?
- Are the benefits reasonable in light of the expected harms and costs?
- How have similar ethical problems been approached in the past?
- Have community representatives been involved in developing this activity, and if so, how does the community view this activity?
- Am I violating the real or perceived rights of anyone in carrying out this activity in the way I propose to do it? If so, have I taken steps to minimize the adverse impact on individual rights and maximize the benefits to society from the activity?
- How should I carry out this activity to respect persons and assure that the benefits, harms, and costs are distributed equitably in the population?
- What virtues should I demonstrate?

PROFESSIONAL STANDARDS OF CONDUCT

Several professional societies have developed, or are developing, guidelines for epidemiologists and statisticians to deal with ethical issues frequently encountered by members of their professions. We call the reader's attention to the *International Guidelines for Ethical Review of Epidemiological Studies* developed by the Council for International Organizations for the Medical Sciences (CIOMS) (*28*), *Ethical Guidelines for Epidemiologists* developed by the Industrial Epidemiology Forum (IEF) (*29*), and *Guidelines for Good Epidemiology Practices for Occupational and Environmental Epidemiologic Research by the Chemical Manufacturers Association* (*30*). At the time of this writing, ethical guidelines are being drafted by the American College of Epidemiology (ACE) (*31*) and the American Statistical Association (ASA) (*32*).

These ethical guidelines generally offer a prescription for what epidemiologists should do. Although these guidelines may not address surveillance explicitly, many of the ethical issues confronting public health surveillance are similar to those of other epidemiologic activities (e.g., data collection and storage). Hence, the following overview of the content of these guidelines should provide the surveillance practitioner with a sense of the ethical issues likely to be encountered and with advice from professional societies for dealing with those issues.

The greatest emphasis in the guidelines is placed on the professional duties of epidemiologists and statisticians. Most guidelines place a heavy emphasis on research ethics and less emphasis on other aspects of public health practice. Thus, there are usually extensive discussions of minimizing risks and protecting the welfare of research participants, providing them benefits, ensuring an equitable distribution of risks and benefits, protecting confidentiality and privacy, obtaining the informed consent of participants, and submitting proposed studies for ethical review. However, the new draft guidelines of the ACE include discussions of the virtues epidemiologists should exhibit; maintaining public trust; adhering to the highest scientific standards; involving community representatives in research; avoiding conflicts of interest and partiality; communicating ethical requirements to colleagues, employers, and sponsors; confronting unethical conduct; and carrying out obligations to communities (*31*). In addition, the draft guidelines of the ASA (*32*) explicitly address concerns about the burden of data collection on respondents, privacy and confidentiality, data ownership issues, obligations related to data release, conflict of interest (*33*), and work on interdisciplinary teams that directly relate to public health surveillance practice.

THE OBLIGATIONS OF EPIDEMIOLOGISTS

On the basis of the ethical frameworks presented above and the ethical guidelines of professional societies, we offer the following comments about the obligations of those who conduct surveillance and related epidemiologic activities.

Minimizing Risks and Protecting the Welfare of Participants

Epidemiologists should consider and weigh any known or potential risks (e.g., disclosure of information) that individuals or populations may encounter as a result of their participation in surveillance activities. Consideration of risks includes attention not only to physical risks but also to psychological, economic, legal, and social risks (34). Specifically, surveillance practitioners should be aware of possible stigmatization of groups as a result of categories used for surveillance data (35).

For the routine practice of surveillance, the need to preserve the common good may outweigh the individual right of autonomy and the need for informed consent (e.g., surveillance for acute, communicable diseases). However, when the principles and practice of surveillance extend into the research arena, practitioners should consider the need to obtain the informed consent of participants, disclosing any known or unknown risks, and ensuring that risks are reasonable in relation to anticipated benefits.

Providing Benefits

In addition to minimizing harm to participants, epidemiologists have obligations to maximize the potential benefits of public health surveillance and other epidemiologic projects to participants and to society. The potential benefits of public health surveillance apply to the community: preventing further cases of disease, providing information to initiate control and prevention activities, and ensuring efficient use of resources by evaluating programs and providing cost-effectiveness data (36). The individuals who participate in surveillance projects also may derive benefit from the activity, such as when a previously unrecognized disease is detected during health examinations and individuals are then referred for treatment, or when community interventions are instituted.

Protecting Confidentiality and Privacy

Privacy refers to the right of individuals to refuse to provide information about themselves except to those to whom they choose to reveal this information. *Confidentiality* refers to obligation to the party maintaining the data to keep information about an individual restricted to those to whom the person who was the source of that information agreed to permit access. Except under unusual circumstances (e.g., when there is a need for follow-up counseling or treatment, or when release of information is mandated by a court of law), information obtained about participants in a surveillance project should be kept confidential. Protection of confidentiality is not only required by the ethical principle of respecting persons (autonomy), but also because the disclosure of certain information to third parties or subsequent use of the data for a purpose other than that which motivated its initial collection may cause harm to an individual, e.g., discrimination in employment, housing, and health insurance coverage (37). Development of surveillance systems should involve provisions for maintaining confidentiality and consideration of potential uses of data that contain personally identifying information.

The use of a unique study number often permits updating and revision of the data for surveillance participants. Surveillance practitioners should restrict access to personal information and store this information in secure environments (e.g., locked file cabinets). To further ensure confidentiality of information (including self-reported and biologic data), data should be gathered, stored, and presented in such a manner so as to prevent identification of study participants by third parties (38). Confidentiality can be violated even without the release of personal identifiers such as names or social security numbers. For example, the release of surveillance information from a small town could indirectly identify an individual patient in that community even though no name or social security number was given. Release of data with birthdate and location, when matched with other data sets such as drivers' license files, can lead to the identification of individuals. Therefore, it should be standard surveillance practice to aggregate numbers in such a way that individual identities cannot be released indirectly (39).

Informed Consent

Informed consent is intended to ensure that participants fully understand the purpose and nature of the data collection, the potential risks and benefits, and who the investigators and sponsors are. For most surveillance activities conducted as part of mandated public health activities by government agencies, collection of data involves minimal risk of possible harm and violation of confidentiality, and benefits to the community outweigh these. In addition, states have laws in place to protect data collected as part of mandated public health surveillance activities. Thus, informed consent is not required in these circumstances.

However, when the surveillance activity becomes research, investigators are obligated to disclose information that patients or other individuals usually consider important in deciding whether to participate. Information should be provided about the purposes of the data collection system, the procedures that will be used, any anticipated risks and benefits, any anticipated inconveniences or discomfort, and the individuals' right to refuse participation or to withdraw from the data collection activity at any time without repercussions. Additional disclosures may be necessary and steps should be taken to ensure that the participants (including minors) understand the disclosures; obtaining informed-consent is a process and informed consent statements must be understandable to a lay person. Although participants sometimes receive compensation for their participation in studies (for example, reimbursement for transportation costs), they must voluntarily consent to the planned intervention without undue incentives for participation, coercion, or manipulation.

Peer Review

An important aspect of public health surveillance practice is the dissemination of data from the system as soon as possible. The timely publication is important to guarantee usefulness of the data for prevention and intervention. Peer review plays an important role in improving scientific reports and thereby contributes directly to the potential benefits of surveillance to the scientific community and to society (40). Publications based on data from surveillance activities conducted collaboratively should involve those partners in the authorship and review processes.

Maintaining Public Trust

Public trust is essential if epidemiologic functions (e.g., surveillance and research) are to continue to be supported by the public. Trust is an expression of faith and confidence that epidemiologists will be fair, reliable, ethical, and competent. To promote and preserve public trust, epidemiologists should adhere to the highest ethical standards and follow relevant laws and regulations concerning the conduct of epidemiologic research and practice activities (including the protection of human research participants), confidentiality protections (41,42), and disclosure or avoidance of conflicting interests.

Objectivity, Conflicts of Interest, and Partiality

Epidemiologists must ensure that objectivity prevails at every step of the study. All scientists bring interpretive biases to problems; however, partiality can arise when such preconceived notions unduly affect the conduct or reporting of a study. Maintaining honesty and impartiality in the design, conduct, interpretation, and reporting of findings is an essential professional duty and a virtue. Reports should include sufficient data (in aggregate form) and sufficient information about the surveillance methods to ensure that interpretations and conclusions made from the findings can be corroborated independently by others. Full information should be reported about the representativeness, completeness of coverage, and other potential sources of bias.

Partiality can arise when pressure is brought to bear by any parties that have an interest in seeing the research results favor their particular interests. Epidemiologists conducting surveillance or research studies should not enter into contractual obligations that are contingent on reaching particular conclusions.

Investigators should disclose any conflicts of interest to appropriate persons (e.g., collaborators, sponsors, participants, employers, scientific colleagues, and journal editors). Full disclosure can help ensure the identification of conflicts of interest. Epidemiologists should distinguish perceived conflicting interests from actual conflicting interests. Perceived conflicts must be addressed but are not a reason to disqualify oneself from participation in an epidemiologic project.

Communicating with Trainees, Colleagues, Employers, and Sponsors about Ethical Requirements and Confronting Unacceptable Misconduct

Epidemiologists should convey and model the values and obligations of a professional epidemiologist to trainees, colleagues, employers, and sponsors. This dissemination of information may occur informally during discussion of issues (e.g., confidentiality, authorship, informed consent, and interpretation and communication of results) or in formal lectures. Epidemiologists should demonstrate appropriate ethical conduct to colleagues and students.

Confronting and alleging unacceptable conduct (e.g., scientific misconduct) is unpleasant but important to the individuals concerned, the profession, and society. Sponsoring institutions and funding agencies must have appropriate procedures in place to investigate allegations of misconduct as well as to protect whistle-blowers (see Office for Research Integrity (ORI) Web site: http://grants.nih.gov/grants/oprr/oprr.htm). The rights of the accused to due process should be respected and protected.

Obligations to Communities

Obligations to communities are central to any account of the professional role of epidemiologists. Epidemiologists meet their obligations to communities by undertaking public health practice (e.g., surveillance) and research activities that address causes of morbidity and mortality or utilization of health-care resources, and by reporting results in a timely fashion so that the widest possible community stands to benefit. The optimal time to disseminate the findings of surveillance systems and epidemiologic studies is not always easy to discern. Both premature and unnecessarily delayed release of data can be harmful to individuals and to society.

Although epidemiologists cannot always prevent the media or other parties from sensationalizing research results, epidemiologists should strive to ensure that, at a minimum, surveillance and research findings are interpreted and reported on accurately. The goal should be to communicate data to allow full use of the information for the public good (43).

In confronting public health problems, epidemiologists sometimes act as advocates on behalf of members of affected communities. Care must be taken to ensure that such advocacy does not impair scientific impartiality. Public health advocacy should be clearly distinguished from professional roles relating more directly to scientific research or public health practice.

CLINICIANS AND THE PUBLIC HEALTH COMMUNITY

Physicians, laboratorians, and other health-care practitioners play a critical role in reporting infectious diseases to local and state health departments (44). Reporting traumatic events (e.g., gunshot wounds and child abuse) is also required in some states (45). Fulfilling these duties may prevent further infection or trauma. Although reporting selected diseases and injuries is mandatory for physicians and others in all states, completeness of reporting ranges from 6% to 90% for many notifiable diseases, and reporting laws are seldom enforced (46).

Investigators have a duty to report findings to clinicians, since data from surveillance systems and research studies may also have implications for patients in general or for patients with certain conditions (47).

LEGAL PROTECTIONS TO SAFEGUARD PARTICIPANTS IN EPIDEMIOLOGIC ACTIVITIES

Although most behavior in surveillance and research depends on voluntary adherence, legal protections for participants in data collection activities (both surveillance and research) are relevant. Here, we will discuss briefly federal regulations governing research involving human subjects and laws, and regulations for maintaining the confidentiality of private information held by researchers.

Federal regulations promulgated by the Office for Protection from Research Risks (OPRR) of the National Institutes of Health (NIH), apply to institutions that use federal funds to collect data involving human subjects (9). These regulations apply to research, which is defined as a systematic investigation designed to develop or contribute to generalizable knowledge; human subjects are defined as living individuals about whom individually identifiable information will be obtained through intervention or interaction with the individual or through use of private, identifiable information (e.g., medical records). Since surveillance activities may extend into the research arena, we briefly summarize these regulations here.

The OPRR's regulations require that each institution that conducts research on human subjects have an assurance of compliance on file at OPRR. This assurance is: *a*) a commitment to OPRR that the institution will conduct research according to principles espoused in the Belmont Report (*15*); *b*) a pledge that the institution will follow federal regulations (or an equivalent code, guideline or regulation) for the protection of human subjects, *c*) a description of how it will do so, and *d*) an identification of who will be responsible for ensuring that the regulations are being followed (including a listing of institutional review board [IRB] members). Most institutions which conduct much research have a multiple project assurance (MPA) that permits them to conduct many different research projects for several years (usually five) before resubmitting another application for an assurance. Institutions which rarely conduct research involving human subjects usually obtain a single project assurance (SPA) for each research project. When a surveillance activity becomes a research activity, investigators should find out if the institutions to be involved in their project have an assurance on file.

Federal regulations also require that proposed federally funded research involving human subjects be reviewed by an IRB (*27*). The purpose of the IRB is to ensure that research involving human subjects is designed according to relevant ethical standards. The IRB is charged with focusing on the rights and welfare of the subjects as well as on the equitableness in the selection of subjects. The IRB members will examine the protocol, including study design (since a poorly designed study cannot answer the research question and is therefore unethical), participant consent form, appropriateness of interventions, and measures for safeguarding records and maintaining confidentiality. Appendix 9A provides an example checklist for surveillance projects which may include research components.

In addition to OPRR regulations, privacy and confidentiality laws and regulations affect surveillance and other epidemiologic activities (*48*). In the United

States, public health surveillance activities conducted under the sponsorship of the Executive Branch (including the Department of Health and Human Services [DHHS] and the Bureau of the Census) are regulated by the Public Health Service Act (49) and by the Privacy Act of 1974 (50). Both acts can be applied, whether the data collection activity is surveillance or research, to regulate contractors of federal agencies as well as the agencies themselves, and address "systems of records ... from which information is retrieved by the name of the individual or by some identifying number, symbol or other identifying particular assigned to the individual," and covers data held at the federal level (51). Records without identifiers, such as data in many surveillance systems, may be exempt from these regulations, and data held by other federal agencies as a result of a federally funded program may not be covered.

Individual states (counties and local agencies) use surveillance information primarily for their own disease- and injury-control programs. As major surveillance agencies, the states have been critically concerned with issues of confidentiality (52). Although all states have provisions for complying with freedom of information requests and maintaining confidentiality of information, they vary in specific regulations and their enforcement. Twenty-five states have general confidentiality requirements with little specific definition; 7 require written consent for release of information; 7 exclude surveillance information from subpoena; and 10 have penalties for unlawful disclosure of information on some or all reported infectious diseases (53). The states are concerned with the protection of the confidentiality of data released for federal surveillance systems and, in collaboration with CDC, have established confidentiality guidelines for the release of data from the notifiable disease surveillance systems (54).

Although the Privacy Act focuses on the disclosure and dissemination of information already collected, the act also restricts surveillance information that may be collected by stipulating that records may contain only "such information about an individual as is relevant and necessary to accomplish a purpose of the agency." This enforces the ethical obligation to conduct surveillance on issues with identifiable public health benefit, as opposed to issues that might be of interest purely from a research or academic perspective. In addition, the Privacy Act prohibits use of surveillance (or other information) "for any purpose other than the purpose for which it was supplied unless such establishment or person has consented ... to its use for such other purpose" (49).

The Privacy Act gives individuals the right to obtain their own records, to correct errors in the record, and to receive an accounting of how the record has been disseminated. Exemptions to individual access include the use of records maintained for statistical purposes only rather than for administrative use (e.g., census information). The Act requires that federal agencies train and regulate personnel with access to record systems and that agencies maintain physical means of protecting records from unwarranted access. Agencies are also required to describe their record systems and to report procedures used to comply with requirements in the Federal Register. Criminal penalties and fines may be imposed on persons who violate the stipulations of the act. Finally, the Privacy Act requires that potential participants in record systems be informed of the authority under which the data are collected, the purposes of the information, the routine uses of the information, and the consequences of not participating.

The Privacy Act forbids the disclosure of information in which individual identity is ascertainable, unless the subject has agreed to disclosure. This principle thus protects the confidentiality of individuals and affects the dissemination of surveillance findings. Records protected by the Privacy Act are exempt from Freedom of Information Act (FOIA) requests. Specifically, FOIA exempts "personal and medical files and similar files, the disclosure of which would constitute a clearly unwarranted invasion of personal privacy" and matters "specifically exempted from disclosure by statute" (55).

Other confidentiality concerns may be addressed by requesting certificates of confidentiality from the DHHS agency that funded the research (or, if the research is not federally funded, from the NIH) (see also Chapter 10). Subsection 301(d), added to the Public Health Service Act in 1988 (42USC§§241[d] and 242m[d]), provides authority for the issuance of certificates of confidentiality for health projects. The certificate relieves the holder (for example, investigators carrying out genetic testing as part of a research protocol) from the obligation to comply with compulsory legal demands such as court subpoenas for individual research records. Public health practitioners working with a Public Health Service agency may be able to obtain even stronger protection of their data under subsection 308(d) of the Public Health Service Act.

In addition, states have legislation that may apply to surveillance activities. In the United States, this system represents 54 different sets of legislation which generally cover medical records and vital statistics, but may not address other types of surveillance information and almost never extend to computerized data systems or data transmitted electronically (53,56).

Despite these ethical and legal protections, recent advances in computer technology, the development of large data sets, and the ability to link different data sets with or without personal identifiers have created great concern about confidentiality of information about individuals. In addition, recent developments in genetics also have heightened concern about the confidentiality of, and the inappropriate use of, genetic information. In response to these developments, some states have strengthened their laws regarding the confidentiality of health information. Laws are being proposed now to restrict how genetic information can be used. In addition, Congress is considering federal privacy legislation. Epidemiologists should be alert to and comply with state, provincial, and national (federal) laws regarding confidentiality and privacy, including those pertaining to data sharing or pooling of data and the use of genetic information.

EXAMPLES OF ETHICAL ISSUES IN SURVEILLANCE

Surveillance for AIDS

The AIDS epidemic that results from infection with HIV illustrates the ethical problem of labeling of populations groups. Since 1985, AIDS has been reportable to the National Notefiable Diseases System (NNDSS) of the United States. Early reports of cases were from populations of young, homosexual or bisexual men (57). Because of this clustering, surveillance for the disease developed to include information on risk factors (including sexual orientation and practices). Case investigations resulting from early surveillance indicated that the syndrome was linked to homosexuals and that concurrent increases in the incidence of sexually transmitted disease and of drug use among men could explain the emergence of this syndrome (58). However, continued surveillance revealed cases among hemophiliacs with little reported drug use, intravenous drug users without homosexual activity, and others (59). Thus, the labeling of AIDS as "a gay disease" proved inappropriate and inaccurate. Similarly, at one point, persons from Haiti were identified as having an increased risk for AIDS, but later data showed that certain behaviors were the major determinants of risk, not country of origin.

Labeling of specific population groups as being at risk was a double-edged sword. As surveillance and research continued, affected communities began using the data generated from these activities to demand research and access to care (60). Subsequently, such activities were in part a motivating factor for a change in the surveillance case definition (61) and expanded surveillance activities to study the spectrum of HIV disease (62). This use of labeling for either discriminatory or enhanced treatment points to the importance of maintaining confidentiality of surveillance data and emphasizes that care must be taken in choosing labels for groups at risk for certain diseases.

State-Based Fire Injury Surveillance

This example illustrates a surveillance activity that evolved into a research project. In 1995, residential fires accounted for an estimated 3,600 deaths and approximately 18,600 injuries; property damage and other direct costs were estimated to exceed more than $4 billion annually (63). To address this public health problem, surveillance data from fire-related injuries was used to show that fire deaths occur disproportionately in the South; during winter months; at night; and among poor, minority, and rural populations. The surveillance program was expanded to include information on smoke detector usage, and a program was implemented to provide funding to states to study the effectiveness of approaches to promoting residential smoke detectors in high-risk populations. Thus, the original surveillance activity evolved into a research project and IRB determinations were sought.

The scale and significance of public health surveillance demand scrupulous and ongoing attention to ethics as well as to science (64). Ethics should not be regarded as an afterthought, or worse, an obstacle, to professional practice, but as an element vital to its foundation and goals (65).

Appendix 9A
Example of a Protocol Checklist
for Surveillance

Surveillance System Overview

Summarize the main idea and identify the variables included in the surveillance system.

Abstract

Give a concise overview of the surveillance system. Describe the purpose of the system, the importance of the health problem under surveillance, the population, and the methods that will be used.

Investigators, Collaborators, and Funding Sources

Include the names and degrees of all surveillance staff and their roles in the project. Note any conflict of interest for each investigator and acknowledge all funding sources.

Introduction

Literature Review and Current State of Knowledge about the Surveillance Topic

Discuss relevant information about the surveillance activity (including quantifying data) based on a review of the literature. In the References section, attach a bibliography of the sources used.

Justification for Surveillance System

Explain the public health significance and the scientific importance of the problem under surveillance. In the context of existing surveillance systems, describe the contribution of an additional surveillance activity.

Objectives

Clearly and concisely list the objectives for the surveillance system.

Hypotheses

List the clear and focused questions that the data from the surveillance system will answer.

Surveillance Population

Description of Surveillance Population

Demographically and in terms of the specific public health condition(s) under surveillance, define the population that will be included in the system and the population to which inferences will be made. Describe the number of cases expected per reporting period and compare the number of cases during epidemic and nonepidemic periods.

Procedures and Methods

Description of How Surveillance System Design Will Meet Objectives and Address Hypotheses

Explain the appropriateness of the surveillance system design to the research project, to the objectives, and to the hypotheses previously outlined.

Complete Description of Data and Data System

Describe the sources of data, the type of data, and its representativeness. Give the case definition and explain whether the surveillance system is active or passive. Specify methods used to identify aberrations in the data.

Clinical and Laboratory Procedures

Explain any clinical and laboratory processes necessary to the surveillance system.

Catchment Area

Explain where cases will come from and whether there is more than one source for this data. If there are multiple sources, explain overlaps in collection and whether the same definitions and standards are used by each source. Explain the frequency of reporting and the length of and justification for delays in reporting. How were sentinel sites selected? Are any clearances required (federal or state)?

Quality Control and Quality Assurance Procedures

Describe the steps to ensure that the methods result in no unintended consequences that could affect the quality of the data. Those steps might include determining methods to capture all reported data exactly as received; assuring logical consistency among all parts of a record; and ensuring that manipulation of the data produces no unintended changes.

Data Entry, Editing, and Management

Describe the process for entering, editing, and managing the data collected.

Procedures for Avoiding Bias in Data Collection, Measurement, and Analysis

Describe separately the kinds of bias that may occur in collecting the data, in the measurement, and analysis phases of the research, and the steps that will be taken to avoid, minimize, or adjust these biases. Include factors in the population or in surveillance personnel that could bias results as well as the steps that will be taken to assure valid self-reporting, if applicable.

Surveillance Data Collection Methods

Describe the procedures for collecting the data. Include information related to electronic transmission and procedures for confidentiality protection.

Description, Explanation and Justification for Variables Collected and Primary Variables and Outcomes To Be Analyzed

List and briefly describe the variables to be collected and explain the primary variables/outcomes to be analyzed. If sensitive information, such as illicit drug use, is to be collected, provide a clear justification for why it is needed.

Description and Usage of Study Instruments Including Surveillance Data Forms, Laboratory Instruments, and Analytic Tests (Specificity and Sensitivity/Reproducibility/ Reactivity/Validity and Reliability/Completeness of Reporting)

Describe the surveillance study instruments and explain their use. Include a description of the quality of those instruments in terms of their known validity and reliability.

Describe How and How Often the Surveillance System Will Be Evaluated

What criteria will be used to determine that the system is functioning as intended?

Description of Training Methods for All System Personnel

Describe training (e.g., interviewer techniques, data collection and handling methods, or informed consent) provided to study personnel.

Plans for Responding to New or Unexpected Findings or to Changes in the Surveillance Environment

Describe procedures for identifying and handling new or unexpected findings.

Provisions for Identifying, Managing, and Reporting Adverse Events

Describe the types of adverse events that might be encountered and how surveillance personnel will be trained to react. Describe methods that will be used to track adverse reactions and their potential impact on the surveillance system.

Procedures for Notifying Participants of Surveillance Findings

Explain whether the participants will be offered the option of receiving surveillance study findings and the form they will take.

Limitations of Surveillance System

Explain factors that might reduce the applicability of results.

Plans for Disseminating Results
Self-explanatory.

Surveillance System Time Line—Key Activities or Milestones
Self-explanatory.

Data Analysis

Data Analysis Plan (Including Statistical Methodology)
Describe the surveillance methods, information collection procedures, methods to maximize coverage, and statistical procedures in sufficient detail that the methods are reproducible.

Records Management

Procedures for Handling Data Collection Forms, Specimens, and Computer Files Including Location of Storage Area
Describe how surveillance materials (including questionnaires, statistical analyses, unique reagents, annotated notebooks, computer programs, and other computerized information) will be maintained to allow continuous and future access for analysis and review. If non-CDC persons have been involved in the system, state who owns the data and any rights to (or limitations upon) access. Document the manner in which confidentiality will be preserved during transmission, storage, analysis, and dissemination.

Procedures for Storing and Protecting Data and Specimens from Degradation and Breeches of Confidentiality
Self-explanatory.

Final Disposition of Study Records and Specimens
Describe the manner in which surveillance materials and data (including observations not leading to publication) will be stored and what the final disposition will be. Include a statement about confidentiality and criticality and name the person/position responsible for stewardship.

Statement about Need or Lack of Need for Assurance or Certificate of Confidentiality
This refers to formal assurances and certificates of confidentiality as described in Public Health Service Act, subsection 308(d) or 301(d).

Protection of Human Participants

Description of Risks (Physical, Social, Psychological) to the Individual or Group
Discuss possible discomforts and risks, including risks to confidentiality, to participant or group, based on results of previous studies or other evidence, when

applicable. Define the nature, magnitude, probability, and duration of harm that a person may receive by participating in this surveillance activity and the steps that have been taken to minimize risks. Describe alternative procedures or treatments that might be advantageous to the participant.

Description of Potential Benefits to the Research Participant or Others

Discuss benefits to participants, to the group with which they are identified, or to society. Describe the steps that have been or will be taken to maximize benefits.

Procedures for Implementing and Documenting Informed Consent

Describe procedures for informing participants and methods to document consent. If informed consent will not be obtained, describe the justification for waiver.

Provisions for Protecting Privacy and Confidentiality

Explain provisions for protecting participants from being identified either directly or indirectly. If for any reason data identifying subjects will be published or released to persons outside of the project, explain why this is necessary.

Justification for Collecting Personal Identifiers

Explain why personal identifiers are needed, if applicable.

References

Appendix Materials

Include all relevant supplementary materials. All materials for use by participants must be written in lay language.

> Surveillance Data Collection Forms
> Medical Records and Other Abstraction Forms
> Request and Authorization for Release of Medical Records
> All Manuals for Training Surveillance System Personnel
> All Consent Forms
> Other IRB Approvals

If this surveillance study involves other institutions, and/or will be conducted in a country other than the United States, include IRB approvals from the participating institutions and/or countries as well as evidence of approval by the awarding organization.

RECOMMENDED READING

Beaglehole R, Bonita R. Public health at the crossroads: achievements and prospects. New York: Cambridge University Press, 1997.

Bond GG. Ethical issues relating to the conduct and interpretation of epidemiologic research in private industry. *J Clin Epidemiol* 1991;44(suppl 1):29S–34S.

Booker MJ. Compliance, coercion, and compassion: moral dimension of the return of tuberculosis. *J Medical Humanities* 1996;17:91–102.

Brandt AM, Rozin P (eds.). Morality and health. New York: Routledge, 1997.

Callahan D. Public health and personal responsibility. In: False hopes: why America's quest for perfect health is a recipe for disaster. New York: Simon & Schuster, 1998.

Calman KC. Ethical issues in public health. Leeds, England: Nuffield Institute for Health, University of Leeds, 1993.

Cassel J. Ethical principles for conducting fieldwork. *Am Anthropologist* 1980;82:28–41.

Cole P. The epidemiologist as an expert witness. *J. Clin Epidemiol* 1991;44(Suppl 1): 35S–9S.

Coughlin SS. Ethics in epidemiology and clinical research: annotated readings. Chestnut Hill, Massachusetts: Epidemiology Resources, 1995.

Coughlin SS. Ethics in epidemiology and public health practice: collected works. Columbus, Georgia: Quill Publications, 1997.

Coughlin SS, Soskolne CL, Goodman KW. Case studies in public health ethics. Washington, DC: American Public Health Association, 1997.

Faden RR, Kass NE (eds.). HIV/AIDS and childbearing: public policy, private lives. New York: Oxford University Press, 1996.

Faden, RR, Kass NE. Bioethics and public health in the 1980s: resource allocation and AIDS. *Annual Review in Public Health* 1991;12:335–60.

Feinleib M. The epidemiologist's responsibilities to study participants. *J Clin Epidemiol* 1991;44(suppl 1):73S–9S.

Fletcher J. Morals and medicine. Boston: Beacon Press, 1960.

Gostin LO. The resurgent tuberculosis epidemic in the era of AIDS: reflections on public health, law, and society. *Maryland Law Review* 1995;54:1–131.

Henig RM. The people's health: a memoir of public health and its evolution at Harvard. Washington, DC: Joseph Henry Press, 1997.

Lake LT. A partnership for public health. *Minnesota Medicine* 1997;80:20–4.

Lappe M. Ethics and public health. In: Maxcy-Rosenau public health and preventive medicine. Twelfth edition. Norwalk, Connecticut: Appleton-Century-Crofts, 1986:1867–77.

Last JM. Obligations and responsibilities of epidemiologists to research subjects. *J Clin Epidemiol* 1991;44(suppl 1):95S–101S.

Leeman E. Misuse of psychiatric epidemiology. *Lancet* 1998;351(9116):1601–2.

Lupton D. The imperative of health: public health and the regulated body. London: Sage Publications, 1995.

Morone JA. Enemies of the people: the moral dimension to public health. *J Health Politics, Policy and Law* 1997;22:993–1020.

Nikku N, Eriksson BE. Preventive medicine. In: Chadwick R (ed.). Encyclopedia of applied ethics. Volume 3. San Diego, California: Academic Press, 1998:643–8.

Porter D (ed.). The history of public health and the modern state. Amsterdam: Rodopi BV, 1994.

Rothman KJ. The ethics of research sponsorship. *J Clin Epidemiol* 1991;44(suppl 1):25S–8S.

Soskolne CL. Ethical decision-making in epidemiology: the case study approach. *J Clin Epidemiol* 1991;44(suppl 1):125S–30S.

Taylor CE. Ethical issues influencing health for all beyond the year 2000. *Infectious Disease Clinics of North America* 1995;9:223–33.

US Preventive Services Task Force. Guide to clinical preventive services: an assessment of the effectiveness of 169 interventions. Baltimore: Williams & Wilkins, 1989.

Weed DL. Preventing scientific misconduct. *Am J Public Health* 1998;88:125–9.

Wikler D. Bioethics and social responsibility. *Bioethics* 1997:11:185–92.

REFERENCES

1. Coughlin SS, Beauchamp TL. Ethics and epidemiology. New York: Oxford University Press, 1996.
2. Epstein A. Impure science: AIDS, activism, and the politics of knowledge. Berkeley: University of California Press, 1996.
3. Cairns J. Matters of life and death: perspectives on public health, molecular biology, cancer, and the prospects for the human race. Princeton, N.J.: Princeton University Press, 1997.
4. Cunningham GC. A public health perspective on the control of predictive screening for breast cancer. *Health Matrix: Journal of Law-Medicine* 1997;7:31–48.
5. Holtzman NA. Editorial: genetic screening and public health. *Am J Pub Health* 1997;87:1275–7.
6. Little M. Assignments of meaning in epidemiology. *Soc Sci Med* 1998;47:1135–45.
7. McCormick J. Medical hubris and the public health: the ethical dimension. *J Clin Epidemiol* 1996;49:619–21.
8. Last J. Professional standard of conduct for epidemiologists in ethics and epidemiology. Coughlin SS, Beauchamp TL (eds.). New York: Oxford University Press, 1996.
9. Office for Protection from Research Risks, National Institutes of Health. Protection of human subjects. Washington, D.C.: U.S. Department of Health and Human Services, National Institutes of Health, 1991. (Code of Federal Regulations Title 45, part 46) (Revised June 18, 1991).
10. National Commission for the Protection of Human Subjects of Biomedical and Behavioral Research. The Belmont report: ethical principles and guidelines for the protection of human subjects of research. Publication no. (05)78-0012. Washington, D.C.: U.S. Department of Health, Education, and Welfare, 1978.
11. Frazier EL, Okoro CA, Smith C, McQueen DV. State- and sex-specific prevalence of selected characteristics—Behavioral Risk Factor Surveillance System, 1992 and 1993. In: CDC Surveillance Summaries (December 1996). *MMWR* 1996;45(SS-6); 1–34.
12. Krieger N, Birn AE. A vision of social justice as the foundation of public health: commemorating 150 years of the spirit of 1848. *Am J Public Health* 1988;88:1603–6.
13. Last JM. A dictionary of epidemiology. Second edition. New York: Oxford University Press, 1988.
14. Beauchamp DE. Public health as social justice. *Inquiry* 1976;13:3014.
15. Beauchamp TL, Childress JF. Principles of biomedical ethics. Third edition. New York: Oxford University Press, 1989.
16. Bruntland GH. Reaching out for world health. *Science* 1998;280:2027.
17. Mann JM. Medicine and public health, ethics and human rights. *Hastings Center Report* 1997;6–13.
18. Kalman KC, Downie RS. Ethical principles and ethical issues in public health. In: Oxford textbook of public health. Detels R, Holland WW, McEwen J, Omenn GS (eds.). New York: Oxford University Press, 1997.
19. Mill JS. Utilitarianism. In: Collected works of John Stuart Mill. Volume 10. Toronto: University of Toronto Press, 1969.
20. Weed DL, McKeown RE. Epidemiology and virtue ethics. *Intl J Epidemiol* 1998;27: 343–9.
21. Warren SD, Brandeis LD. The right to privacy. *Harvard Law Review* 1890;4:193–220.
22. Lomas J. Social capital and health: implications for public health and epidemiology. *Social Science and Medicine* 1998;47:1181–8.

23. Mooney G. "Communitarian claims" as an ethical basis for allocating health-care resources. *Soc Sci Med* 1998;47:1171–80.
24. Maciak BJ, Moore MT, Leviton LC, Guinan ME. Preventing Halloween arson in an urban setting: a model for multisectoral planning and community participation. *Health Educ Behav* 1998;25:194–211.
25. Parker EA, Schulz AJ, Israel BA, Hollis R. Eastside village health worker partnership: community-based health advisor intervention in an urban area. *Health Educ Behav* 1998;25:24–45.
26. Levine RJ. The institutional review board. In: Ethics and epidemiology. New York: Oxford University Press, 1996:257–73.
27. Roush S, Birkhead G, Koo D, Cobb A, Fleming D. Mandatory reporting of diseases and health conditions by health-care professionals and laboratories. *JAMA* 1999;282:164–70.
28. Council for International Organizations of Medical Sciences. International guidelines for ethical review of epidemiological studies. Geneva: CIOMS, 1991.
29. Soskolne CL. Light A. Towards guidelines for environmental epidemiologists. *Science of the Total Environment* 1996;184:137–47.
30. The Chemical Manufacturers Association's Epidemiology Task Group. Guidelines for good epidemiology practices for occupational and environmental epidemiologic research. *J Occup Med* 1991;33:1221–9.
31. International Epidemiological Association. Guidelines on ethics for epidemiologists. American Public Health Association, Epidemiology Section Newsletter, Winter 1990.
32. American Statistical Association. Ethical guidelines for statistical practice. (Available at http://www.tcnj.edu/Çasaethic/asagui.html.)
33. Stolley PD. Ethical issues involving conflicts of interest for epidemiologic investigators. A report of the Committee on Ethical Guidelines of the Society for Epidemiologic Research. *J Clin Epidemiol* 1991;44(Suppl 1).
34. Charlton BG. Public health medicine—a different kind of ethics? *Journal of the Royal Society of Medicine* 1993;86:194–5.
35. Plant AJ, Roshworth RL. Death by proxy: ethics and classification. *Soc Sci Med* 1998;47:1147–53.
36. Spencer BD (ed.). Statistics and public policy. Oxford: Clarendon Press, 1997.
37. Seltzer W. Population statistics, the Holocaust, and the Nuremberg Trials. *Pop Dev Rev* 1998;24:511–52.
38. Greenawalt K. Privacy. In: Reich WT (ed.). Encyclopedia of bioethics. New York: Free Press: 1356–63.
39. Federal Committee on Statistical Methodology. Report on statistical disclosure limitation methodology. SPWP 22: (available at: http://www.bts.gov/fcsm/methodology).
40. Hogue CJR. Ethical issues in sharing epidemiologic data. *J Clin Epidemiol* 1991;44 (Suppl 1):103S–7S.
41. Jabine TB. Procedures for restricted data access. *J Official Statistics* 1993;9:537–89.
42. National Center for Health Statistics. NCHS staff manual on confidentiality. Hyattsville, Md.: Centers for Disease Control and Prevention, 1997.
43. Cohn V. News and numbers: a guide to reporting statistical claims and controversies in health and other fields. Des Moines: Iowa State University Press, 1989.
44. Teutsch S, Berkelman RL, Toomey KE, Vogt RL. Reporting for disease control activities. *Am J Public Health* 1991;81:932.
45. Vernon TM. Confidential reporting by physicians. *Am J Public Health* 1991;81:931–2.
46. Osterholm MT, Birkhead GS, Meriwether RA. Impediments to public health surveillance in the 1990s: the lack of resources and the need for priorities. *J Public Health Management Practice* 1996;2:11–5.

47. Cole P. The moral bases for public health interventions. *Epidemiology* 1995;6:78–93.
48. Lako CJ. Privacy protection and population-based health research. *Soc Sci Med* 1986;23:293–5.
49. Public Health Service Act (as amended). Washington, D.C.: U.S. Government Printing Office, 1944.
50. The Privacy Act. Washington, D.C.: U.S. Government Printing Office, 1974.
51. Grad FP. Public health and the law. Philosophy of the law of public health. In: Reich WT (ed.). Encyclopedia of bioethics. Revised edition. New York: Simon & Schuster Macmillan, 1995;2173–8.
52. Vogt RL. Confidentiality: perspectives from a state epidemiologist. In: Challenge for public health statistics in the 1990s. Proceedings of the 1989 Public Health Conference on Records and Statistics. National Center for Health Statistics, July 17–19, Washington, D.C.
53. Gostin LO, Lazzarini Z, Neslund V, Osterholm, M. The public health information infrastructure: a national review of the law on health information privacy. *JAMA* 1996;275:1921–7.
54. Koo D, Wetterhall SF. History and current status of the National Notifiable Diseases Surveillance System. *J Public Health Management and Practice* 1996;2:4–10.
55. US Department of Justice. Available at http://www.usdoj.gov/04foia/referenceguidedec98.htm.
56. Beauchamp DE. Legal moralism and public health: public health and the law. In: Reich WT (ed.). Encyclopedia of bioethics. Revised edition. New York: Simon & Schuster; Macmillan, 1995:2178–81.
57. Centers for Disease Control. Pneumocystis pneumonia—Los Angeles. *MMWR* 1981; 30:250–2.
58. Altman D. AIDS in the mind of America. Garden City, N.Y.: Doubleday, 1986.
59. Centers for Disease Control. Opportunistic infections and Kaposi's sarcoma among Haitians in the United States. *MMWR* 1982;31:353–61.
60. Cohen CJ, Iwane MK, Palensky JB, Levin DL, Meagher KJ, Frost KR, Mayer KH. A national HIV community cohort: design, baseline, and follow-up of the AmFAR observational data base. *J Clin Epid* 1998;51:779–93.
61. Centers for Disease Control and Prevention. Current trends: trends in AIDS diagnosis and reporting under the expanded surveillance definition for adolescents and adults—United States, 1993. *MMWR* 1994;43:826–31.
62. Heyward WL, Curran JW. The epidemiology of AIDS in the U.S. *Scientific American* 1988;259:72–81.
63. Centers for Disease Control and Prevention. Deaths resulting from residential fires and the prevalence of smoke alarms—United States, 1991–1995. *MMWR* 1998;47 (38):803–6.
64. Beauchamp DE. Philosophy of public health. Volume 3. Reich WT (ed.). Encyclopedia of bioethics. Revised edition. New York: Simon & Schuster; Macmillan, 1995.
65. Beauchamp TL, Cook RR, Fayerweather WE et al. Ethical guidelines for epidemiologists. *J Clin Epidemiol* 1991;44(Suppl 1):151S–69S.

10

Public Health Surveillance
and the Law

GENE W. MATTHEWS
VERLA S. NESLUND
R. ELLIOTT CHURCHILL

The people's good is the highest law.
        Marcus Tullius Cicero

Public health surveillance and the law are joined by so many interconnecting links that virtually every aspect of a surveillance program is associated with one or more legal issues (for a more detailed discussion of law-related surveillance issues, see Chapter 4). In the United States, and throughout the world, many surveillance efforts have been effected through mandates enforced by statutes or regulations. By the same token, reports derived from the interpretation and application of data from surveillance programs have been used to drive legislation relating to public health.

It may be useful to have a working definition of the law to meld with the definition of surveillance. In essence, as Wing observes, the law is "the sum or set or conglomerate of all of the laws in all of the jurisdictions: the constitutions, the statutes and the regulations that interpret them, the traditional principles known as common law, and the judicial opinions that apply and interpret all these legal rules and principles" (*1*).

However, that is by no means all. The law is also the legal profession, and, in order to understand the law, we must try to understand the lawyers—how they think, how they speak, and what roles they play in the legal process. In addition, from a very practical point of view, the law is also the legal process—legislatures and their politics, as well as the time, efforts, and costs associated with changes in legislation. Finally, the law is what it is interpreted to be. This takes us back to the lawyers, as well as to the judges in the legal system.

We cannot avoid what Wing describes as "the traditional barrier" between the legal profession and the rest of the world. He continues with the observation that "the legal profession has for centuries done many things to surround the practice of law with a quasi-mystical aura. Much as the medical profession would have us believe that there is something almost sacred about medical judgment and that only a physician can understand it, lawyers have perpetuated the only partially justified myth that there is something called legal judgment that only someone with the proper mix of formal education, practical experience, and appropriate vocabulary can make" (1).

"The basic function of the law is to establish legal rights, and the basic purpose of the legal system is to define and enforce those rights. . . . Legal rights [are the] relationships that establish privileges and responsibilities among those governed by the legal system" (1). This concept of "legal rights" does not purport to cover freedoms or interests given unconditional, global protection, but rather it covers the protection of carefully specified interests against the effects of other carefully specified interests. Finally, some rights are protected, not by statute or regulation, but by an understanding and application of the prevailing ethics in an area. In general, ethics are regulated through whatever sanctions are imposed against censured behavior by peers or colleagues (see also Chapter 9).

This orientation is pivotal in our discussion of legal issues associated with surveillance because the reader must continue to be alert to the fact that everything in this chapter is subject, first of all, to different interpretations in different legal settings, and, second, to amendment of both statute and practice.

The task of surveillance as an applied science could be simplified considerably by avoiding any discussion of legal issues. Although this observation is probably valid, we have already pointed out that surveillance very often takes place under statute. Beyond this fact, the relevance of the definition of the police powers of a state must be acknowledged, i.e., "powers inherent in the state to prescribe, within the limits of state and federal constitutions, reasonable laws necessary to preserve the public order, health, safety, welfare, and morals" (2). That describes a sweeping scope of authority and certainly covers anything that would be dealt with under the heading of "public health surveillance."

In other words, one cannot look at surveillance and claim to have created an accurate picture without considering the legal constraints and processes that accompany it—particularly since, for public health surveillance, we have added the component of "timely dissemination of the findings" to our definition of surveillance. How information is collected, from and about whom it is collected, how it is interpreted, and how and to whom the results are disseminated all must be scrutinized under the umbrella of "accepted practice" and "the law." The sections that follow contain information specific to the United States, but for an international orientation, the issues and concerns remain basically constant, while the written body of the law and the process through which the law is enacted and enforced vary widely.

If the reporting component of public health surveillance is treated as a requirement, one can assert that such surveillance began in the United States in 1874 in Massachusetts, when the State Board of Health instituted the first statewide voluntary plan for weekly reporting of prevalent diseases by physicians. By the turn of the century, the forerunner of the Public Health Service (PHS) had been established, and laws in all states required that certain communicable diseases be reported to local authorities (3).

SURVEILLANCE AND LEGAL ISSUES
IN THE EARLY YEARS (1900–1930)

With the development and growth of surveillance in the United States in the early 1900s came the inevitable disagreements created when the interests of one human being conflict with those of another individual or political unit. Much of the debate took place because of the problem the United States was experiencing with sexually transmitted diseases—which became even more acute with the participation of American troops in World War I. The major issues were

- the moral dilemma created by not reaching consensus on the purpose of information obtained through surveillance (i.e., whether to direct control efforts toward sexual behavior of the individual or toward the disease agents),
- the debate surrounding the duty of the physician to his/her patient and to society, and
- the disagreement about whether government provision of health services comprised unfair competition to the private practitioner.

Since these concerns still have not been completely resolved in the United States today, we examine them in more detail in the sections that follow.

Social Hygiene versus the Scientific Approach

By the early 1900s, the epidemiology of syphilis was reasonably well-documented. This understanding was not an unmixed blessing. As William Osler told his students at the Johns Hopkins Medical School in 1909, "In one direction our knowledge was widened greatly. It added terror to an already terrible disorder" (4). Aside from the scope of the destructive powers of syphilis, physicians were just beginning to appreciate the fact that many "innocent victims" were contracting this disease. The prevailing wisdom of earlier years of "reaping what one sowed," as well as other statements of poetic and moral justice, was no longer adequate when women of "good family and unblemished reputation" were known to have contracted syphilis from their spouses, and when children suffered severe effects from congenital syphilis.

What medical and public health officials apparently had the most difficulty reconciling was how to direct their efforts to deal with the growing problem of syphilis. Both surveillance and treatment efforts could be directed toward a) people, a focus on behavior modification through education as a control strategy or b) the disease vector, a focus on the organism that caused the disease and how to eradicate it from individuals and society at large. Neither approach to syphilis control was ever agreed to be the ideal, and, in fact, the two in combination have still not proved totally effective. The tensions represented by the "moralistic" and the "scientific" approaches are, moreover, still quite evident in public health practice and surveillance in the 1990s.

One only has to review the popular press for the past several years to see how the moral versus scientific dilemma relates to public health in the context of such currently serious problems as HIV/AIDS and the re-emergence of multi-drug-resistant strains of tuberculosis.

Duty of Physicians

The concept of the confidential nature of communication between patient and physician is clearly stated in the Hippocratic oath and has continued to be emphasized in legal and social settings. In the context of the syphilis epidemic in the United States in the early years of the 20th century, this concept became a crucial point of debate in efforts to control the spread of the disease. Physicians did not wish to breach the confidence relied on by their patients by reporting cases of syphilis to the authorities; by the same token, if they did not report the occurrence of syphilis—if not to the authorities at least to the patients' spouses—they were tacitly participating in the continued transmission of the disease to "innocent victims." The entire issue boils down to whether a physician's primary responsibility is to an individual or to society. Although this issue clearly has not been resolved, it constitutes an important component of the success or failure of present-day surveillance efforts.

Economic Competition

Also still unresolved is the problem created for public health officials and for practicing physicians in the early 1900s by, on the one hand, the need for physicians to report all cases of sexually transmitted disease and to establish public health clinics to provide prompt treatment and education to patients and, on the other hand, the need for public health officials to protect the financial interests of physicians by not infringing on their turf and removing paying customers to free or financially subsidized facilities. At the same time, it did not seem reasonable to expect the physicians to make such reports and refer such patients for treatment elsewhere when it would mean, in essence, taking money out of their own pockets. For surveillance efforts, this dilemma guaranteed under-reporting of cases, with the selective reporting of cases representing patients who could not pay, and the withholding of reports of cases representing patients who could pay.

Early in the HIV/AIDS epidemic, physicians may have chosen not to report cases of HIV positivity for fear their patients might be discriminated against in a work or social setting. Problems with insurance during those early years may also have to to such under-reporting.

ERA OF GRADUAL GROWTH IN MANDATED SURVEILLANCE (1940S–1970S)

From the 1940s through the 1970s, states added many diseases to their mandatory reporting lists. Even in states that did not enact legislation to require additional reporting, surveillance and reporting efforts were broadened during this period through state regulation or directive from the state health commissioners (5).

In contrast, surveillance and reporting to agencies in the federal government were—and continue to be—voluntary. The resulting discrepancy in data obtained on a particular disease at the state and federal levels leads to problems in analysis and interpretation. However, several professional organizations including the Association of State and Territorial Health Officers (ASTHO) and the Council of State and Territorial Epidemiologists (CSTE) have been instrumental in setting up a patchwork system to coordinate and improve the quality and completeness of surveillance data.

In 1976 the Federal Protection for Human Subjects Regulations were instituted. One of the most well-known of the regulations states the requirement that "informed consent" be obtained from any person who is asked to participate in a medical research project. In addition, the regulation covers compensation for persons injured during the course of a project and confirmation of the ethics of the research being conducted.

LEGAL ISSUES RELATING TO SURVEILLANCE (1980–1994)

There is little dispute that biomedical research and surveillance activities of the 1980s were greatly affected by concerns and reactions associated with the HIV/AIDS epidemic. All the old issues from early in the 20th century reemerged at critical levels: Do we want to treat persons for the disease, or do we want to modify their behavior in control and prevention efforts? Is the physician's primary duty to protecting a patient's privacy or to the greater good of society? Is the public health machine treading on the physician's turf by advertising and providing medical treatment more inexpensively than the physician can?

Although these questions still need to be answered fully, public health action cannot wait until consensus is reached before constructing and applying interventions. The sections below examine four key legal issues that relate to these questions and have a major impact on surveillance today.

Personal Privacy

The right of an individual to have his/her privacy protected under the law is a vast gray area. The U.S. Constitution does not specify a right to privacy, although particulars relating to the protection of privacy under particular circumstances are included in the Bill of Rights (e.g., protection from "search and seizure"). As noted earlier in this chapter, the issue of right to privacy and the physician's role in protecting that privacy through the concept of privileged communication emerged as a hotly debated issue during the war on sexually transmitted diseases in the United States in the early years of the 20th century. The concept of the so-called *medical secret* (6) involved the dilemma that faced a physician whose male patient had a sexually transmitted disease (for which there was no sure cure), whose reputation the physician wished to spare, but whose spouse or future spouse was at risk of having the disease if the physician did not step forward and report it. Many physicians opted to remain within the accepted double standard of behavior of the day and, according to Prince Morrow, became "accomplices" in the further transmission of infection (7). The medical secret was described by one physician as a "blind policy of protecting the guilty at the expense of the innocent," and a New York attorney ventured the opinion that "a physician who knows that an infected patient is about to carry his contagion to a pure person, and perhaps to persons unborn, is justified both in law and in morals, in preventing the proposed wrong by disclosing his knowledge if no other way is open" (7).

Unfortunately, the right-to-privacy issue was no more resolved in the early-20th-century United States than was the public health problem created by the nation-wide problem of sexually transmitted diseases. Public health officials continue to struggle with questions associated with privacy and the rights of the individual versus the good of society to this day.

The landmark case relating to the right of an individual to privacy was *Griswold v. Connecticut,* 381 U.S. 479 (1965), which resulted from the arrest of the director of the Planned Parenthood League of Connecticut (Griswold) on the grounds that she had provided information, instruction, and medical advice about contraception to married people. In Connecticut at the time, the law stated that the use of contraceptives was punishable by law. Subsequently, the U.S. Supreme Court declared the Connecticut law to be unconstitutional and reversed the criminal convictions in the case. In the majority opinion written for the Court by Justice William Douglas, there are references to the so-called *penumbras* or auras of privacy that radiate out from the specific rights to privacy stated in the Bill of Rights. He observed that "various guarantees create zones of privacy" (8). He went on to say that the Connecticut law exceeded its bounds by seeking to regulate the *use* of contraceptive devices rather than their manufacture and/or sale. The only means he could postulate for enforcing the law as written involved the invasion of the clearly defined zone of privacy represented by marriage. Lest anyone misunderstand his meaning, he observed: "Would we allow the police to search the sacred precincts of marital bedrooms for tell-tale signs of the use of contraceptives? The very idea is repulsive to the notions of privacy surrounding the marriage relationship" (8).

Later courts would refer to this constitutionally recognized right of the individual to privacy in certain contexts as a "fundamental interest." In the precedent-setting abortion case of *Roe v. Wade,* 410 U.S. 113 (1973), a single woman challenged the constitutionality of a Texas law forbidding abortion (except when the pregnant woman's life was in jeopardy). She claimed that this law denied her constitutional right to privacy and cited the earlier opinions of the Supreme Court relating to birth control. Justice Blackmun observed that "the state does have an important and legitimate interest in preserving and protecting the health of the pregnant woman . . . [and] it has still another important and legitimate interest in protecting the potentiality of human life. These interests are separate and distinct. Each grows in substantiality as the woman approaches term and, at a point during pregnancy, each becomes 'compelling' " (9).

The link between the right to privacy and surveillance is also related to the Freedom of Information Act (amended 1986). In essence, the act spells out the situations and conditions pertaining to the right of the U.S. taxpayer to obtain information s/he has paid for from agencies within the federal government. Clearly, there is the potential for conflicting interests in such situations, if information about taxpayer *A* is released to taxpayer *B*. The Act takes this point into consideration in its statement that "to the extent required to prevent a clearly unwarranted invasion of personal privacy, an agency may delete identifying details when it makes available or publishes an opinion, statement of policy, interpretation, or staff manual or instruction" (*10*).

An essential aspect in designing a surveillance program is the assurance to the persons (agencies) who report and those being reported upon that the privacy rights of the persons whose health information is of interest will not be violated. Virtually all states have statutes or regulations that provide some level of privacy protection for individual medical records and for heath-related data maintained by the government (*11*). The conflict created by the "right to privacy" versus the "need to know" represents an area that must be monitored by the managers of a surveillance program as diligently as they monitor the health conditions to be reported. To illustrate: One of the most important court decisions the CDC has obtained in recent years related to litigation arising out of the epidemic of toxic-shock syndrome of the late 1970s and early 1980s. The attorneys representing the manufacturer of the tampon that had been strongly statistically associated with the occurrence of toxic-shock syndrome wanted to obtain not only data about women who had toxic-shock syndrome and from whom CDC had collected information, but the names of the women as well. The agency argued (through district court and up to the Federal Court of Appeals) that participation in federal surveillance is voluntary and that participants in such programs have a reasonable expectation that their confidentiality will be protected by the federal government. The Appeals Court ruled in CDC's favor, but this position will continue to be challenged on a need-to-know basis, and persons who are designing and operating surveillance systems should always keep in mind the specter of the forced divulgence of information they have assured participants would be confidential. This is particularly likely in situations involving litigation, because of the courts' strong bias to make available the same information to legal representatives for both plaintiffs and defendants.

The final observation in this section is that the manager of a surveillance program, at least within a federal agency, is always in danger of being accused by the popular media or the legal community of hiding something deliberately—not to protect the privacy of individuals—but for sinister reasons that are usually hinted at but not stated. This sort of accusation may have no basis in fact, but it must be taken seriously and generally requires, at a minimum, an undesirable outlay of energy and worry on the part of the surveillance program manager.

Right of Access

If the taxpayers support the gathering of information, they have a right to that information (*12*). This statement forms one basis for the right-to-access position. Both the Privacy Act and the Freedom of Information Act reflect the post-

Watergate era, with its focused concern on the potential for the government to keep secret files containing information on individuals. Beyond that is the "reasonable-man" position, which maintains that a person has a right to any information that is about him or her. Unfortunately, giving information to an individual about himself or herself can sometimes have the effect of providing information that assigns liability to another person (or organization) in the data set. So even the process of providing personal information to the person in question is not without its hazards.

In addition to the individuals who wish to obtain information about themselves, there are the so-called third-party inquirers. These individuals call for information on a need-to-know basis and may range from members of the U.S. Congress through attorneys and special-interest groups (e.g., "right-to-life" or "pro-choice" groups) to representatives of the news media.

A major point for the surveillance program manager to ponder is when to make a public-use data set. Once the first paper has been published about a data set, it is probably prudent to place that data set in the public domain if there is a reasonable expectation that is will be used in the future. Although this creates the risk of extra work and having others preempt publication, it obviates accusations about willful withholding of information, or the danger that forced release of data before they are properly prepared for public use will allow some subjects to be identified.

Product Liability

This heading could be "Research Institution Discovers Corporate America—and Vice Versa." The issue has been around for many years but rose to prominence in the United States with the emergence of toxic-shock syndrome in the late 1970s and early 1980s. It is not unusual for investigations to show that a product is contaminated, that someone used a machine incorrectly, or even that someone deliberately tampered with a medication or device and caused illness or death. What was not familiar was that a "good" product—one that met all its quality-control specifications and did what it was advertised to do—could also cause harm. Thus, no one was ready to deal with the situation in which an efficiently designed tampon apparently led to a life-threatening illness. The scientists had to accept the findings because scientists deal in fact (probability), and the media had grist for their mills, but the manufacturer of the tampon (and its employees, stockholders, and legal representatives) did not have an easy time coping with "the facts." In fact, they underwent a classic grief reaction—which the staff at CDC and other health science agencies have since learned to anticipate and to recognize—involving the stages of denial, anger, depression, acceptance, and resolution. Human nature was applied with a vengeance, and the first three stages were immediate, intense, and enduring. The last two stages took some time and extensive effort to induce.

Ideally, one should assure that surveillance programs are flawless and that all the information reported is unassailable. In the world of public health practice, such utopian standards can rarely be met. And public health practitioners must continue to be prepared to deal with issues on a mixture of levels—including public health, legal, ethical, socio-cultural, and emotional components.

Litigation Demands

Under litigation demands, the issue is to what extent an agency is responsible for providing its staff to testify in litigation relating to findings it obtained through surveillance or research. Of course, there is no simple answer, just as there have not been any simple answers to the other questions posed in this chapter. Clearly, it is not responsible to refuse to provide expert testimony in any instance in which it is solicited. In some cases, agency scientists may be the only ones who have worked in the area in question and have facts to cite. By the same token, in situations in which there are massive numbers of suits being conducted over a period of several years (as with toxic-shock syndrome or transfusion-associated HIV infection), all of the scientific resources of an agency could be expended on time in court and, therefore, none of them on the science that is their primary business. Somewhere, there is a correct answer for each agency and each health issue, and this problem may need to be faced when planning surveillance activities.

CURRENT ISSUES THAT LINK SURVEILLANCE AND THE LAW (1995–PRESENT)

Department of Health and Human Services Privacy Regulations

Congress recognized the need for minimum national health-care privacy standards to protect against inappropriate use of individually identifiable health information by passing the Health Insurance Portability and Accountability Act of 1996 (HIPAA), Public Law 104–191, which called for the enactment of a privacy statute within three years of the date of enactment on August 26, 1996. In the law, Congress addressed the opportunities and challenges presented by the health-care industry's increasing use of and reliance on electronic technology. Sections 261 through 264 of HIPAA are known as the Administrative Simplification Provisions. Pursuant to various parts of these sections, the Department of Health and Human Services (DHHS) has already published proposed standards concerning electronic exchange of information regarding financial and administrative transactions and security of electronic information. (See 63 Fed. Reg. 43242 [August 12, 1998]; 63 Fed. Reg. 32784 [June 16, 1998]; and 63 Fed. Reg. 25272 [May 7, 1998]).

In addition, Section 264 of HIPAA called for the Secretary of Health and Human Services to develop and send to Congress recommendations for protecting the confidentiality of health-care information. On September 11, 1997, the Secretary presented to Congress her recommendations for protecting the "Confidentiality of Individually Identifiable Health Information." In those recommendations, the Secretary called for new federal legislation to create a national floor of standards that provide fundamental privacy rights for patients, and that define responsibilities for those who obtain identifiable health information. These recommendations are available on the DHHS Web site at http://aspec.os.dhhs.gov/admnsimp/pvcrec.htm.

Within the provisions of HIPAA, the U.S. Congress further recognized the importance of such standards by providing the Secretary of Health and Human Services with authority to promulgate health-privacy regulations if Congress did not enact a privacy statute before August 21, 1999. In the fall of 1999, after extensive consultations with other federal agencies, professional associations, and representatives of state and national organizations, the Secretary of Health and Human Services published draft health privacy regulations in the *Federal Register* that included many of the Secretary's 1997 recommendations (*Federal Register* 59918-60065 [November 3, 1999]. See also Web site *http://aspe.hhs.gov/admnsimp*). To the extent permitted under the HIPAA legislative authority, this draft regulation, which is scheduled to be finalized sometime in 2000, is an elaboration of the Secretary's recommendations. It includes new restrictions on the use and disclosure of health information, the establishment of new consumer rights, penalties for misuse of information, and redress for those harmed by misuse of the information.

Model State Public Health Privacy Act

In 1998, CDC, in collaboration with CSTE, provided funding for Georgetown University Law Center to draft a model state public health privacy act. The purpose of the model privacy act project was to develop a model state law that addresses privacy and security issues that arise from the acquisition, use, disclosure, and storage of identifiable health information by public health agencies at the state and local levels. Although the model law project was initiated at the time CDC announced that it would begin comprehensive surveillance for HIV, the model act was intended to protect all health-related information.

Lawrence O. Gostin, Professor of Law at Georgetown University Law Center, served as the principal investigator and drafter of the model law. In 1998 and 1999, Gostin convened two meetings of consultants who represented public health organizations, professional associations, state legislatures, federal government agencies, advocacy groups, and the legal profession in order to review and edit the model act. The model act was finalized in August 1999 and was posted on a special Web site sponsored by Georgetown. The model act includes regulation of the acquisition, use, disclosure, and storage of identifiable health-related information by public health agencies without substantially limiting the ability of agencies to use such information for legitimate public health purposes.

The Model State Public Health Privacy Act is divided into eight articles, summarized as follows:

ARTICLE I, FINDINGS AND DEFINITIONS, sets forth legislative findings and purposes, as well as key definitions in the context of the act, including *a*) what it means to *acquire, use, disclose,* and *store* information; *b) protected health information*—to include only identifiable information regarding an individual's health status; and *c) legitimate public health purposes*—referring to those

population-based activities or individual efforts primarily aimed at the prevention of injury, disease, or premature mortality, or the promotion of health in the
community. Other key terms frequently mentioned in the Act are also defined,
including *non-identifiable health information, public health agency,* and *public
health official.*

These and other definitions underlie the scope of the Act. Specifically, the Act
protects the privacy and security of identifiable health-related information about
individuals through various measures concerning the acquisition, use, disclosure,
and storage of such information by public health agencies or public health officials. Critical to these objectives is the definition of *protected health information.* For the purposes of the Act, this term means any information, whether oral,
written, electronic, visual, pictorial, physical, or any other form, that relates to
an individual's past, present, or future physical or mental health status, condition, treatment, service, products purchased, or provision of care, and that *a)* reveals the identity of the individual whose health care is the subject of the information, or *b)* where there is a reasonable basis to believe such information could
be utilized (either alone or with other information that is, or should reasonably
be known to be, available to predictable recipients of such information) to reveal
the identity of that individual. Since non-identifiable health information does not
implicate serious privacy and antidiscrimination concerns at the individual level,
information which cannot freely be identified or linked with the identity of any
individual is not subject to the Act's provisions.

ARTICLE II, ACQUISITION OF PROTECTED HEALTH INFORMATION, sets forth fundamental requirements concerning the acquisition of protected health information
by public health agencies. Sections within Article II: *a)* restrict the acquisition
of protected health information to that information which is directly related to
achieve a legitimate public health purposes; *b)* prohibit the secretive acquisition
of protected health information; *c)* require public notice and comment accomplished in a confidential manner, prior to acquiring protected health information;
and *d)* require that public health agencies meet the same requirements for acquisitions of existing protected health information between agencies.

ARTICLE III, USES OF PROTECTED HEALTH INFORMATION addresses the uses of protected health information by public health agencies. Uses of such information must
be *a)* directly related to the legitimate public health purpose for which the information was acquired; or *b)* for public health, epidemiological, medical, or health
services research provided that several requirements as stated in Section 3-101 *c)*
of the Act are met. Subsequent uses of the information are allowed provided the
agency can justify them under the standards for acquisition stated in Article II.
The Act encourages the use of non-identifiable information whenever possible
and requires the minimum amount of information to be used in the judgment of
the public health official. Commercial uses of protected health information are
prohibited. Protected health information whose use no longer furthers any legitimate public health purpose must be expunged in a confidential manner.

ARTICLE IV, DISCLOSURES OF PROTECTED HEALTH INFORMATION, generally concerns the disclosure of protected health information by public health agencies to
persons outside the agency. Protected health information is deemed non-public

information, which cannot be disclosed without the informed consent of the person who is the subject of the information (or the person's lawful representative) unless otherwise allowed via narrow exceptions stated in the Act.

The act specifically defines informed consent for the purposes of disclosures of protected health information from public health agencies. Protected health information shall be disclosed for any purpose and to any person for which the disclosure is authorized via informed consent. Unless specifically authorized via informed consent or pursuant to the Act, non-identifiable health information shall be disclosed. When protected health information must be disclosed, it shall be limited to the minimum amount of information needed in the reasonable judgment of the person making the disclosure. Any disclosure of protected health information, with or without informed consent, must be accompanied by a written statement of the public health agency's policy on disclosures.

While the Act generally prohibits disclosures without informed consent, such disclosures may be allowed for narrow exceptions including *a*) to individuals who are the subjects of the information; *b*) to appropriate federal agencies pursuant to federal or state law; *c*) to health care personnel in the event of an emergency to protect the health or life of the individual to whom the information relates; *d*) pursuant to a court order authorizing the disclosure through subpoena, compelled testimony, in a civil, criminal, administrative, or other legal proceeding; *e*) to health oversight agencies to perform oversight functions concerning the public health agency; or *f*) for the purpose of identifying a deceased individual, the deceased's manner of death, or provide necessary information about a deceased person who is a donor or prospective donor of an anatomical gift.

The dilemma of *secondary disclosures* of protected health information by persons who receive the information from public health agencies is resolved by prohibiting the subsequent disclosure of the information to other persons unless authorized by the Act. Finally, public health agencies are required to establish written records of disclosures of protected health information.

ARTICLE V, SECURITY SAFEGUARDS AND RECORD RETENTION, imposes the general duty on public health agencies to acquire, use, disclose, and store protected health information in a confidential manner. Specific security measures concerning protected health information are set forth, including a requirement that CDC security recommendations concerning HIV/AIDS information be followed. The Act proposes the appointment of a new or existing public health official as a public health information officer in each public health agency. This individual is responsible for overseeing the administration of security and privacy issues inherent in government collection and use of identifiable protected health information. This individual is also responsible for preparing and circulating reports concerning the status of protected health information privacy on at least an annual basis.

ARTICLE VI, FAIR INFORMATION PRACTICES, sets forth basic fair information practices designed to allow individuals the opportunity to inspect and copy their protected health information in the possession of public health agencies (subject to minimal limitations), as well as request that information that is erroneous, incomplete, or false be corrected, amended, or deleted. Denials of rights to inspect, copy, or revise incorrect or incomplete information by the public health agency must be in writing. Individuals may appeal such determinations.

ARTICLE VII, CRIMINAL SANCTIONS AND CIVIL REMEDIES, sets forth various criminal penalties and civil enforcement mechanisms to protect individuals who are harmed by violations of the Act by public health agencies, public health officials, and other persons. Several forms of immunity are provided. The State's Administrative Procedure Act generally applies to actions taken by public health agencies pursuant to this Act.

ARTICLE VIII, MISCELLANEOUS PROVISIONS, includes *a*) the short title of the act (the Model State Public Health Privacy Act); *b*) a uniformity-of-the-law provision; *c*) a severability clause; *d*) a clause for repeals of existing state law; *e*) a saving clause concerning preemption; *f*) a provision concerning unintended conflicts with federal and existing state laws; and *g*) a provision setting forth an effective date of the Act if passed.

COMMENTS explaining the various provisions of the Act follow Sections of each Article where appropriate. These Comments are explanatory, but not legally binding.

CONCLUSION

Public health surveillance systems operate in the massive fishbowl that encompasses both public health practice and the law. For those who set up and run surveillance programs, it is important to note the following summary comments.

- Plan and design surveillance systems so that they are most likely to provide all the information and only the information actually needed.
- Include as few personal identifiers as feasible.
- Analyze and publish data in a responsible and timely fashion.
- Be prepared to stand behind the results (and hope your agency will stand behind you).
- Be prepared to place each data set in the public domain as soon as the first results are published.
- If the findings are revolutionary, be prepared for a hostile reaction rather than a medal.
- Finally, remember that the individual has rights (to privacy, to access information, to participate or not to participate in surveillance programs, and the like). The public health practitioner, at least in the role of public health practitioner, has no rights—only responsibilities.

Public surveillance constitutes one of the bridges between what we think is happening and what is actually happening. As such, it is one of the most valuable tools of the public health practitioner. With surveillance data as the light bulb and the law as a rheostat that stimulates change and regulates behavior, the two areas can work in concert to improve the quality of the public's health.

REFERENCES

1. Wing KR. The law and the public's health. Ann Arbor, Mich.: Health Administration Press, 1990:1–50.
2. Friedman LM. A history of American law. New York: Norton Press, 1986:1–8.
3. Thacker SB, Berkelman RL. Public health surveillance in the United States. *Epidemiologic Reviews* 1988;10:165.
4. Osler W. Internal medicine as a vocation. In: Aequanimitas: with other addresses to medical students, nurses and practitioners of medicine. Third edition. Philadelphia: W.B. Saunders, 1932:131–46.
5. Hogue LL. Public health and the law: issues and trends. Rockville, Md.: Aspen Systems Corporation, 1980:10.
6. Brandt AM. No magic bullet: a social history of venereal disease in the United States since 1880. New York: Oxford University Press, 1985:157–8.
7. Parran T. The next great plague to go. *Survey Graphic* 1936:405–11.
8. 381 U.S. at 484–6.
9. 410 U.S. at 162–4.
10. The Freedom of Information Act (as amended). Washington, D.C.: Government Printing Office, 1986.
11. Gostin LO, Lazzarini Z, Neslund VS, Osterholm MT. The public health information infrastructure. *JAMA* 1996;275:1921–7.
12. Abraham HJ. Freedom and the court: civil rights and liberties in the United States. New York: Oxford University Press, 1988:23.

11

Computerizing Public Health Surveillance Systems

ANDREW G. DEAN

Everything should be made as simple as possible. But to do that you have to master complexity.

Butler Lampson

This chapter on informatics will first explore what technically might be the content and function of an ideal public health surveillance system that computerization makes possible, assessing the gap between this and one of the best of today's actual systems. The barriers to optimal use of computers in surveillance—mostly social, organization, and legal—are described. Then some of the technical problems that must be confronted in thinking about microcomputer-based surveillance are discussed. The chapter leans heavily on examples from the National Notifiable-Disease Surveillance System (NNDSS) in the United States.

AN IDEAL SURVEILLANCE SYSTEM: GENERAL-PURPOSE COMPREHENSIVE SURVEILLANCE

An ideal surveillance system might be expected to produce, for all diseases and injuries or any other selected category, quantitative data on:

- deaths—years of life lost
- disability—years of full and fractional disability
- medical-care costs—in dollars or years of average personal income
- behavioral and environmental risk factors
- denominators for all of the above
- medical and public health resources and interventions

These data should be current and available for any desired time period and geographic location. The results should be displayed in graphic form so that trends and unusual findings in huge masses of data command instant and appropriate attention.

In the ideal system, risk factors for both ill and well persons would be obtainable, and relative risks (risk ratios [RR]) would be obtained directly from surveillance data. Today, RRs are available mainly from research studies, and may have to be estimated from odds ratios that have been obtained through case-control studies. Research results or meta-analysis of such results (combined data from many studies) can be used to model the relationship between risk factors and outcomes. An ideal surveillance system would produce and continually adjust RRs from data in the system, so that it would no longer be necessary to assemble them from research studies.

AN IDEAL SURVEILLANCE SYSTEM: RAPID-RESPONSE SURVEILLANCE

Surveillance for rapid response has different objectives from that directed toward assessing long-term trends and relationships as described above. Rapid response may require focusing on conditions of special interest, such as those that suggest bioterrorism is likely to develop during such international events as the Olympic Games (1). Rapid-response systems may require tapping diverse data sources, such as emergency room and hospital records; pharmaceutical, food manufacturing, or water-quality data, and conducting personal interviews with selected individuals. The example below suggests how a local rapid response surveillance system in the future might operate.

Ideally, the epidemiologist of the future will have a computer and communications system capable of providing management and surveillance information that is also capable of being connected to individual households and medical facilities in order to obtain additional information. Suppose that he or she has a computer with automatic input from all inpatient and outpatient medical facilities, including standardized records for each office or clinic visit and each hospital admission. The epidemiologist chooses to compare data from today or this week with those from a desired period, perhaps the past 5 years, and the computer produces a series of maps for all conditions with unusual patterns. One of the maps seems interesting, and the epidemiologist may point to a particular area and request more information. A more detailed map of the area appears, showing the data sources that might provide the desired information and growing estimates of the cost of obtaining the items desired. A few clicks of the mouse button select the sources, types of data, and format for a display, and the computer spends a few minutes interacting with computers in the medical facilities involved—extracting information and paying the necessary charges from the epidemiology division's budget. Soon the more detailed information is displayed on the epidemiologist's computer screen.

A pattern of hospitalizations and outpatient visits for asthma stands out, and the epidemiologist requests a random sample of specified size of persons who have ever had asthma in the same area, matched by age and gender, to serve as controls for a case-control study. The video-cable addresses of these controls and of the case-patients are quickly produced through queries to appropriate local medical-information sources. The epidemiologist formulates several questions about recent experiences, types of air conditioning, visits to various public facilities, and the like, then adapts these to a previously tested video questionnaire format and requests that video interviews be performed for case-patients and controls. Each household is contacted or left a FAX-like voice mail request to tune to a particular channel and answer a 5-minute query from the state health department on a matter of importance to public health. The video version of the interview is included as an attachment to the e-mail or voice mail. Eighty-five percent of the subjects respond to the first query, and the computer automatically follows up with the rest, bringing the response to 92%, with half of the remaining 8% reported as being absent from their homes for at least 2 days.

While waiting for the interview results, our epidemiologist uses the search capabilities of the Internet to look for similar outbreaks, and s/he downloads considerable information on the relationship of asthma to weather, air contamination, and industrial products. A search for epidemics of asthma turns up many relevant articles in the MEDLARS data base of the National Library of Medicine. Full-text versions are available for those that seem interesting, although some of the full-text downloads incur a small charge.

The case-control study yields an odds ratio significantly higher than 1.0 for persons recently hospitalized for asthma and who work in or visit in a particular neighborhood. In such cases, the epidemiologist connects via local-area network to the state occupational surveillance system to request a display of all factories in the relevant area. Selecting those that deal with potentially allergenic materials, s/he issues a request for a more detailed investigation of activities at designated factories in a selected time interval. The epidemiologist also requests information from the weather bureau on temperature, rainfall, and wind direction and velocity.

Within a short time, a factory is identified that is in the process of moving a large pile of by-products with a bulldozer. A request is issued that the by-product be sprayed with water to prevent its particles from becoming airborne, and the plant manager readily agrees when shown maps that depict hospitalization rates for asthma and emergency-room visits for persons working or visiting downwind from the plant. To monitor progress and widen the investigation, the epidemiologist asks the computer to do similar studies for conjunctivitis and coryza, or hay fever, over the previous and next 2 weeks. Selecting several maps and tables to include in the report, the epidemiologist asks the computer to write a description of the studies performed and the findings, and then dictates a brief summary of the problem and several follow-up notes to the voice port of the computer.

At the end of 2 weeks, the number of cases of asthma has fallen to normal for the area. The computer calculates on the basis of the number of medical visits during the outbreak that $55,000 has been saved at a total cost of a few hours of the epidemiologist's effort, a site visit to the plant, and charges of $9,500 for the data and communications facilities used to perform the interviews.

BARRIERS TO THE IDEAL SURVEILLANCE SYSTEM

Obviously, we are a long way from implementing the system described above. It may be helpful in thinking about the future to explore what barriers must be surmounted before this scenario can be enacted. Strangely enough, few of them are technical; all of the necessary systems could be built today with fairly conventional equipment and software, with the exception of the two-way interactive video connection with each household. This hook-up with the individual household is more likely to be available within the next 10 years than is the connection between the physician's record files and the health department. In fact, the two-way interactive video link between household and the outside world is simply awaiting the government's or the marketplace's decision on what format will be used. Entrepreneurs, public telephone companies and cable television providers are rapidly beginning to offer fast, 24-hour Internet connections for private homes making it practical to send modest-size video segments to many homes, within the near future.

However, there are other, more difficult problems to be solved before the "ideal system" can be implemented. In the United States, for example, there is a profusion of computerized systems for inpatient and outpatient records, as well as for insurance and other purposes. Most medical records remain only partially computerized and existing systems contain a plethora of different variables and use a variety of formats. Until a simple core public health record of age, gender, geographic location, diagnosis, and a few other items is created for each outpatient visit and each hospitalization, and until it is available in a standard format without delay, the responsive interactive system described above will remain an unrealistic pipe dream.

The barriers to establishing standardized public health output from computerized medical records are primarily political and administrative; most large retail organizations create records for each item sold, and the average item carries, on average, a much lower price than the cost of a visit for medical care. Once there is the will to establish a national computerized medical records system, the technical hurdles will be readily overcome. The needs include standard but suitably flexible record formats and codes, solutions to problems associated with confidentiality, incentives to create the records (including the assurance of appropriate and cost-effective use of the records), and voice input.

Another problem is the lack of recognition that information about patients, except for legally designated reportable diseases, is useful in public health and should be available to public health agencies. The level of awareness could be heightened if technical solutions to problems of confidentiality were publicized and understood by the public and their legislative representatives. Such solutions as one-way encoding of algorithms could provide solutions to matching and follow-up problems, and at the same time allay fears on the part of the public that public health agencies will turn into "Big Brother."

A common problem is the pervasive feeling among those in charge of data that their database must be clean before anyone else can use it. Months or even years are consumed while corrections and updates are made to make data as accurate as possible. Quality control is necessary and important, however there must be a realization on the part of everyone concerned—including the media and the public—that the concept of surveillance includes rapid turnaround. It must be understood that data are preliminary, that in order to look at today's data today, one must be willing to accept today's imperfections. Several kinds of mental shifts, as well as corresponding technical developments, will be necessary before a computerized system can be used to examine automatically a time slice of disease and injury records that originate in clinics and hospitals. Imperfections will be many and methods must be found to cope with reality—even if it includes warts—on an immediate basis.

THE TECHNOLOGY OF THE FUTURE

As stated above, today's technology, given enough social and organizational development, is adequate to allow the creation of miracles in public health information and communication. Nevertheless, it seems likely that development in technology will continue to be more of a driving force in public health computing than progress in political and social organization. Technologic developments over the next decade will probably include the areas discussed below.

High-Capacity Storage Devices

Compact disks with read-only memory (CD-ROMs), similar to those used for music, make it possible to have access to large bibliographic data bases wherever electricity is available. The MEDLARS data base of the U.S. National Library of Medicine can be searched from a clinic in Africa. Once there are lower prices for books available on CD-ROM that include needed illustrations, it will be possible to take a medical library anywhere in a briefcase. Past data bases from the United States and elsewhere will become available on CD-ROM or on the Internet, although the process of cleaning them up for this purpose often reveals gaps and inconsistencies that reflect changing definitions and diminish their value as consistent anchors for comparison.

Local- and Wide-Area Networks

A local area network (LAN) is a system linking microcomputers, terminals, and workstations within an office or building to each other and perhaps to a mainframe computer to facilitate sharing of equipment (e.g., printers), programs, data, and other information. Servers—usually microcomputers—provide central memory and processing capability to support the network software. LANs have transformed the way many agencies do business. The most noticeable effect is the transmission of written memoranda that could or would not have been typed, packaged, and sent through a paper system. The cost of installing and supporting a LAN is not small, particularly in terms of support personnel. Uses for surveillance include entering data at multiple computers connected by a LAN. This requires special-functions ("record-locking") software to protect against errors if several people enter data in the same file at the same time. Special precautions to protect confidentiality are also necessary in a network if several people enter data in the same file at the same time. Often, LANs are connected together in a wide-area network (WAN) serving an agency or corporation. Such systems can be made relatively private, since they depend on direct connections.

The Internet

During the past few years, the Internet has assumed worldwide importance comparable to that of piped water, electric power, or the telephone. Since it is designed for communication in network, rather than hierarchical fashion, the Internet has many advantages for public health work. Search engines permit almost instant identification of data or people with similar interests anywhere in the world, so that one can publish information to the world, or query the worldwide knowledge base in a matter of minutes and with very modest resources. The Internet protocols that allow e-mail, Web pages, and files to be transmitted offer standards for uniting systems that could never have emerged from public health alone. Future surveillance and information systems will increasingly be built around evolving Internet technology and will provide access to diverse information sources of types not previously available. With a modest computer, a thin piece of cable, and an Internet service provider, anyone can search and use the world's largest library of information (and misinformation) at little or no cost.

Currently, all 50 U.S. states and six territories have web pages, which differ considerably in organization, level of detail, and amount of surveillance data displayed. More than 80% provide some surveillance data, but fewer than 10% appear to use the Internet in collecting the data they report. It appears likely that future surveillance systems will increasingly be built around Internet technology. They will provide access to information sources not previously available, and, we hope, will provide innovative ways of initiating and monitoring actions based on surveillance and will be a source of rapid collection of data to facilitate investigations of identified surveillance aberrations.

New User Interfaces

The parts of programs that interact with users have become easier to understand and more attractive, with pull-down menus, windows, and pointing devices such as the mouse. This elegance comes with costly requirements,—including faster computers, more memory, and, particularly, greater skill to produce such programs. Some new programs cause unexpected problems when run with older programs or on older computers. All in all, the trend is toward a standard set of screen controls, like those in modern cars, but the path in that direction is replete with experiment and minor failures.

New Programming Tools

It is widely recognized that software production is the narrow point in the implementation of new ideas in computing. Useful software still requires hundreds of thousands of lines of handwritten and highly personal coding. Many new tools such as fourth-generation improved data bases, computer-assisted software design (CASD) tools, and object-oriented design have made programming more productive, but this area of new tools is one in which major advances would create revolutionary changes. Methods of linking diverse and non-standard data bases are particularly important in public health.

Higher-Capacity Processors and More Memory

The almost miraculous advances in computer speed and memory capacity in the last decade have removed many of the limits that required use of mainframe computers or minicomputers rather than microcomputers. Today, given sufficient motivation, almost any project—even those involving millions of records—can be done on a microcomputer or several microcomputers connected by a LAN.

Video and Computer Integration

Photographs and fully functional video will soon be appearing on our computer screens. Although this has the greatest impact in pathology, radiology, and education, it also increases opportunities to use color and three-dimensional dynamic displays for epidemiologic data. The possibilities for computer interaction via ordinary television sets are exciting. Whether computers become television sets or television sets acquire computer features, the two are becoming one, and television cables are providing fast Internet connections to private homes. Every epidemiologist (and market researcher) can savor the possibility of interviewing citizens via cable television with the results captured immediately in computerized form. The medium offers new challenges in filtering responses that result from the various stages of humor, exasperation, or intoxication that citizens may undergo in the privacy of their homes.

Voice and Pen Input

Systems are now available that identify thousands of spoken words and can transcribe continuous speech with reasonable accuracy, particularly if the context is well defined and a specialized dictionary is provided (2). Palmtop computers that recognize handwritten text of reasonably structured type are currently being sold. Presumably, the rather elementary state of computerization of medical records will undergo a quantum leap once such systems allow medical staff to dictate to the computer without typing and preferably without being near a computer. When medical handwriting is replaced by voice dictation into a lapel microphone, real progress may occur in the use of computers in both clinical medicine and public health settings. As stated above, however, realizing real public-health benefit from such technology will require dramatic social and legal changes.

Notifiable Disease in the United States: An Example of Computerized Public Health Surveillance Today

The NETSS in the United States is one example of a computerized surveillance system. Beginning in 1985, CDC and state health department staff installed customized disease-surveillance software in 40 state and territorial health departments, and in a number of county, district, and territorial departments. The software in has been based on DOS versions of *Epi Info,* a public-domain word-processing, data-base, and statistics package for IBM-compatible microcomputers that is a joint product of CDC and the WHO's Global Programme on AIDS (*3–5*). These systems have made possible the participation of all 50 states in the NETSS (*6,7*). Benefits cited in a recent evaluation include improved access to data and improvement in both quality of data and access associated with decentralized entry of data (*8*).

Much of the rest of this chapter is based on CDC's experience with reportable-disease surveillance using *Epi Info* in NETSS. Although reportable-disease systems are a specific kind of surveillance system and *Epi Info* is only one type of data-base and statistics program around which a system can be built, many of the principles of computerization apply to other systems. The information is directed to those considering computerization of a disease-surveillance or similar records system, whether they plan to do their own system design or work with professional computer-systems designers.

Computerizing a surveillance system for disease is not easy. Since the success of computerization depends as much on the administrative and epidemiologic environment as on the software, it is vital that public health practitioners understand the details of a new system and participate in its design.

An important step in developing a computerized surveillance system is identifying the public health objective for the system. In some cases, the objective will have been clear for decades in a manual system (e.g., "Identify, treat or isolate cases of *x* and evaluate results," or "Assess results of immunization programs and identify new cases for special control efforts"). Computerization can then be directed toward accomplishing the same task more efficiently or in greater volume or detail.

The most successful computer systems, however, are those that change methods by which an agency operates rather than those that merely automate a manual task (*9*). In establishing a new surveillance system or reexamining an existing system, it may be useful to address the following question: "What key pieces of information do I want to see on my desk (or computer screen) every day, week, month, or year that will make my work easier or more effective?" The same question can be asked at several levels of management—from epidemiologic technician to epidemiologist to director of a public health agency.

If a surveillance system that is already in place has a public health goal and to some extent achieves the goal, why computerize? Sometimes the answer is obvious—the annual report takes a host of clerks 2 years to process, or like the graphs that the neighboring health department turns out so easily with a computer. Potential benefits relate to quality of data and reports, quantity of data that can be processed, and speed of processing. Easier transmittal (copying) of surveillance records to another site is one reason disease reports in all 50 states are computerized.

We were unable to find systematic studies on the benefits of computerizing public health surveillance systems, although numerous articles describe individual systems that have been computerized, and Gaynes *et al.* describe methods for evaluating a computerized surveillance system (*10–14*). In literature about the commercial world, benefits of computerization have been examined from the viewpoint of financial savings. Savings by automating a manual information process may amount to 20% or so, but the real benefits are achieved if computerization transforms the entire process concerned, giving a competitive advantage in the commercial world—which would correspond to a new order of service in the public health world (9). So far, most public health applications have automated manual systems, although some—such as the spreadsheet calculation of the impact of smoking on populations—verge on establishing new and previously unknown styles of doing business (15). Quantum leaps in benefits, however, are more likely to result from access to new sources of data, or the ability to process information too voluminous to be included in previous surveillance systems (16).

One problem associated with developing a computerized surveillance system also occurs in other vertical markets (industries with specialized practitioners) such as the construction, meat-packing, and real estate industries. With only 7,000 epidemiologists in the United States, relatively few commercial developers feel that it is financially worthwhile to develop software for this market alone, since applications such as spreadsheets, languages, and word processors may sell millions of copies to the general public (17).

Basic Needs

The first requisite for computerization is a paper system or operational design that works reasonably well or would do so if the process were speedier and more accurate. Chaos computerized is not necessarily an improvement over what is already in place, although the process of computerization offers a chance to rethink some of the features of a system and to make improvements. If the surveillance system is new, it may be desirable to evolve the computer facilities in small stages with minimal investment until the system proves to be useful and well-conceived. This requires careful planning (including provision for changing the plan if necessary), but will minimize the expense of adaptation as the epidemiologic design of the system undergoes the inevitable adaptation to external reality. Once the bare-bones system has proven its worthiness and the probability of expensive changes is lower, the details can be added later.

Personnel to do the collection of data, data entry, analysis, and system maintenance are important contributors to the system. Many of the tasks can be learned by current employees, particularly if they welcome this challenge. If possible, those chosen should be long-term employees to assure stability of the system, although they may be aided by students and other temporary employees. The epidemiologist who will use the results should participate in the planning of the system and should understand how it is constructed. A staff member with programming skills or aptitude for microcomputing should be involved in designing and setting up the system, even if an outside consultant does the actual programming.

If several computers are to interact and share data, a set of standards is necessary (e.g., just as humans carrying on a conversation need a common language). In the United States, the states and CDC chose a standard record format for NETSS so that computers of different types could reformat data to a set of standard records and send these to the central agency. This standard, first devised in 1984 and revised in 1991, has served the purpose well, without placing unnecessary restrictions on the type of hardware or the format of records kept within each state. One state may maintain 20 times more information for local use than do other states, but all export data in the same standard record formats to the national level. The new standard record format allows for standard demographic and diagnostic information, attachment of variable-length detailed reports for selected diseases, mixture of summary with individual records, and automatic comparison of state and national data bases with each transmission. Since the record format specifies only the location and content of each field on a 60-character line of text, records can be produced by any type of computer from desktop to mainframe, and no particular type of software is required.

Recent industry and health-sector developments in data transmission have provided protocols for electronic commerce (such as X12) and medical record information (such as HL7). A new universal protocol called XML provides tags like those that underlie the display of Internet pages via HTML. These tags can be used as "metadata" to identify data elements. Programs can use the labeled elements for display or processing as defined in other files. Producing a language for describing public health data in any of these formats, however, requires many decisions and definition, and agreement by those creating and using the data to use the same standards. Committee efforts are now under way at many levels of government and in the health-care industry to develop such standards.

Purchasing

Most government settings have an organization in charge of computer programming, approval of new systems, and purchasing of computers and software. Functions such as Year 2000 compliance and control of computer security and access require such centralization. It is important to maintain liaison with this organization and to arrange its assistance ahead of time with difficult areas such as purchasing computers. In some organizations, purchases are limited to particular types of computers—occasionally with unique characteristics—or to centrally administered systems. We recently encountered a network of diskless workstations that presented numerous problems in trying to load or run software or to back up files from a particular station without a removable storage device. If requirements that result in problems or delays are present, it is prudent to discover and, if possible, to surmount and minimize them at an early stage through patient negotiation and collaboration, or other methods if necessary. The technical difficulties that arise in setting up a computer system are usually the easy problems; the difficulties that lead to months and years of delay and unhappiness usually reflect misunderstanding and miscommunication among individuals or organizational entities.

Files, Records, and Fields

Computerized records are stored in files or data bases. A file (or a table within a data base) is a collection of records, usually one record per case, that has a name (e.g., GEPI.REC or EPI.MDB, for general epidemiology) and can be manipulated as a unit. Files and tables, like books, can be opened, closed, read, written to, or discarded. They are stored on nonvolatile media such as hard or floppy disks (magnetic tape) or on CD-ROMs, which have the advantage of resisting magnetic fields and a greater degree of permanence with storage.

Records correspond to one copy of a completed questionnaire or form, such as a disease-report card. Usually, one disease report or questionnaire is stored in a file as a single record. Records can be displayed on the screen, searched for by name or some other characteristic, saved (written) to a disk, or marked as deleted. Many records can be stored in each file.

A field (or variable) is one item of information within a record. NAME, AGE, and DATEONSET might be fields within a disease-report record. Records in a particular file all have the same fields. Each field has a name, a type (text, uppercase text, numeric, date, etc.), and sometimes a length, such as 22 characters for NAME or three digits for AGE. In *Epi Info* 2000, text fields are of variable length, up to 128 characters, or may be declared as multiline for essentially unlimited blocks of text. During analysis, fields may be called variables, and commands such as TABLES DISEASE COUNTY are used to instruct the system to process a particular file and construct the desired table by tabulating the fields or variables called DISEASE and COUNTY. In this case, the result in *Epi Info* would be a table that lists DISEASE down the left side and COUNTY across the top, with numbers of reports by county indicated in the cells of the table.

Hardware: What Size Computer Is Appropriate?

With microcomputers that cost around a few thousand dollars, it is possible to process more than 100,000 records in a reasonable time period. Processing time tends to reflect the record length as well as the number of records, however, and the size of each record should be kept short if large numbers will be processed. Since the total number of disease reports for the United States is several hundred thousand per year, states and counties should find it possible to build most systems on a microcomputer, if desired. A hard disk capable of storing 200 million 60-character records (13 gigabytes) can be purchased for a few hundred dollars.

Minicomputers and mainframes can serve as the basis for surveillance systems if available at reasonable cost and if programming and support staff are available to work creatively with staff of the surveillance system. The greater technical skill required to run and program such computers often resides in an organization other than the one running the surveillance system, and close coordination becomes much more important than in the do-it-yourself situation with a microcomputer.

Systems that seem to require processing of millions of records, such as hospital discharge or Medicare records for a state, can be reduced to a manageable size for the microcomputer by sampling. A mainframe can be used to select a sample of records (e.g., particular age groups, diseases or every tenth record). Files are then exported for processing on a microcomputer that is more responsive to the epidemiologist's wishes. Epidemiologists are usually acutely conscious of sample size when performing interviews but sometimes fail to recognize how unnecessary it is to process 6 million records to estimate a simple proportion.

Software

The type of software used to perform the computerization is often less crucial than the skills of those who program and run it. Usually, there are several types of data base or statistical packages that will do a given task well if properly programmed. Beware the indispensable programmer syndrome, in which a single expert programmer writes a system in his or her favorite language and then departs for greener pastures, leaving the users without resources for further support and modification.

Data-base packages such as dBASE, Paradox, Foxbase, Clipper, Oracle, Sybase, and SQL Server are designed to allow data input, storage, retrieval, and editing. Most will count records but do not easily do such statistics as odds ratios or confidence intervals. They require a skilled programmer to produce a customized system.

Statistics packages, such as Statistical Analysis System (SAS) and Statistical Package for the Social Sciences (SPSS), focus on producing statistical reports, usually from single files of data. They are less convenient for data entry. Both SAS and SPSS now have mainframe and microcomputer versions. They contain statistical functions routines rarely used by epidemiologists and those in other fields, such as the social sciences that occupy large amounts of disk space (tens of megabytes for SAS).

Epi Info fits on a single 1.4 megabyte diskette for DOS or Windows and provides a combination of data-base and statistical functions, allowing relational linking of several files during data entry or analysis. Questionnaires or forms may be up to 500 lines, which contain hundreds of numeric or text fields, and the number of records is limited only by disk storage space. *Epi Info* 2000 can also store large text fields, images, and tables. Frequencies, cross-tabulations, customized reports, and graphs can be produced through commands contained in a program file or interactively from the keyboard. Commonly used epidemiologic statistics are part of the statistical output. Although it takes little experience to use *Epi Info* for investigating outbreaks, producing a complete surveillance system from the beginning takes both skill and time. It is, however, simpler to modify the surveillance software supplied with the program.

It is important to realize the limitations of software packages before they are used. Both statistical and data-base packages typically cost at least several hundred dollars and therefore are not as likely to be feasible for classes of students or large numbers of computers as a public-domain program. Some data-base packages limit the number of fields in a record or the number of records in a file, and few do statistics without advanced programming or purchase of a supplementary package. Statistics packages, on the other hand, may have limitations in handling textual (alpha) data, and most allow processing of only one file at a time. A complete surveillance system may require the functions of both data base and statistical programs.

Compatibility with the Internet and other data–base and file systems that may be used in related systems is an important feature to investigate. *Epi Info* for DOS comes with programs for importing and exporting files in a number of formats. *Epi Info* 2000 is built around the Microsoft Access file format, and therefore offers considerable potential for exchanging files as well as having import and export functions for other file formats. Some current systems and many future systems use the Internet for either data entry or dissemination of results. *Epi Info* 2000 produces results in Internet format (HTML) to facilitate such efforts.

The current version of *Epi Info* (5.0 1.b) has limitations on the number of records that can be sorted or relationally linked at one time (tens of thousands). Since text fields are limited to 80 characters, the current version of *Epi Info* would not be a good choice if large amounts of text need to be stored, as in a complete clinical system containing dictated notes.

Designing Entry Forms

In a surveillance system, data items are usually entered in a standard format (e.g., a questionnaire or report form). The information is usually stored in files containing one record per individual or per episode. In *Epi Info,* the format of the data-base file is specified by developing a questionnaire or form in the word processor. The result resembles a paper form, with prompts or questions and entry blanks indicated by special symbols (e.g., underlined characters for text fields and number signs for numeric fields). The computer reads the form and constructs a file data base in the proper format.

The amount of data entry and computer storage required may be minimized by computerizing only information that will actually be used. If follow-up information such as name, address, and telephone number is on the paper form, there may be no need to enter it into the computer. If contact tracing is recorded, the computer record may summarize the number of contacts named and the number found or treated, with the details on each and progress of the follow-up efforts relegated to the paper forms used by field investigators. When including an item on the input form, it is helpful to ask how it will be analyzed and how it will look after processing. Computers around the world are full of data items that someone entered "just in case we need it." Most are never needed, or, when needed, are useless because of the large amount of missing data.

Identifiers

In designing a form, it is useful to include a unique case identifier as a number or combination of letters and digits. This may include meaningful information, such as the year, but should not include any item that may need to be changed, such as a disease code. It must be designed so that a new and unique number will always be available for each record.

In a simple data collection system, each record might represent an event rather than a person, and there might be no need to correct or update records after submission. Such a system would not require identifiers, since every event would be considered unique, and there would be no need to link new records with older ones.

This situation might occur in a one-time survey or investigation, but in most real-world situations, records are updated, merged, searched, sorted, deleted, or otherwise managed in ways that require matching of related records based on a unique identifier. Even simple rechecking of data entry against paper source forms requires identifiers.

Various kinds of identifiers can be used, such as name, date of birth, and arbitrary identification numbers. People's names alone are generally inadequate, as there are too many Joneses, Lees, and Garcias to make attribution of diagnosis by name alone a safe procedure. Adding date of birth can help, but there is often at least one incorrect digit. The same person may have different names over time, or use different first names with different agencies. Social security numbers have no check digit for verifying accuracy, are legally protected for many government purposes, and often are inaccurately recorded.

The ideal identifier for most health systems would be assigned to each person at birth, readily recalled by the owner without error, contain verification information, and would not change in the individual's lifetime. At some point legislation in the United States may provide such a number, as it has in many European countries; or biological markers such as fingerprints, iris image patterns, or even DNA structure may become practical identifiers.

Until such identifiers are available, however, unique numbers can be assigned for a given system when a person enters the system, as is done by hospitals, insurance companies, and credit card companies. A health department, for example, could assign a client number for each person encountered. A central registry would be used to look up each client at the beginning of a visit or on receipt of a specimen or report and ascertain whether an ID number has already been assigned. If so, the number and previous records are retrieved; if not, a new number is assigned.

It is important to consider the scope of such identifiers. Imagine a health department with separate laboratory and epidemiology divisions. Each may receive information or specimens from individuals with a reportable disease—not necessarily under identical names or numbers. If laboratory and epidemiologic results are to be matched, however, this can be done manually by a technician, who decides that Jack Jones and John Jones are the same person because they have the same county and disease and arrived within a few weeks of one another; but one has an address and an age, and the other has a post office box number and a date of birth. A computer would require a very sophisticated algorithm to do the same thing, and a certain percentage of matches would be incorrect or missed.

Alternatively, a technician in each division of the health department could consult a central registry common to the two divisions when receiving a report or specimen. Identification of the data belonging to either an old or new client would be made at that time, and a unique identifying number would be assigned, much as a patient's hospital record number is retrieved on admission to the hospital and used for identification of the patient's records and specimens thereafter. Identifiers, such as the Lab/Epi number proposed here or hospital record numbers, are of sufficient scope to accomplish their intended task, but are less threatening or politically sensitive than universal identifiers such as a national health registration number. Effort is required to accomplish the initial identification of the report or specimen as unique or belonging to a previous client. The reward is that no manual effort is required to match specimens between the Lab and Epi data bases, once the identification numbers have been correctly assigned in the data-base records. Performing a probabalistic match is not necessary to perform matching or merging of records.

Of course there are many other aspects of identifiers to be considered, but this scenario illustrates the crucial importance of unique identifiers in maintaining and sharing computer records. Design of computerized record systems requires careful thought about the scope, nature, verification, and maintenance of identifiers, as well as provisions for maintaining confidentiality to allow their proper use.

Conceptualizing Data Entry Items

Data for surveillance systems should be structured for easy analysis. Textual material can be captured, stored, retrieved, and printed from a computer file, but it is usually difficult or impossible to process such entries as "Pen, Strep, and Ampicillin," to produce meaningful tabulations. For serious analysis a more usable format would be:

Penicillin	⟨Y⟩
Streptomycin	⟨Y⟩
Ampicilin	⟨Y⟩

Each "⟨Y⟩" (in the DOS versions of *Epi Info*) represents a single yes or no answer.

A common problem in designing entry forms is that several data items may be similar. Suppose you want to record name and treatment (RX) status for up to 12 contacts of each patient with a sexually transmitted disease. One possible approach is to create fields called NAME1 through NAME12 and RX1 through RX12. This approach allows the data to be entered, although it creates a very large data-entry record (say 12 by 22 characters for NAME and 12 by 1 characters for RX, or 276 characters, even if no information about contacts is entered). However, analyzing the information becomes a programming nightmare, as determining the number of contacts or their treatment status requires examining at least 12 different fields in each record to see whether they have been filled in and keeping a running tally of the results. In computer data-base jargon, the record is not "normalized." These repeating groups of fields should be placed in separate records—one for each contact—linked to the main file as described below in the section on linking special-purpose records. A patient with one contact has one record in the case file and one record in the contact file, rather than the equivalent of these plus 11 empty records in a single file.

This problem is resolved by rethinking what is really the best unit around which to build an individual record. After deciding what kind of record should be the "parent" or main record, other records can be related to the main record by assigning a "key" or ID number common to both types of records. The simple answer is that if you intend to tabulate cases, the parent builds a case record; if you tabulate contacts or follow-up visits, then you need a contact or follow-up as a "child" record. If both are necessary and the system is large or permanent, records should be placed in separate files or tables and linked using relational data-base features as described below.

Data Entry

The details of data entry should be determined and documented, including who will prepare the paper records (if needed) for entry, who will enter them, and at what intervals. The status of the report as suspected or confirmed may determine whether it is entered, and this must be determined at the outset. Most disease reports are entered in batches—once a week, for example—and in many states not more than an hour or two is needed to enter the data for a week, although the number of records and time required to enter data varies greatly among states.

Records linked to more extensive specialized forms can be sent as partial submissions and revised later to avoid delays in reporting caused by the slower progress of data collection for the more detailed forms. This issue needs to be considered and resolved in advance.

Cleaning and Editing the Data

Errors or duplications inevitably occur during data entry, and additional information may arrive that requires changes or additions. The data can be cleaned during data entry or with the help of analytic programs that display "outliers", (nonsense or extreme data values), and data can be checked visually by browsing through records in the ENTER program or by scanning a list printed by the ENTER or ANALYSIS programs. Records can be viewed and corrected in a spreadsheet format in ANALYSIS. Finally, a program called VALIDATE can be used to compare files entered in duplicate by different operators. Records showing differences in the two files are printed out for reconciliation.

Epi Info allows extensive programming of error checks on data entry. Each field can be set to accept only specified codes, and, if necessary, multiple fields can be checked for inconsistencies such as gynecologic conditions recorded for males. Unfortunately, not all errors can be caught by such systems and wrong codes can still be entered for a less gender-specific disease. They can eliminate male pregnancies and female prostatectomies, but incorrect entries for diarrhea or coronary insufficiency are harder to catch. Another method involves running a special checking program after all records have been entered.

Error checking can also be done by

- dual entry of data by different personnel, followed by computerized comparison of the duplicate files and reconciliation of any differences
- entering data a second time in "key-punch verification" mode, in which any differences are reconciled as soon as each field is entered
- having one person read data from the original form while another reads from the screen or from a printout
- doing frequencies on a completed data file to look for outliers

Regardless of the method used, errors should be caught and corrected as near the time of data entry as possible, since they can create much larger problems if left for the end of the year. The choice depends largely on the orientation and number of personnel available, and perhaps on their preferences after trying different methods.

Analysis of Data

The type of output desired should be planned in advance, since the inputs and outputs usually specify fairly precisely what kind of processing is needed to achieve the results. Dummy tables and graphs should be sketched on paper. *Epi Info* and many other data-base programs can be programmed to print a table or mixture of text and tables in almost any format, using a feature called the report generator.

It is not necessary to design reports to cover all possible needs, since ad hoc queries are an important part of any system, and additional reports can be added later if they are deemed useful. In *Epi Info,* an epidemiologist can learn to do simple queries (READ GEPI; TABLES RACE COUNTY) in a short time and to limit these to particular time periods (SELECT REPORTWK = 34) almost as easily.

Sometimes a simple report, such as a list of this week's entries sorted by disease, may be as useful as a large table with very small numbers in each cell. The number of records should be considered in designing reports and in determining how often they will be produced.

Distributed Data Base: The Architecture of Surveillance Systems

A surveillance system may be maintained in a single microcomputer. As more community health departments obtain computers, however, the trend is toward more integrated software protocols, with networks of computers within a state, connected by Internet, Intranet, WANs, modems, or other means. In ways analogous to those used in the NETSS, for example, such an integrated system may have more than 50 state and territorial participants, and similar processes are followed by interacting cities, countries, and participating state health departments. Each participating site enters data and sends records periodically to a computer at the next higher level.

This process would be simple if all data were entered at the local level and sent to the state level, and if no changes were made later. However, in practice, not only are changes made, but in some states records are entered at both state and local levels. Some method must be in place to see that all levels of staff eventually have the same records.

Ideally, only one copy of records would be considered the master copy, and each user would know its location and provide updates only at the designated time. The best way to accomplish this objective is still being worked out, and experiments of several types are likely. Designating only one source as the "owner" and rightful editor of the data is one possibility. Creators of records indicate the site in which the record was created. Only the site that "owns" the record is allowed to make changes, which are transmitted weekly to the other sites to update their copies of the records.

In NETSS, state health departments use the latest software to transmit year-to-date summary information on the state data base to the national level each week. These summaries are compared automatically with the contents of the national data base, and any discrepancies are reported.

Future surveillance systems may be designed as

1. Client-server systems, in which data resides on a central server, perhaps at the state level, and clients (cities and counties) enter and query data via an Internet browser or other client program over a network or the Internet, using a secure connection similar to those for personal banking or credit card transactions.
2. "Replicated data bases," in which copies of an empty standard data base created at the state level are loaned to cities and counties. Each locality is responsible for maintaining data in a portion of the data base. Periodically local files are transmitted to the central level for automatic reconciliation with the main data base, after which updated copies are transmitted to the local level. Providing the rules for automatic reconciliation is the challenge for this method.
3. Truly distributed data bases, in which data is maintained locally and only accessed when needed by more central levels. This could be done with an Internet system, for example, in which each agency "publishes" summary or individual data to authorized users. Security would be maintained by encryption to provide a "virtual private network." At intervals, perhaps once a week, a central search engine or program with a list of participants would automatically assemble and publish current data from all participating sites. The degree of possible automation is attractive, as is the presence of only one copy of the "gold-standard" data, but such a system is completely at the mercy of human error and procrastination at the participating sites. Maintaining confidentiality on a public network also presents a serious challenge.

Transmitting Data

In the NETSS, most states transmit reports each week through a commercial telecommunications network, to a microcomputer at CDC. The 50-plus reports stay in the network computer until they are picked up on Tuesday morning by CDC staff, stripped of comments and address material, and joined together in a single file for processing on the CDC mainframe computer. Error checking is done to test for invalid codes and other problems, and error notices are sent back to the states.

Another method that eliminates errors caused by telephone noise involves transmissions directly from computer to computer by means of modems and software that retransmits if errors are caused by noise. Several states are using this method to connect with CDC microcomputers that, in turn, send the files to the CDC mainframe computer. Internet browsers and most other communications software provide this service automatically.

A third, less elegant but often practical solution is physical transfer of floppy diskettes by mail or messenger at intervals. This allows large files to be transferred with minimal inconvenience, and may be appropriate if the additional trouble of setting up modems and software is not yet warranted or in developing countries where telephones are unreliable or unavailable.

In any case, the result is that a copy of a file of records from the peripheral site arrives at the central site. The records must then be merged into the main data base. If all are new records, this task is straightforward. If the incoming records contain updates for records previously transmitted, the process is more complex, and the integrity of unique identifiers becomes an important issue.

Computer Security and Confidentiality

Anyone familiar with the daily newspaper knows that these are important public issues. Surveillance systems must deal with sensitive data in a responsible way, and even data that is not sensitive must be protected from corruption or misinterpretation. Amalgamation of different data sets should not reveal identifying details. Such issues are covered in more detail elsewhere in this book (see Chapters 3–6).

Special precautions in computer systems must be taken to prevent or recover from corruption by hardware or software failures or by computer viruses. Commercial virus protection software should be employed at the least, and most organizations now provide "firewalls" that protect computers inside the organizational network.

In the NETSS, the microcomputers that receive files from reporting states and territories each week are isolated from the main CDC network on a separate LAN, and are automatically rebooted before being accessed from CDC. Special precautions are taken to assure that the computers dialing in and connecting to the NETSS hub are actually those in health departments. Commands to upload files are issued by the CDC computers, not by the computer that dialed in. The files being transmitted are encrypted.

Correcting and Updating Records from Another Site

In the NETSS, only state participants are allowed to update records; CDC staff do not do so, although they may enter temporary telephone reports. Updates are sent as records with the same identification number as that for the original record. If a new record has the same identification number as a record in the data base, the existing record is updated so that all non-blank fields of the new record prevail. To change an age, for example, a state would send a record containing the case identification number and the new age. To delete a record, the state, year, and identification numbers are sent in a special "delete" record. When errors are found at CDC, the information is transmitted to the state staff, who then correct the errors and transmit update records the following week. This system is quite dependent on adequate staffing and attention to detail. Future systems hopefully will require less manual oversight.

Individual and Summary Records

Many surveillance systems function with a record for each individual case report. In some, however, there is a need for summary records, each of which represents a number of case reports. This is helpful if large numbers of similar records (e.g., cases of gonorrhea in a big city) are processed, or if only summary numbers are available. It also allows records from entire years to be summarized in condensed format, so that a 5-year trend can be calculated without reading and processing each record for the previous 5 years.

A summary record is similar to a case record, but it contains an additional field called COUNT, which contains a number. The number indicates how many records with the same information are represented by the summary record. *Epi Info* for DOS contains commands called SUMTABLES and SUMFREQ to process summary records. *Epi Info* 2000 allows a field to be designated as a Weight—COUNT, for example. These commands sum the contents of the COUNT field rather than counting individual records. Since a record with COUNT equal to 1 is an individual case record, files that are mixtures of summary and individual records can be processed as a single unit.

Linking Special-Purpose Records to the Main Data Base

As mentioned above, sometimes it is necessary to link related records in different files in order to allow easy processing (for example, patients and contacts who are related to patients). This requires that a common identification number be included in each record. *Epi Info* and other data-base programs, such as dBASE, allow automatic linking of records through such a common identifier. On data entry, answering "Y" to the question "Contacts (Y/N)?" might cause another form, representing the contact file, to appear on the screen. The operator can then enter one or many contact forms for this case, pressing a function key (F10) to return to the main form. A separate record is created for each contact.

In *Epi Info*'s ANALYSIS program, the CONTACT file is READ, and the CASE file is linked (related) to it. Each contact record then contains information about the patient as well as about the contact, and questions such as how many contacts of female case-patients were treated can be answered easily. The CASE file can also be processed alone to answer questions such as how many cases of syphilis there were.

In the NETSS, disease-specific forms are linked to the main data base of reports through the same mechanism. Hepatitis, for example, requires a full page of extra information used to define further the epidemiology of a report. By linking a hepatitis file to the main case file, records are created only if the disease is hepatitis, thus saving a great deal of storage space over the single-file method, in which all the questions on hepatitis would be left blank in a non-hepatitis record. Current systems, including the one distributed as an example on the *Epi Info* disks, contain related files for hepatitis, meningitis, and Lyme disease, each of which only appears if a relevant disease code is entered.

Dissemination of Data

Dissemination of results is an important element of the surveillance cycle. Computerization can assist by making new methods of analysis or presentation practical. Using tabular or graphics software in conjunction with desk-top publishing technology can make the preparation of results not only faster but more accurate and meaningful. A graphic method for comparison of current results with those for the past 5 years has been introduced to the *MMWR* in the United States (see Figure 5–12) (*18*). This method would have been too cumbersome for manual processing.

Computer software greatly simplifies and improves the production of maps and graphs. *Epi Map,* a public-domain companion to *Epi Info* released in 1993, made mapping available to anyone with an IBM-compatible microcomputer. Mapping functions are provided for *Epi Info* in a program called *Epi Map.* The Windows version of Epi Map is compatible with high-end geographic information systems such as ArcView and ARC/INFO.

Tables, maps, graphs, text, and data files may be made available either online via modem connections or by distributing floppy or CD-ROM disks. The latter are particularly useful in remote areas or for large volumes of data that cannot easily be sent over low-speed modems. Increasingly, surveillance results are made available on Internet Web sites. This can increase the speed and possible breadth of dissemination greatly. It also raises new problems by making preliminary data available to a wide audience.

Data Disasters

Destruction or damage of data on hard disks should be expected and planned for. During the first 4 years of the NETSS (and during the 3-year tenure of its predecessor, the Epidemiologic Surveillance Project), a number of hard disks have crashed. In most cases, back-up files on floppy diskettes had been properly prepared and stored, and they were used to restore the data once the disk had been replaced.

Early in the evolution of the NETSS, some state programs began to reuse case identification numbers from several years ago, not realizing that the new records would overwrite the old records in the national data base. It is important to be clear about the time period for which updates will be accepted. Recycling of identification numbers should be avoided if at all possible.

Upgrading either hardware or software is a frequent cause of problems, when the new items have unexpected features, occupy more memory space, or require that protocols for functions, such as communications, be changed. Conflicts between programs are common in the increasingly complicated environment of Windows and on the Internet, where not all upgrades are under the control of the user, or are even known to the user.

Computer viruses are an increasing cause of problems. They can cause a variety of difficulties ranging from erratic behavior of software to complete loss of files. They may be introduced from networks, by accessing other computer bulletin boards, or by loading copied software from unknown sources. Programs to detect and eradicate computer viruses are available commercially. It is essential to install one of these and to be sure that any disk from an external source is scanned for viruses before it is copied or used as a source of new programs.

Back-Up Methods

Methods for disaster prevention and recovery center on regular back up of data files onto floppy diskettes (or tape if available, but beware of tape back ups with only one compatible tape drive in the same institution). Write-once CD-ROMs are excellent for backup because of their permanence and immunity to magnetic fields. The standard (640-megabyte) format CD-ROM can be read by most modern computers. The back-up copies should be rotated so that several circulate in turn and so that the one overwritten has at least two more-recent relatives. To protect against fire, water damage, and damage by panic-stricken personnel (including oneself), it is wise to keep at least one back up in a site remote from the computer. Setting the write-protection feature on the diskettes after making the back up provides an additional protection.

Upgrading hardware or software should be done at a time when use of the system is least critical, and care should be taken to allow for replacing the old system exactly as it was if problems occur with the new one. Thus, before installing a new version of software, the old one should be thoroughly backed up or, preferably, left in place in another directory so that it can be used if necessary.

Training of Staff and Transition Techniques

The most effective staff training occurs by having potential operators participate in the design of the system and receive short demonstrations and hands-on lessons at the time the system is installed. Usually installation of a system takes 2 or 3 days for planning and decision making, 2 or 3 days for programming, and a similar period for staff training, trial runs, and revisions.

National meetings and training sessions for operators of state surveillance systems have been helpful in providing extra training and motivation and in revealing both problems that need to be addressed and new ideas for software improvements.

During the transition from a paper to a computerized system, both systems are run in parallel for a period until the results are satisfactory and staff members feel comfortable with the new system.

DISCUSSION

The old image of the computer expert in an expensive suit, handing the client the keys to the new turn-key system perfectly adapted to his needs, was probably always a fantasy. With modest budgets, small data bases, and a desire for hands-on access to data, such an image has little relevance to public health needs. Although in some ways centralized computers and instant interactivity for updating records would present fewer problems than the distributed systems we have described, public health workers usually do not require and cannot afford the instant updates needed for law enforcement, banking, or airline reservations. Microcomputers and local data bases can maintain the data and analytic results closer to the professionals primarily responsible for prevention and control.

Participation of all 50 state health departments in the NETSS would have been difficult without *a*) software for states that allows customization for use of local forms and procedures, *b*) participation of each state epidemiologist's staff in designing a system unique to the state, and *c*) a standardized record format. The record format for transmission was chosen as a necessary and least restrictive type of standard. Each state has a different input form from which records sent to CDC are restructured and assembled with variable values and recoded by *Epi Info* or other programs so that they are in the uniform standard national transmission format.

As systems become more complex, however, it is important to standardize as many features as possible from state to state so that a thoroughly debugged core system can be used by all. We are gradually achieving this with a new *Epi Info*–based system that has a series of standard modules, accompanied by other modules that are highly customizable.

As pointed out in this chapter, there is an enormous gap between what is technologically possible with the use of computers in public health and what is actually going on at the grass-roots level of public health practice. Until the keeping of medical records in clinical practice is computerized to a much greater extent, our scenario of the future cannot become reality.

Other key issues remaining to be resolved include *a*) the balance between confidentiality and free access to clinical data records for public health purposes; *b*) the cost of data access, programming, and processing; *c*) the ability of both professionals and the public to deal with incomplete and preliminary data; and *d*) methods for unifying data with diverse formats.

Many of these issues have both technical and social solutions. A great deal of work in both realms remains to be done before computerized public health surveillance can be said to have achieved its full potential.

Thanks to Dr. George Allen Tindol, Public Health Informatics Fellow, Epidemiology Program Office, CDC, for examining the web sites of the U.S. state and territorial health departments.

REFERENCES

1. Meehan P, Toomey KE, Drinnon J, Cunningham S, Anderson N, Baker E. Public health response for the 1996 Olympic Games. *JAMA* 1998;279(18):1469–73.
2. Zafar A, Overhage JM, McDonald CJ. Continuous speech recognition for clinicians. *JAMIA* 1999;6:195–204.
3. Dean AD, Dean JA, Burton AH, Dicker RC. *Epi Info*. Version 5. A word-processing, data-base, and statistics program for epidemiology on microcomputers. Atlanta: Centers for Disease Control, 1990.
4. Dean AD, Dean JA, Burton AH, Dicker RC. *Epi Info*: a general-purpose microcomputer program for public health information systems. *Am J Prev Med* 1991;7:178–82.
5. Harbage B, Dean AG. Distribution of *Epi Info* software: An evaluation using the Internet. *Am J Prev Med* 1999;16(4):314–7.
6. Graitcer PL, Burton AH. The epidemiologic surveillance project: a computer-based system for disease surveillance. *Am J Prev Med* 1987;3:123–7.
7. Centers for Disease Control. National Electronic Telecommunications System for Surveillance—United States, 1990–1991. *MMWR* 1991;40(29):502–3.
8. Odell-Butler ME, Ellis B, Hersey JC. Final report for task 8, an evaluation of the National Electronic Telecommunications System for Surveillance (NETSS). Arlington, Va.: Battelle, 1991:49–50.
9. The big pay-off (benefits of computerizing a business) (node supplement). *IBM System User* 1990;(March)S20.
10. Mary M, Garnerin P, Roure C *et al.* Six years of public health surveillance of measles in France. *Int J Epidemiol* 1992;21:163–8.
11. Centers for Disease Control. Surveillance of influenza-like diseases through a national computer network—France, 1984–1989. *MMWR* 1989;38(49):855–7.
12. Watkins M, Lapham S, Hoy W. Use of a medical center's computerized health-care data base for notifiable disease surveillance. *Am J Public Health* 1991;81(5):637–9.
13. Bernard KW, Graitcer PL, van der Vlugt T, Moran JS, Pulley KM. Epidemiological surveillance in Peace Corps volunteers: a model for monitoring health in temporary residents of developing countries. *Int J Epidemiol* 1989;18(1):220–6.
14. Gaynes R, Friedman C Copeland TA, Thiele GH. Methodology to evaluate a computer-based system for surveillance of hospital-acquired infections. *Am J Infec Control* 1990;18:40–6.
15. Shultz JM, Novotny TE, Rice DP. Quantifying the disease impact of cigarette smoking with SAMMEC II software. *Public Health Rep* 1991;106(3):326–33.
16. Gates B. Business at the speed of thought. New York: Warner Books, 1998.
17. Call B. The ones that got away: why some industries have not yet computerized. *PC Week* June 24, 1986;3:25.
18. Centers for Disease Control. Proposed changes in format for presentation of notifiable disease report data. *MMWR* 1988;38(47):805–9.

12

State and Local Public Health Surveillance

GUTHRIE S. BIRKHEAD
CHRISTOPHER M. MAYLAHN

All surveillance is local (paraphrased).
Tip O'Neill

Public health surveillance as discussed in this book was first defined by Alexander Langmuir in the 1960s (*1*). He expanded the traditional concept of "surveillance" as the reporting of individuals who had or had been exposed to disease so they could be monitored or quarantined to the monitoring of health and disease in whole populations in order to guide population-based public health measures. Langmuir redefined surveillance as the ongoing, systematic collection of public health data with analysis and dissemination of results and interpretation of these data to those who contributed them and to all others who "need to know." He added, "The concept, however, does not encompass direct responsibility for control activities. These traditionally have been and still remain with the state and local health authorities"(*1*).

Langmuir's definition and its accompanying caveat highlight several features of public health surveillance at the state and local level that differ from surveillance at the national level in the United States. First, the legal authority for many surveillance activities resides at the state or local level. Second, the impetus for these legal requirements is the need to prevent and control specific health problems in the local community—functions that are often better carried out by state and local public health departments because of their proximity to the population. The primary purpose of surveillance at the state and local level, and the primary justification for new surveillance activities and public health reporting requirements, is usually the need to address specific health problems. Generating data to monitor trends or to suggest research hypotheses, although an important purpose of surveillance at the national level, is usually not the primary purpose of surveillance at the state and local level. Finally, and most importantly, surveillance activities at the state and local level are closely linked to the public health programs that protect and improve the health of the community. *Surveillance* is synonymous with *control* to many public health professionals, policy makers, and legislators at the state and local level, and to members of the public. Therefore, both the historical definition of surveillance—reporting linked directly to control—and Langmuir's broader definition apply at the state and local level in ways that they may not apply at the national level.

There are substantial barriers to carrying out surveillance at the state and local level. Human and monetary resources are usually limited and often are not specifically dedicated to surveillance as distinct from public health program efforts. Few local and state health departments have the funds to employ epidemiologists trained in surveillance across the spectrum of diseases and health-related issues. Specific training on surveillance may not be available or viewed as a priority. Many health departments are therefore unable to access or fully utilize health-related data on their populations in a timely way. The tendency of federal and state public health programs and funding to be organized along categorical disease lines, with independently developed surveillance methods and computer software, has also led to fragmentation and inefficiency in surveillance at all levels, but especially at the state and local level (2).

A key issue for state and local surveillance is the ability to integrate surveillance activities and data along a number of axes (3). This integration may lead to more efficient and effective disease control activities, better understanding of how diseases are affecting local populations, or simply a reduced reporting burden on local practitioners. Examples include a) integrating laboratory and clinical data on individual cases of reportable conditions; b) integrating the flow of data from a single source, for example the clinical laboratory, for use by multiple programs (e.g., infectious disease, cancer, lead poisoning); c) interpreting community or individual data longitudinally along the natural history of disease (e.g., HIV infection, AIDS, death); and d) integrating community and individual data (e.g., cholesterol-screening programs, behavioral data on diet and exercise, and data on the incidence of cardiovascular disease).

The landmark 1988 Institute of Medicine report, *The Future of Public Health,* affirmed that assessment, including surveillance, is a core function of public health agencies at the state and local level. "An understanding of the determinants of health and the nature and extent of community need is a fundamental prerequisite to sound decision-making about health," the report stated. "Accurate information serves the interests both of justice and the efficient use of available resources. Assessment is therefore a core governmental obligation in public health." State responsibilities include "assessment of health needs within the state based on statewide data collection" and "establishment of statewide health objectives, delegating power to localities and holding them accountable." Responsibilities of local public health units include "assessment, monitoring, and surveillance of local health problems and needs and resources for dealing with them" (4).

In this chapter, we discuss those features that characterize public health surveillance at the state and local level and highlight where they may differ from surveillance at the national level. Because the purposes of surveillance vary at the national, state, and local levels, the methods used by practitioners of surveillance may differ as well. This chapter presents the current challenges that face public health surveillance at the state and local level and discusses some underlying principles and efforts under way to address these challenges.

HISTORY OF STATE AND LOCAL SURVEILLANCE IN THE UNITED STATES

Reporting of diseases of public health interest began in the United States at the local level as early as 1741 when Rhode Island instituted requirements for tavern keepers to report patrons with smallpox, yellow fever, and cholera to local authorities (5). Later, the U.S. Constitution left issues related to health to the states. Therefore, organized public health surveillance activities began at the state and local government level in the mid- to late 1800s, when the reporting of certain communicable diseases to newly established departments of health was required in some cities and states. For example, in 1874 the Board of Health in Massachusetts asked physicians to report 14 communicable diseases weekly by postcard (6) on a voluntary basis. Michigan instituted a similar system in 1883 to require, by law, the reporting of smallpox, cholera, diphtheria and scarlet fever. These initial efforts at disease reporting were later expanded to include typhoid fever, tuberculosis, and syphilis, for which isolation and quarantine—the only public health measures of the day thought to prevent further cases—could be applied. Registration of vital events (births and deaths) in the United States is, like disease reporting, a state and local function.

In the United States, a partnership between states and the federal government in the conduct of public health surveillance began in the late 1800s. States began to submit data from communicable disease reports to the federal government in 1878 when Congress authorized the Marine Hospital Service to collect such information. These reports were made by states on a voluntary basis. The first national summary of notifiable diseases was not published until 1912. The uniformity of these national surveillance efforts was improved by the development in 1913 of a model state statute for disease reporting of 53 diseases to state health departments, and then forwarded to the Surgeon General. This model law divided conditions of interest into infectious, occupational, and venereal diseases and injuries. Again, the underlying principle for selection of diseases was the ability or need to undertake public health measures, often directed at individuals with disease and their direct contacts.

An important milestone in the state/federal collaboration around public health surveillance came in 1951 with a national meeting of a group of state and territorial epidemiologists, convened through the efforts of Alexander Langmuir at CDC (7). This group established the Conference (now Council) of State and Territorial Epidemiologists (CSTE). The CSTE was designated by the Association of State and Territorial Health Officials (ASTHO) to have responsibility with CDC for determining those diseases recommended for states to list in their reporting requirements and to report voluntarily, without identifying information, to CDC. This was named the National Notifiable-Disease Surveillance System (NNDSS). Since its founding, CSTE has provided a forum to discuss surveillance issues for epidemiologists working in states, United States territories, and local health departments. The CSTE also designated state epidemiologists as surveillance consultants, in content areas such as infectious diseases and environmental health, to CDC and other federal and international agencies. In addition to CSTE, other professional organizations representing state surveillance inter-ests have worked collaboratively with the federal government to coordinate sur-veillance efforts within and across the topical areas of public health. Examples include the National Association for Public Health Statistics and Information Sys-tems in the area of vital registration; the National Association of Central Tumor Registrars on issues on cancer registries; the Association of State and Territor-ial Chronic Disease Program Directors on issues related to chronic disease sur-veillance; and the State and Territorial Injury Program Directors Association on issues related to injury prevention and control.

Federal/state surveillance coordination remains a dynamic activity as the pub-lic health and health-care systems continue to change. Recent milestones in sur-veillance coordination efforts include the 1994 National Surveillance Conference, co-hosted by CSTE and CDC, which was the first national surveillance confer-ence since the 1951 meeting (8). The conference sought to develop a blueprint for surveillance into the next century (9). In 1989, and again in 1995, CSTE and CDC jointly developed and approved the first sets of standard surveillance case definitions for public health surveillance of diseases on the NNDSS list (10,11). Efforts to standardize surveillance recommendations for states and localities have continued. In 1998, for example, CSTE and CDC sought input from more than 60 other professional organizations in developing a list of 56 indicators related to chronic diseases, risk factors, and related disease outcomes recommended for state and national surveillance. These recommendations were endorsed unanimously by CSTE members at their 1998 annual meeting (see Web site http://www.cste.org). Recent milestones in surveillance policy that affect state and local surveillance activities are summarized in Table 12–1.

Table 12–1 Recent Milestones in Surveillance Policy That Affect State and Local Surveillance Activities

Year	Milestone	Organizations
1986	CDC 5-year surveillance plan (12)	SCG/CDC
1988	Surveillance evaluation guidelines (13)	CDC
1990	Surveillance case definitions (10)	CDC/CSTE
1990	Compendium of state reporting requirements (14)	CDC
1992	Formation of CSTE national office	CSTE/CDC
1994	National surveillance conference (8)	CSTE/CDC
1995	*Integrating public health information and surveillance systems* (15)	CDC
1995–1996	Blueprint for a national public health surveillance (9)	CSTE
1996	Foundation of the Health Information and Surveillance Systems Board	CDC
1997	National list of 56 chronic diseases, risk factors, and indicators adopted*	CDC/CSTE/ASTCDPD

SCG = Surveillance Coordination Group, CDC
CSTE = Council of State and Territorial Epidemiologists
CDC = Centers for Disease Control and Prevention
ASTCDPD = Association of State and Territorial Chronic Disease Program Directors
*www.cste.org

DISTINGUISHING FEATURES OF STATE AND LOCAL PUBLIC HEALTH SURVEILLANCE

Legal Basis of Surveillance

Surveillance activities at the state and local level are usually based on specific state and local public health laws, rules, and regulations which authorize and require them (see also Chapter 10). The legal basis for surveillance is often found in the specific requirements for health-care providers and others to report to the health department persons with diseases of public health importance, and also in the general authority of state and local health commissioners (health officers) to protect the public health, including broad powers to act in emergency situations. Reporting requirements are generally placed either in statute, requiring legislative action to amend, or in rule or regulation, which health departments and boards of health may amend through administrative procedures. State laws are the basis for most surveillance activities, but large cities and counties may add additional reporting requirements. States often share surveillance data with CDC and other federal agencies on a voluntary basis or as a condition of receiving federal funds, but surveillance data with individual identifying information is almost never forwarded to CDC or other federal agencies.

Surveillance and control activities are authorized in state statute as part of the "police powers" of states (16). They balance the needs of society to protect public health and realize benefits for society that individuals acting alone could not, with the right of privacy of individuals (17,18). This tension between the need to protect the public health and individual privacy is ongoing. Recent examples include the controversy about HIV reporting (19).

Most states have laws requiring reporting of some or all communicable diseases, vital events, cancer, and environmental and occupational conditions and injuries. Although other surveillance activities, such as the use of administrative hospital discharge data or periodic health surveys for surveillance, may not have a specific legal reporting requirement, these activities may be justified by the general charge to, and powers of, state and local public health agencies to protect the public health. In general, regulated health-care providers are required to provide information on persons with reportable conditions to the health department for surveillance purposes, but the individual citizens are not required to provide information about themselves. Data gathering directly from individuals is usually voluntary.

Purposes of Surveillance

The primary purposes of surveillance at the state and local level are to trigger disease control activities and to plan, implement, and evaluate health promotion and disease prevention programs. It is primarily at the state and local level that society can "expeditiously implement interventions to prevent disease" (20). This may involve identifying cases that require specific public health follow-up, as well as collecting population-based data to direct public health programs. While the relationship between surveillance and public health interventions for chronic diseases, which develop over months or years, may be more complex than for acute diseases, the fundamental purposes are similar. The close link between surveillance and disease prevention/control activities undertaken by state and local health departments can be illustrated at four levels.

Accurate Diagnosis and Treatment

One purpose for surveillance is assuring the accurate diagnosis and appropriate treatment of an individual with a disease or condition of public health importance, and determining the source and route of infection (or how it was acquired). For example, botulism is a rare disease often linked to contaminated food. Suspicion of the diagnosis of botulism is based on symptoms and medical history (21). Since it is rare, clinicians may need assistance in making the diagnosis and accessing specific treatment (botulinum antitoxin). Therefore, reporting of cases has several purposes. Public health workers have the expertise to advise physicians on diagnosis. State public health laboratories may perform laboratory diagnostic tests for botulism which are not commonly available in clinical laboratories. Antitoxin, which is available in limited supplies, is stored at federal quarantine stations and released to physicians only after a request from state health officials. This further encourages surveillance reporting. A second example of the benefits to the individual cases of surveillance activities is in sexually transmitted disease control. Sexually transmitted diseases are also relatively rare in clinical practice, and clinicians may not be familiar with the latest treatment guidelines or antimicrobial resistance patterns in their community. Reporting to the surveillance system enables appropriate diagnosis and treatment (22).

Management of Persons Exposed to Disease

Identifying contacts of cases of disease and assuring that prevention or prophylactic measures are applied is a second purpose of surveillance. Following up with contacts of ill persons is also a case-finding mechanism for surveillance. One example is identifying close contacts of cases of meningococcal meningitis in a household or child day-care setting for the purpose of administering antibiotic prophylaxis (23). This must occur very quickly following the report of a case to prevent additional cases from occurring, making the timeliness of surveillance reporting important. Similar efforts occur following the report of cases of sexually transmitted diseases such as syphilis or gonorrhea, often referred to as "partner notification." Information about recent sexual partners is solicited on a voluntary basis from reported cases. Partners are notified of their exposure and encouraged to undergo testing and prophylaxis to prevent disease (22). Rapid reporting to the surveillance system can result in the treatment of partners during the incubation period of disease before they become infectious, thus breaking the chain of transmission. These partner notification activities may also identify the sources of infection for index cases and allow them to receive treatment. A third example is the surveillance of cases of occupational pesticide poisoning to identify the source and remove co-workers (contacts) from further exposure.

Identify Disease Outbreaks

Identifying and removing the source of transmission in disease is a third purpose of surveillance. In the botulism example discussed above, local health officials undertake an investigation in cases of confirmed or suspected botulism to determine the source of infection. This often involves collecting food samples and having them analyzed at the public health laboratory. Reporting serves the additional purpose of identifying contaminated food items, leading to a recall of such items, and can also alert other practitioners to heighten diagnostic suspicion to detect other cases as part of an outbreak. A second example is identifying clusters of farm injuries related to new farming equipment or farming practices and alerting the farming community to avoid exposure to these risks (24). Surveillance can lead to the identification of clusters of injuries, such as an unusual pattern of teen suicide attempts, prompting a community response to prevent further attempts and potential fatalities (25).

Guide Population-Based Prevention Programs

Monitoring the health status and disease trends in the community and determining the need for and effectiveness of public health programs at the community level is a fourth purpose of surveillance. Surveillance monitors disease outcomes and can measure determinants and risk factors for communicable and noncommunicable diseases. Examples include surveillance of vaccine coverage and vaccine-preventable disease morbidity to evaluate immunization programs; screening rates (e.g., mammography, cholesterol, Pap smears) and disease morbidity and mortality to evaluate cancer and cardiovascular disease screening and prevention programs; smoking prevalence by age to inform smoking prevention programs (26); and pregnancy rates to evaluate teen pregnancy prevention programs.

This section highlights disease prevention and control functions as key purposes of surveillance at the state and local level. Purposes like developing hypotheses or conducting research are of secondary importance at this level and alone are usually not sufficient to justify population-based public health surveillance activities, especially those that involve mandated reporting. At the federal level, the purposes for surveillance are more general: to determine national trends and monitor them over time, to detect emerging health problems, to demonstrate the need for resources and monitor their use, and to establish national health policy (e.g., routine vaccination recommendations).

Surveillance Is Not Research

Surveillance is not generally viewed as a research activity by public health practitioners (27). In recent years, there has been discussion among state/local and federal public health professionals about whether surveillance constitutes research in some cases (28,29). Research is defined in the federal code of regulations as a "systemic investigation . . . designed to develop or contribute to generalizable knowledge" (30). Activities which meet this definition should be reviewed and receive approval from an institutional review board (IRB). If information identifying individuals is gathered, informed consent is often required. Public health surveillance as practiced at the state and local level usually does not meet the definition of research because the purposes (see above) are not to contribute to generalizable knowledge but rather to undertake prevention and control steps among ill or at-risk persons or their communities. These direct purposes should be spelled out in laws or in supporting materials. The fact that surveillance is often not research does not lessen the need to maintain individual confidentiality or to make individuals aware that their providing information about themselves and their disease risks to public health officials is voluntary. Interestingly, surveillance data collected at the state or local level with a specific disease control purpose may be subsequently used for more general purposes. In these cases, IRB review may become necessary, especially if identified individuals are to be re-contacted or their data linked to data about them from other sources. Meanwhile, CDC and CSTE are developing guidelines defining what public health activities constitute research.

The Methods of Surveillance

Since the purposes of surveillance at the state and local level may differ from those at the national level, the preferred methods of conducting surveillance may differ as well. In 1992 and 1993, CDC and CSTE undertook an activity to identify the purposes and methods of surveillance at the federal, state and local levels (CSTE unpublished data) (9). A process of developing and modifying a list of possible purposes and methods was developed by a modified Delphi technique involving interested epidemiologists at CSTE and CDC. An example of how surveillance purposes and methods for *Haemophilus influenzae* type b (Hib) disease may differ at the local, state and national level is given in Table 12–2. At the local level, immediate disease control activities are the primary purpose of surveillance. Characterizing the epidemiology of Hib is the primary goal at the national level, which, because of the rarity of Hib, is the only level where sufficient numbers of cases to study may be present. The purposes and methods of state surveillance activities encompass some aspects from both the local and national level.

The immediate disease control purposes of surveillance at the local and state level call for universal and rapid systems of reporting. State- or locality-wide surveillance is often required, rather than sample-based or sentinel surveillance, because of the jurisdiction-wide disease control responsibilities of the public health department. Because of the small geographic areas and populations often involved, surveillance methods focusing on small area analysis are often needed. Passive surveillance systems are the norm at state and local levels. In some cases, because of the need for universal data from all communities, risk assessment, disease detection and monitoring of outcomes are performed as a secondary purpose of data collected for other reasons. The lack of resources for active systems may also explain why public health often relies on passive surveillance. Passive systems, however, may not provide all the information nec-

Table 12–2 Purposes, Methods, and Desired Attributes of Public Health Surveillance at the Local, State, and National Public Health Governmental Levels for *Haemophilus influenzae* Type B (Hib)

Purposes	Surveillance Attributes	Methods
Local Health Department Level		
• Proper diagnosis and treatment of cases • Prophylaxis of contacts	• Timeliness • Sensitivity	• Case reporting by physicians and emergency rooms • Laboratory reporting of clinical isolates to detect on reported cases
State Health Department Level		
• Monitor and assure appropriate local surveillance and control • Detect intercounty clusters • Assess Hib vaccination programs • Obtain resources and institute regulatory action to control disease	• Completeness of reporting • Positive predictive value of reports	• Collect data from local health department • State public health laboratory confirmation of diagnosis • Review hospital discharge and mortality data for unreported cases • Assess vaccine usage and coverage
National Level		
• Monitor nationwide trends • Characterize epidemiology of Hib (vaccine efficacy; risk factors for disease • Detect interstate outbreaks • Obtain resources	• Complete demographic and risk data • Positive predictive value • Comparability • Flexibility	• Collect data from state health department • Special studies and surveys

essary to make informed public health decisions. More active, targeted surveillance may be necessary in these cases, or the information may simply not be available.

Since direct provision of disease control activities is usually not a federal function, reporting of individual cases of disease does not occur directly to the national level. For example, notification, or disease reporting, is an important method for surveillance at the state and local level (see below). The methods of surveillance employed at the national level include aggregating local and state data (see descriptions below for NNDSS and Behavioral Risk-Factor Surveillance System (BRFSS)) and conducting surveys of nationally representative samples. This latter method usually can not be used to provide estimates for each state or locality. Examples of national surveillance methods that may not provide state/local-specific estimates include the Hepatitis Sentinel Counties Surveillance System, the National Nosocomial Infection Surveillance System, the National Electronic Injury Surveillance System, and the National Hospital Discharge Survey.

Selection of Surveillance Measures

The choice of measures used to describe health status, population characteristics, or community attributes related to health is a distinguishing characteristic of disease surveillance at different levels of the population. At the local level, collection of data directly related to the control efforts is a priority. For example, collection of name and address is important to locate individuals for follow-up or to eliminate duplicate reports. This information may not be needed at the federal level or even the state level. On the other hand, information on race, ethnicity, etc., is very useful in monitoring national trends and comparing one area of the country with another. However, most states and local communities do not have sufficient heterogeneity in these variables to justify devoting limited resources to their measurement.

Measures appropriate for state and local surveillance fall into several different classes: health *status measures* include the number of people with a given risk factor, health condition, or disease; *sociodemographic measures* include population characteristics such as educational attainment, income, and marital status; and *community-level measures* include characteristics of the community that influence health such as policies, ordinances, and environmental supports for healthy behavior. Cheadle *et al.* (*31*) have described a class of community-level measures, called *environmental indicators,* which derive from observation of the community environment. The term *environment* is used broadly to include anything external to individuals that is shared by members of the community, such as the legal, social, and economic environments, as well as the physical one. Environmental indicators measure an important intermediate step in community-based interventions, namely environmental factors that influence health and behavior. Examples of measures in each of these classes, at different levels of population, that pertain to tobacco use, are given in Table 12–3.

Whether they can be measured, their robustness, and their relevance to the health condition or issue of interest judge the importance of these indicators for state/local surveillance. They must be actionable, that is, amenable to change through public health approaches, sensitive enough to reflect often subtle and incremental changes, and timely. The need to link action to outcome has led to an increasing emphasis on measuring proximal versus distal indicators and to use surveillance for performance measurement. In this context, proximal indicators reflect changes that are closely linked in time, space, and causality to the actions taken. For chronic disease surveillance, proximal indicators are especially useful because the changes that result from interventions may take a long time to manifest, or because actual changes in behavior or health status may be difficult or too expensive to measure.

The issue of performance measurement for public health programs was recently addressed by the National Research Council, which published two reports on performance measures (*32,33*). The authors acknowledge that performance measurement presents the opportunity to focus attention on defining and using evidence-based best practices to achieve desired outcomes. The second of these reports focused on recommended improvements to existing local, state, and fed-

Table 12–3 Integrated Surveillance Matrix Using Tobacco Control as an Example

Levels of Surveillance	Background Variables (Contributing Factors)	Input Variables (Pro-Tobacco and Tobacco Control Influences)	Intermediate Outcome Variables	Primary and Secondary Outcomes Variables	Goal Outcome Variables
Individual	Level of education	Exposure to direct tobacco marketing	Attitudes, beliefs, program awareness and support	Maintenance of tobacco-free lifestyle, average number of cigarettes smoked	Number of upper respiratory infections over time
Family/household	Income	Parental tobacco use, number of members using tobacco	Family rules, family enforcement policies	Family exposure to tobacco smoke, number of new smokers	Exacerbations of childhood asthma
Community	Social capital (readiness to change)	Advertising, media	Support for tobacco control policies	Reduce tobacco use prevalence	Rates of emphysema, lung cancer, CVD
Organization	Health promotion infrastructure	Program funding, Tobacco control policies	Incentives for reducing tobacco use	Reduce employee tobacco use prevalence, number of quit attempts	Rates of absenteeism among smokers/former smokers
Geopolitical	Political climate, existing tobacco-related ordinances	Political contributions	Support for tobacco control policies	New tobacco control ordinances, legislation	Funding for tobacco control programs

eral data systems that would facilitate the collection of data for performance measurement. These improvements would simultaneously benefit disease surveillance since the necessary investment in data collection systems, and their coordination, would likely lead to more efficient measurement of health outcomes.

One class of measures that has been receiving increasing interest includes the so-called composite measures of health, such as quality-adjusted life years (*34*). These measures provide governmental agencies and others with a set of estimates of current patterns of health, disease, and disability for national and international comparisons. Their potential value in policy development and allocation of resources is great; yet the ability of state and local public health departments to obtain or produce the data needed for their calculation is still highly variable.

SURVEILLANCE SYSTEMS AND METHODS OF IMPORTANCE AT THE STATE AND LOCAL LEVEL

The following sections describe six of the major state and local surveillance systems and provide a practical example of each.

Notification (Reportable-Disease Surveillance)

Notification was one of the earliest forms of surveillance and is still employed especially for communicable and other acute diseases where public health action may be triggered by an individual case or where an individual case may be the indication that a disease outbreak is occurring. Physicians and hospitals have historically been required to report, but reporting of diagnostic test results by laboratories is becoming an increasingly important source, and many states now require reporting from laboratories for appropriate diseases and conditions (*35*). If action is to be taken on each individual case, it is important to strive for complete reporting (e.g., meningitis or lead poisoning). Otherwise, completeness of reporting is often poor.

Example: Communicable Disease Surveillance

Surveillance Methods
States develop legal reporting requirements using as a guide the list of communicable diseases recommended to be under surveillance as part of the NNDSS (*36*), as well as based on local public health priorities. The NNDSS list is developed and revised periodically by CDC and CSTE. The current list of state reporting requirements was recently published (*34*) and is available in updated form at Web site http://www.cste.org. Surveillance case definitions for each disease or condition are established and revised periodically by CSTE and CDC (*11*). The most current definitions are available at Web site http://www.cdc.gov/epo/phs.htm. Most case definitions require laboratory test results to confirm a surveillance report, but also contain a clinical case definition to enable providers to report cases without or in advance of laboratory confirmation. Funding is usually obtained through a combination of state and local funds, federal block grant funds (e.g.,

Preventive Health Services Block Grant), and federal categorical program funding (e.g., STD, immunization, TB, and HIV categorical program funds). There is no established program of federal categorical funding for general communicable-disease surveillance.

Authorization for Data Collection and Confidentiality
State statutes, rules, and regulations usually require reporting. In some states, the list incorporates the national list by reference to the NNDSS list. State statutes authorizing reporting generally provide for protection of this confidential information, but specificity of these protections varies (*17*). Identifying information is not sent to CDC.

Data Sources and Collection
All states require reporting of selected notifiable disease by physicians. In practice, hospitals often fulfill the reporting function for attending physicians of hospitalized patients with reportable conditions. Increasingly, clinical laboratories also require reporting; managed-care organizations may be required to report as well in some states. In states with local health departments, reporting is commonly to the level at which any immediate public health action would be taken (Figure 12–1). In states without local public health infrastructure, reports may go directly to the state health department. For most of this century and even to some extent today, reporting of notifiable disease from health-care providers and laboratories is done by mail, although many efforts are under way to develop electronic reporting systems.

Initial reports, especially from laboratories, may not contain complete information on demographic variables, exposure and risk factors, treatment, and other information needed for immediate public health action (for example, in sensitive settings like day-care centers for children or commercial food preparation facil-

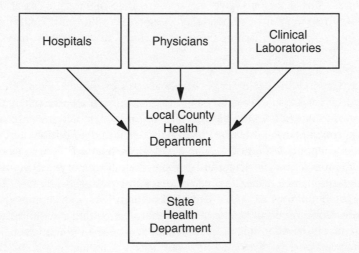

Figure 12–1 The flow of infectious disease surveillance data at the state and local level.

ities). Part of the surveillance protocol, therefore, includes a public health worker (e.g., a public health nurse who contacts the diagnosing physician to obtain missing information). The workload and cost in this step in surveillance are substantial and often underestimated. For this reason, contact with the physician for additional data may not occur in all cases unless the disease in question requires public health action to treat contacts or if an outbreak is suspected. While reporting is legally required, states and local health departments generally rely on the voluntary cooperation of physicians to report, and physicians are rarely sanctioned for failure to report (37,38).

Local health departments forward disease reports to state health departments on a periodic basis (Figure 12–1). Until recently, these reports have been sent through the postal system, but increasingly this, too, is occurring electronically. States forward individual case-level data to CDC weekly in a standard format without identifiers. This transmittal occurs from all states, but on a voluntary basis.

Data Analysis and Dissemination
Currently all states and most local areas are able to computerize communicable disease surveillance data. The CDC has supplied standard data elements, coding, and electronic formats as part of the National Electronic Telecommunications System for Surveillance (NETSS) (39). Program staff at the state and local level should analyze surveillance data on reportable diseases on a regular basis to monitor trends and detect outbreaks, but it is not known how many do so. Automated software programs to monitor trends and detect outbreaks may assist with this process routinely in the future (40). At a minimum, annual summaries and interpretation of surveillance data should be produced and disseminated by all state health departments. National data, by state, for most NNDSS diseases are published weekly and annually in the *MMWR*. Increasingly, Web-based surveillance data on reportable diseases are available at Web site http://www.cdc.gov/epo/phs.htm. These systems give the option of accommodating user-defined analyses with appropriate confidentiality safeguards to prevent identifying individuals in local areas by limiting minimum cell size in cross-table analyses.

Key Surveillance System Attributes
Completeness and timeliness are key attributes of surveillance. Completeness is enhanced by relying on laboratory reporting because there are relatively few laboratories to interact with to ensure complete reporting, and many have electronic systems that make it feasible to automate reporting of positive test results indicating a reportable disease for the health department. Effective laboratory reporting requires that physicians order appropriate laboratory tests so that specific diagnoses can be made. For example, reportable diarrheal diseases may be missed if stool cultures are not ordered and patients receive symptomatic treatment only. Concerns have been expressed that cost-cutting measures in medicine may result in under-diagnosis and under-reporting of conditions of public health interest.

Vital Registration

All states and most major cities require the registration of live births, marriages and dissolution of marriages, and deaths, (usually including fetal deaths), among their residents. The basis for vital registration resides in state and federal statute. Reports are filed by local registrars, hospitals, and attending physicians. The reporting form used is based on the national standard certificate (or standard data set when used in electronic reporting). States have some flexibility in the format and content of this certificate, with the ability to ask for additional information. Fetal deaths, which include spontaneous abortions and induced terminations of pregnancy, are reported on a separate certificate. By comparing births and deaths in a given year, states can perform a more detailed review of maternal characteristics associated with pregnancy. There is under way a transition to electronic registration of the birth and death certificate, which will minimize the reporting burden of births and deaths, accelerate the calculation of birth and death rates, and facilitate the linkage of the two events.

States have found many uses for information on births and deaths, including making population projections, forecasting disease trends, planning needed health services, predicting the need for new schools, etc. Because this information is obtained continuously for all events (not a sample), the data permit calculation of rates for small geographic areas and trends over time. Through analysis of mortality data and mortality reviews, high-risk population subgroups or geographic areas that have experienced excess mortality can be identified. The health-care system uses this information to identify deficiencies in the delivery of services and access to care, and to evaluate health interventions.

Example: Infant Mortality

Surveillance Methods
The infant mortality rate is the number of infant deaths during the year per 1,000 population. Information on births and deaths is usually completed by doctors, hospital staff, nurse midwives, funeral directors, coroners, and medical examiners using the standard certificate or fetal death certificate (not all states require fetal death reporting; some require it only if gestation meets a minimum threshold). All states receive funding from the NCHS to conduct mortality registration. States submit mortality data, including identifiers, to NCHS. In some states, NCHS provides additional funds to obtain more information from case reviews about the circumstances of death.

Authorization for Data Collection and Confidentiality
The requirement for reporting all live births, fetal deaths, and all other types of deaths is found in state statute; the federal government has no jurisdiction in this regard. States require reporting for all events within their respective jurisdictions, not just for their residents. By agreement, states share certificates for non-residents with the state of residence; this process is protected by strict confidentiality safeguards, which vary across the nation.

Data Sources and Collection
Deaths are required to be reported to state or local registrars; the physician who certifies the death completes the death certificate and includes the cause of death. Electronic reporting of these certificates occurs in some states. The calculation of infant mortality requires knowing the number of live births and deaths up to one year of age, using the standard birth and death certificates. States design their own certificates. Most states use the national standard certificates as a model, deleting items of no interest, adding items of local interest, and rewording items as appropriate.

Data Analysis and Dissemination
Infant mortality is a very common and widely used health measure. Fortunately, in many communities or small geographic areas, an infant death is a rare event. Because of small numbers or unexpected circumstances, the rate in local areas may fluctuate widely from one year to the next. Therefore, a multi-year average (e.g., over three years) is often presented. Annual reports, including electronic data tabulations on the Internet, are used to disseminate this information.

Key Surveillance System Attributes
Reporting of births and deaths is a well-established practice and is legally required. Timeliness and completeness are generally good. The information for events occurring in hospitals tends to be more accurate, since for deaths occurring outside the hospital, the circumstances of death and its potential causes may not be fully known.

Disease Registries

Statutory reporting of individuals with specific diseases or conditions, or those who have received immunizations, is employed to study certain public health problems in greater depth. Cancer registration is the most common, with cancer registries now established in many states. Registries have also been established for conditions such as congenital malformations, traumatic brain injury, and Alzheimer's disease. They are often statutorily required. Registries are like disease notification systems, but often are used in chronic disease control where ongoing, longitudinal data are collected on individuals. This enables surveillance of disease at different stages: diagnosis (risk factors for illness, efficacy of screening and prevention programs), treatment (health-care access, treatment success), and mortality (combination of prevention, screening, and treatment efficacy). For some conditions like Alzheimer's disease, academic institutions have established disease registries for research purposes. Without statutory authority of reporting, such registries are often based on consenting clinic populations and are therefore not population based.

Example: Cancer Surveillance

Surveillance Methods
Cancer registries collect information about people diagnosed with cancer. Depending on resources available, the information may include basic demographic

data on the individual and type of tumor, or may encompass detailed data on the anatomic site of the tumor, the stage at diagnosis, the cell type of the cancer, and treatment and follow-up clinical information. When a person is diagnosed with more than one type of cancer, information is obtained for each separate tumor in a case report. Most registries include reports of all malignant cancers. Some skin cancers, as well as basal cell and squamous cell carcinomas, may not be reported because they are rarely fatal and usually do not require hospitalization. Sociodemographic information, such as age, sex, ethnicity, race, residence, and place of birth, as well as date and cause of death, are usually obtained. The methods used for cancer registration have been well-documented (41,42).

The National Cancer Institute (NCI) supports the Surveillance, Epidemiology and End-Results (SEER) program that was mandated to assemble a representative sample of the United States to study cancer. The NCI funds population-based SEER registries in a few states and some cities. In the remaining states and some territories, CDC supports cancer registries through the National Program of Cancer Registries, which has established standards for data collection that guide reporting in states. In 1995, the federal Cancer Registries Amendment Act provided new or additional funding to state cancer registries. Besides federal funding for cancer registries, many states provide funding support for their registries. Most cancer registries are represented in the North American Association of Central Cancer Registries (NAACCR), which sets standards and goals for the member registries to meet and promotes the use of cancer registry data in studies of defined populations and in cancer control programs. Useful Web sites for obtaining more information about cancer registries are www.cdc/cancer/npcr/ and www.seer.ims.nci.nih.gov/.

Authorization for Data Collection and Confidentiality
In most state-based cancer registries, reporting of cancer cases is required in state law. These laws date back to 1940, when New York State passed the first law that required reporting of cancer cases diagnosed in the state, outside New York City, to the state health department; the law was amended in 1973 to include all cancer cases in the state. All information reported to cancer registries is considered confidential, with strict procedures in place to protect the privacy of cancer patients and to limit the release of information to outside investigators. Research studies involving data with patient identifiers must be approved by IRBs. Furthermore, release of individual-level data for small geographic areas is restricted, and when there is a low number of cases in a small area, the exact number of cases is not revealed.

Data Sources and Collection
Each time a patient is diagnosed with a new tumor, a report is sent to the state health department. Frequently, reports are submitted by hospitals, although other types of reporting facilities include pathology laboratories and physicians. With recent changes in the health-care delivery system that have altered the manner in which cancer is diagnosed and treated, reporting occurs increasingly from non-hospital sources such as ambulatory care centers.

Data Analysis and Dissemination

Descriptive information about the cancer registry, such as the reporting sources and data quality and completeness, is useful in evaluating the general quality of the registry and in interpreting differences among them. For incidence registries, the anatomic site- and sex-specific cancer incidence rates are calculated. Mortality rates are also produced. Both of these rates can be calculated for sub-state areas, such as counties, although it is usually necessary to combine years to produce stable rates (e.g., 5-year incidence rates). Both crude and adjusted rates can be calculated, using U.S. or world population counts for standardization. The age adjustment allows cancer rates in communities with different age structures to be compared.

Key Surveillance System Attributes

Because cancer surveillance is legally required and considered a major public health priority, cancer registry data are generally of high quality, relatively complete, and representative of the state's population. Some registries, especially in states that lack the resources to maintain them, are not timely in releasing information and may be incomplete. Most registries do not track clinical outcomes in reported cases.

Sentinel Surveillance

Sentinel surveillance systems involve a limited number of selected reporting sites, reports from which may be generalizable to the whole population. Such systems may be useful for common conditions where complete case counting is not important and where public health action is not taken in response to individual reported cases. Such systems may be cheaper to operate than case-based reporting systems.

Example: Influenza Surveillance

Surveillance Methods

Influenza is a disease of public health importance that occurs in epidemic form each winter in the United States, causing tens of thousands of cases and excess deaths. It is preventable by vaccination, and outbreaks caused by influenza type A strains can be prevented or terminated by use of antiviral therapy (*43*). Despite influenza's public health importance and preventability, individual cases of influenza are generally not reportable in most states because the large number of cases would overwhelm the communicable-disease surveillance system and because public health action is usually not taken in response to each case. In addition, the clinical definition of influenza is not highly specific and laboratory confirmation is not often sought, nor is it widely available, in most clinical settings. Surveillance for influenza is helpful to determine the level of disease activity in the population, to detect outbreaks in sensitive settings like nursing homes, and to inform clinicians and the public about which strains of influenza are circulating. This permits antiviral prophylaxis or treatment of persons at risk for complications. Investigation of selected outbreaks allows determination of the vaccine efficacy of the current influenza vaccine to the predominant circulating strains.

Sentinel surveillance is an appropriate methodology to achieve these purposes. Sentinel physicians or clinics are a selected group who agree to report rates of influenza-like respiratory illness and may obtain nasopharyngeal swabs for viral diagnosis on some ill patients. Reports of aggregate data are usually submitted by sentinel sites to the state or local health department each week. In a recent survey of all states, three-quarters used sentinel physicians for influenza surveillance, the most common method used (CSTE, unpublished data). Many states also conduct other types of sentinel surveillance for influenza such as monitoring rates of absenteeism in selected occupational or school settings or rates of respiratory illness rates in selected clinical practices where clinical specimens to determine strain type may also be collected. Some states receive pneumonia and influenza mortality reports from the vital registrars in cities participating in the national 121 cities surveillance system (44). Data from all these sources, combined with reports of influenza outbreaks, allow state communicable-disease epidemiologists to report to CDC on a weekly basis the level of influenza activity in their states. No specific federal funding is available for state or local influenza surveillance, although some states have used immunization or other categorical funds from CDC to support this activity.

Authorization for Data Collection and Confidentiality
Data collection is usually authorized under the general powers of the state health department or health commissioner, with the cooperation of sentinel reporting sites. Individual cases of influenza may be reportable in some states, but efforts are rarely expended to encourage reporting. Aggregate data without personal identifiers are generally collected from sentinel sites, so data protection and confidentiality are of less concern. Personal identifiers collected in the course of outbreak investigations are not released beyond the health department.

Data Sources and Collection
Aggregate data are usually collected by telephone, fax, or electronic mail on a weekly basis. Clinical specimens are referred to collaborating public health laboratories for identification and typing of influenza strains.

Data Analysis and Dissemination
Because the surveillance data are crude and often in aggregate form, detailed analysis is limited. Data on overall influenza-like illness activity, strain type, and outbreaks are used to determine the level of influenza activities in each state. This information is sent weekly from states to CDC, where it is compiled into a national picture of influenza activity. Maps of influenza activity by state are displayed on television and on the World Wide Web. The *MMWR* usually publishes summaries of influenza activity during the year (45). Local newsletters and press releases also disseminate data.

Key Surveillance System Attributes
Representativeness is the key attribute of sentinel surveillance systems. This ensures that information from a limited number of sentinel sites can be generalized to the whole population.

Periodic Population-Based Surveys

Periodic or ongoing surveys are commonly used to estimate the proportion of people with some particular characteristic (e.g., overweight, immunized with pneumococcal vaccine). Sometimes, population based surveys are conducted to obtain information about an emerging or priority issue, but unless such surveys are repeated at some future interval(s), they are not considered surveillance.

Population-based surveys are conducted using a variety of methods depending on the desired participation or response rate, acceptable levels of validity and reliability of the collected information, and the need for the sample to represent underlying populations. Mailed surveys are usually the least expensive but require having address information for a defined study population. The response rate for mailed surveys is usually lower than that for other types of survey methods.

For population-based surveys to be useful for comparison among different populations—within states, among states, or between a state and the nation as a whole—surveys on the same topic should use a common methodology where possible. A standard protocol should define what information is collected, how each question is worded, how the sample is selected, how the data are weighted to the underlying population, etc. While state and local health departments may wish to customize surveys to their own needs, the loss of comparability may decrease the value of local data.

Example: Behavioral Risk Factor Surveillance System (BRFSS)

Surveillance Methods
The BRFSS is a state-based surveillance system operating in all states and most U.S. territories. It is the primary source of state-based information on risk behaviors among adult populations. In operation since the early 1980s, the BRFSS is a collaboration between CDC and the states in terms of how the survey is designed, conducted, and funded. Adults are asked about their knowledge, attitudes, and practices regarding leading causes of disease and mortality. States select a random sample of adults for a telephone interview. Every state uses similar methods for selecting respondents and the same core questions to facilitate comparisons. After appropriate weighting, the selection process results in a representative sample for each state so that statistical inferences can be made from the information collected. The BRFSS is supported by federal funding and supplemented by state funding in some states. A BRFSS Web site, with descriptive information and data from all the states, is located at http://www.cdc.gov/nccdphp/brfss/.

Authorization for Data Collection and Confidentiality
There is no statutory authority for the collection of data using the BRFSS. Trained interviewers using a computer-assisted telephone interview collect all data. Respondents participate voluntarily and confidentiality safeguards protect their identity. Identifying information is discarded when the survey is completed.

Data Sources and Collection
The BRFSS is conducted by staff located in state health departments or by survey firms hired by the state. The raw, unweighted data from each state's monthly interviews are sent to CDC for processing and analysis. Data collection is continuous throughout the year using a standard questionnaire for the year.

Data Analysis and Dissemination
Annual reports for each state are produced using BRFSS data. States submit final unweighted data to the CDC. The CDC calculates weighted prevalence information and statistical reports for states to use, in hard copy, on CD-ROMs, and on the Internet. The more extensive analyses and dissemination of data are done at the state level with technical assistance from CDC.

Key Surveillance System Attributes
The BRFSS is a flexible surveillance system that provides population-based information on the important precursors and behavioral determinants of disease at the state level. The information is limited by the reliance on self-report and the variable participation and response rates among communities.

Secondary Use of Administrative Data

The most common administrative data systems used for public health surveillance at state and local levels include hospital discharge data, health insurance and Medicaid billing data, managed-care encounter data, pharmacy information systems, and the claims data maintained by the Health Care Financing Administration (HCFA) for Medicare recipients. A limitation of these systems is that they are not designed for pubic health surveillance. Instead, their primary function is usually to pay bills, monitor health-care costs, and assess general patterns of care. The accuracy and completeness of diagnostic information may be uncertain. The advantages of such systems are their relative availability in electronic form, full population coverage, and low cost for secondary uses like surveillance.

Hospital discharge data are the most commonly used for surveillance purposes. Individuals discharged from hospitals are reported to a central location (usually the state health department) and their reason for hospitalization is specified according to the *International Classification of Diseases (ICD)*. More than half the states now have such systems in place. Due to the growing public health interest in preventing injuries, many hospitals have introduced a coding system, called e-codes, to document the circumstances or selected health conditions that may have been related to an injury (e.g., hip fracture).

Example: Asthma

Surveillance Methods

At their 1998 annual meeting, CSTE unanimously endorsed placing asthma under state and national surveillance and recommended enumeration, by review of administrative data (specifically, hospital discharge data or the cause of death recorded on the standard death certificate). A person hospitalized for their asthma can be identified in hospital discharge data using specific ICD codes, which may appear as a "primary" or "secondary" cause on the hospital discharge abstract. Emergency department billing systems, where they exist, may often provide a means to count people who visited the emergency room because of asthma.

Authorization for Data Collection and Confidentiality

In some states, hospitals must report all hospital discharges to the state health department or other state agency. Emergency department visits and use of ambulatory care for treatment of asthma or its exacerbation are not currently reported in most jurisdictions. Recently, there have been at least two unsuccessful attempts to pass legislation requiring the establishment of asthma registries (New York and California).

Data Sources and Collection

Depending on the asthma-related measure, the data source is an existing reporting form or system containing information relevant to the surveillance of asthma. Hospital discharge data are usually reported electronically in a standard format taken from a written discharge summary or abstract. The data usually contain billing information; primary, multiple, and secondary causes of hospitalization; and treatment and procedures employed.

Data Analysis and Dissemination

The information from hospital discharge data systems, for example, is analyzed to produce discharge rates per population in the hospital catchment area or for the population living in a particular geographic area (e.g., counties or census tracts).

Key Surveillance System Attributes

The surveillance of asthma using administrative systems is affected by the access and availability of primary care and of specialty or follow-up treatment for people with asthma. When asthma first manifests in young children, it is often too difficult to diagnose and there is also variability in how local practitioners define asthma. Furthermore, people with asthma often have multiple encounters with the health-care system so the lack of unique identifiers in administrative data systems makes it difficult to eliminate duplicate counts or follow the longitudinal course of individual patients. However, alternative approaches using case reporting by medical providers would pose a huge burden on the public health system, thus making administrative systems a more feasible approach for asthma surveillance.

Other Data Sources

To carry out surveillance activities, state and local health departments use many other sources of data. These include, for example, vector surveillance for mosquitoes and ticks which are capable of carrying disease; environmental surveillance of potable water quality in public water systems; surveillance of zoonotic disease with potential for human impact (e.g., animal rabies, bovine tuberculosis). In the area of injury surveillance, police reports can be a good source of surveillance data on firearm-related injuries at the state and local level (46). Emergency rooms are also a good source of injury data (25).

CONSTRAINTS AND OPPORTUNITIES IN
STATE AND LOCAL SURVEILLANCE

Resource Needs

Lack of dedicated funding for surveillance activities at state and local levels is an ongoing concern. State and local public health budgets have become increasingly constrained with efforts to shrink the size of state governments. Existing resources for surveillance often come from federal categorical monies that primarily fund programmatic efforts, and which may limit states' flexibility to support overall surveillance efforts. For example, a 1992 survey of states in the area of communicable-disease surveillance showed that 85% of all funding for state communicable-disease surveillance and 80% of state and local communicable-disease surveillance personnel were supported by four categorical federal programs HIV/AIDS, STD, TB, and immunization (2). Federal block grants are a common source of funding support for state-based epidemiologists, but over time have become strapped because of cuts in state funding for public health. Consequently, surveillance resources, when they do exist, come piecemeal from individual federal grants.

These funding restrictions have begun to be addressed on a number of fronts. In 1998 CDC and Health Resources and Services Administration (HRSA) announced an initiative to increase flexibility in the use of categorical grant funds for the development of integrated health information systems extending beyond the categorical boundaries. Under this so-called *investment analysis* initiative, states with a plan for integrated health information systems can request the use of a percentage of their federal categorical funds for the purpose of surveillance and information system support (see http://www.cdc.gov/funds). To date, a few states have begun the application process. Another example of the federal government seeking to address this issue is the 1999 funding for state bioterrorism preparedness which allowed states to dedicate funding for support of basic public health infrastructure, including surveillance systems.

Personnel and training are also resource needs. The challenges facing state and local public health surveillance often come down to the common denominator of public health programs, the local public health practitioner. This person, often a public health nurse, sanitary engineer, or baccalaureate-prepared public health worker must often work across several categorical programs because of resource limitations and needs adequate training to carry out surveillance tasks. Because surveillance may take a secondary role to disease control activities, these practitioners may view themselves principally as public health disease control workers. Their role and training as "surveillance practitioners" may be seen as secondary. Caps and hiring freezes on the number of full-time employees (FTEs) are common at many state and local health departments, making hiring difficult.

Definition of Core Public Health Surveillance Capacity

A better definition of core public health surveillance capacity in terms of monetary and personnel resources is a necessary step in increasing the level of understanding of surveillance on the part of policy makers and the general public, and ultimately in obtaining needed resources for surveillance. Although state capacity in communicable-disease surveillance is limited in terms of funding and availability of communicable-disease epidemiologists in all areas (2,47), it often exceeds capacity to perform other surveillance.

A number of surveys of state surveillance capacity in non-infectious disease areas have been reported (48). Before 1990, few state health departments were staffed by an epidemiologist who had responsibility for providing coordinated support across a range of categorical chronic disease programs. By the end of the decade, the number of states with such a person had increased to 28. These staff must cover a large range of issues, often with no local expert with whom they can consult. Even with recent gains, chronic disease surveillance staff are severely strained in most states and territories.

A survey of state environmental health surveillance capacity showed that only one state had surveillance systems covering 12 core environmental health conditions (49). Twenty-three states had systems covering only one or two of the core conditions, and one state had none. In terms of funding, the majority of lead poisoning surveillance systems were completely dependent on federal funding.

A survey regarding state-based asthma surveillance showed that while all states have access to asthma mortality data and 82% have access to hospitalization data, availability was less for other sources of surveillance data. For example, only 31% had access to emergency department data (50). Only 20% reported they had ever done a survey for asthma prevalence. And availability of data did not guarantee its use; only 34% of those with access to hospital discharge data had used it for public health purposes.

The capacity for surveillance of injuries at the state and local level is also low and is largely dependent on federal funding. A series of firearm injury surveillance projects funded by CDC were highlighted in the October 1998 issue of the *American Journal of Preventive Medicine* (46). The CDC also funds about a dozen states for traumatic brain injury surveillance, five states for bicycle safety and 14 for fire prevention programs, all of which use the BRFSS as their primary surveillance tool. Several states are piloting emergency department–based injury surveillance systems. The extent of these activities in states without federal funding is not known. Similarly, only 73% of responding states identified any occupational health activities including surveillance that were not related to the Occupational Safety and Health Administration (OSHA) (CSTE, unpublished data). Even in the area of communicable-disease surveillance there are limitations. A survey of state sexually transmitted disease control programs showed the median number of full-time-equivalent (FTE) epidemiologists working the programs was 0.5 (*51*). One-quarter of the programs had no epidemiologist. Almost half of the programs indicated they had inadequate epidemiological support, including staff resources for surveillance.

Building epidemiologic capacity will require strategies that take into account the availability of trained epidemiologists across these disciplines and the need to identify and coordinate personnel mechanisms and potential sources of funding to fill positions. Because most funding sources are categorically focused, state and local health departments face obstacles in establishing positions that are comprehensive and versatile.

Another facet of the capacity issue is the competencies of existing staff to carry out surveillance functions. In states where epidemiological capacity is limited to one or two staff epidemiologists for all programs, these individuals are required to have a broad range of skills. Through periodic surveys and many anecdotal reports, it is known that staff in state and territorial health departments vary greatly in their knowledge of epidemiology and surveillance methods, especially with respect to chronic diseases, and in their capacity to analyze and use epidemiological data to plan and evaluate community programs. Ongoing training in surveillance is important and must remain a priority.

Surveillance System Design

Surveillance system design must be sensitive to state and local needs and limitations (see also Chapter 2). Much surveillance system design and software development occurs at the federal level. However, state involvement and "buy-in" are necessary for the products of this developmental work to be readily incorporated into public health programs (large states have similar issues with respect to their local health departments). States must be able to directly influence the design and content of the data collection to more effectively address state and local information needs. This encourages the inclusion of relevant data items and should lead to greater use of the data for planning, evaluation, and routine surveillance. The ability to generate local data promotes a sense of ownership. To achieve this, state and local representation is needed in setting national surveillance policy, for example on various federal advisory committees. Flexibility, timeliness, and representativeness are particularly important surveillance system attributes at the state and local level.

Incompleteness of Provider-Based Reporting

There is a common misconception that placing a disease or condition on a list of reportable diseases means that surveillance, or even reporting, will occur. In fact, physicians have historically been poor reporters for most diseases. This is one of the reasons that redundancy has been built into current communicable disease reporting systems over time. Laboratory reporting is useful for conditions which have confirmatory laboratory tests. In addition, acute/severe diseases, which require timely public health action (e.g., meningitis) will often result in hospitalization, where reporting may be improved. Still, nonacute diseases that are based on physician diagnosis will probably continue to be underreported.

The completeness of physician reporting compared to laboratory reporting is poor. In one state study, 71% of initial reports of confirmed cases of notifiable diseases originated from clinical laboratories; only 10% originated from physicians' offices (52). Another study showed that approximately 85% of cases of shigellosis are reported, but laboratories accounted for almost all of the reports received. Laboratories reported 77% of all reported cases, compared with only 6% for physicians (53). Reasons for failure to report cited by physicians in several studies include *a*) lack of knowledge that reporting was required, including not knowing what diseases are reportable or how to report; *b*) concerns about breaching patient confidentiality; *c*) no incentives for reporting; and, *d*) no time to report (52,54–56).

Efforts to improve physician reporting have included active surveillance with regular phone calls to physician offices, which have resulted in two- to five-fold increases in reporting (57–59). In addition, physician education to understand the importance of reporting and feedback from surveillance data may result in improved reporting. Ideally, such education would start in medical school and subsequently include educational mailings, grand rounds presentations, linkage to CME credits or licensing, etc. However, these measures are expensive, time consuming, must be ongoing, and probably are utilized routinely only in rare instances where funding is adequate (e.g. AIDS surveillance). Because health-care providers are poor reporters and the efforts to improve reporting are expensive and must be sustained indefinitely, efforts to collect public health surveillance data should increasingly be directed to sources of data in electronic form such as computerized clinical laboratories, medical record systems, and managed-care data bases. As data from these systems become more accessible for public health purposes, the need to encourage physician reporting will only exist when immediate reporting of clinical syndromes is needed to trigger a rapid public health response (e.g., bacterial meningitis), or for cases where there is not a confirmatory laboratory test.

Harnessing the Health Care and Electronic Data Revolutions

Dramatic changes in the ways that medical care is delivered as well as the increased availability of health-related data in electronic form provide an important opportunity to enhance public health surveillance at the state and local level. Electronic data from clinical laboratories, managed-care organizations, birth and death certificates, and emergency rooms may be the core of future public health surveillance efforts at the state and local level (see also Chapters 4 and 11). State and local health departments must move beyond the U.S. mail for transmission of surveillance data. In addition, innovative surveillance methods and use of nontraditional sources of surveillance data such as newspaper reports for injuries will become increasingly important.

These new data sources bring new issues in surveillance. First, public health surveillance practitioners need to participate in standard-setting processes around electronic medical information systems (60,61). Standardization of definitions and data elements is necessary to achieve integration of surveillance systems. Protection of patient confidentiality will be important as electronic systems containing medical records grow. To effectively use data from different systems for public health surveillance, record linkage across related data systems will be important to achieve, yet not easy to do. Capitation in managed care may create situations where, for example, diagnostic testing is not ordered in order to save costs, resulting in a specific diagnosis not made or treatment not prescribed.

Integration of Surveillance

Increasingly complex community-wide public health interventions increase the need for comprehensive and integrated surveillance data at the state and local levels (3). Integration is needed for efficiency; resources are limited, and public-health-program staff and providers of surveillance data (physicians, hospitals, etc.) may work across categorical public health program areas. In addition, changes in the health-care system with the advent of managed care, the consolidation of clinical laboratory services, and the increased availability of health information in electronic form have provided opportunities for more effective use of health data for public health purposes.

Historically, state chronic disease programs have sought to alleviate the leading causes of mortality (e.g., cardiovascular disease, cancer, and diabetes) through a variety of public health education and screening services for people at high risk. The evolution of these programs has been accompanied by interventions, which target the determinants of health-related behaviors and health outcomes, including social factors and policies, the media and the health-care delivery systems. Consequently, surveillance to document and monitor changes in these factors must be now be performed at multiple levels: the individual, family/household, community, organizational, environmental, and geopolitical levels.

Integration of surveillance systems can occur in other ways: first, integration of the sources of data. For example, emergency rooms can provide data on asthma, diarrheal diseases, and injuries, including occupational injuries. An integrated system would be able to provide data for all of these conditions rather than having separate data systems for each. This makes data collection easier for emergency room staff and more efficient for health department staff. Similarly, integrated surveillance at the level of the clinical laboratory could provide information on laboratory diagnoses of infectious diseases, lead and heavy metal poisoning, cholesterol levels and cancer diagnoses. Integrated surveillance for risk factors can occur with the BRFSS, including cardiovascular disease risk, injury risk, cancer risk, and communicable-disease risk (e.g., STD and HIV). Table 12–4 shows additional examples of integration by data source.

Table 12–4 Matrix of Diseases and Other Conditions of Public Health Interest and Data Sources for Integrated Surveillance

Source	Disease/Condition				
	Infection	Chronic	Injuries	Occupational Diseases	Environmental Conditions
Physicians	✓	✓			✓
Clinical laboratories	✓	✓		✓	✓
Emergency rooms	✓	✓	✓	✓	
Hospital discharges	✓	✓	✓		
Vital records	✓	✓	✓	✓	
Population surveys	✓	✓			✓

A second level of integration involves linking data on the same individual from different data sources (patient-level integration). For example, complete data on the diagnosis, treatment, outcome and the identity of contacts of a case of bacterial meningitis must be collected and combined from physician, laboratory and hospital reports, as well as from public health worker investigative reports to obtain a complete picture of an individual case. Accomplishing this type of integration requires inclusion of standardized data elements (e.g., name, date of birth, medical record number) in each of the medical, administrative, and laboratory data sources that are to be integrated.

Third, integration can link records across the natural history of disease (longitudinal integration). Longitudinal integration in chronic disease surveillance enables analysis of the effects of primary, secondary, and tertiary prevention measures on health-related outcomes and helps direct public health programs aimed at all stages of the disease process. For example, surveillance of cardiovascular disease may monitor each step in the causation–outcome process from risk factors (smoking history, diet, cholesterol levels) to the disease outcomes (stroke, myocardial infarction). Another example relates to surveillance of HIV infection and AIDS, the end stage of HIV infection. Here, the ability to follow individuals and populations from HIV diagnosis to AIDS diagnosis helps to determine how rapidly disease is progressing in the population and how risk factors for disease progression are changing (e.g., access to treatment). The surveillance approach used must take into account the underlying disease causation model which often consists of a complex interplay of factors operating at these different levels, usually over an extended time frame, and with health outcomes occurring over a continuum from clinically manifest disease to disability and death. There may be gaps in the kinds of data needed to describe all stages of disease pathogenesis and to quantify a relationship between risk factors and outcome—gaps that need to be filled.

Finally, surveillance can benefit from integration of data on diseases with the same or similar risk factors. For example, categorical disease control programs have developed around selected notifiable diseases of national importance including STDs, TB, and HIV. Risk factors for STDs are the same as for sexually transmitted HIV; populations at high risk for STDs may predict where HIV may occur in the future. For example, this may be happening now in the southern United States (62). Populations with high rates of HIV should be the focus of intensified TB surveillance efforts because TB occurs more readily in immuno-suppressed persons.

Historically, each national categorical public health program requested different data elements, even for standard demographic variables, and provided states with unique and often incompatible software packages to report data to CDC as a condition of categorical funding. In addition states have maintained NETSS-compatible systems for the purposes of reporting to the NNDSS and for the uniform analysis of all communicable diseases in the state. This has led to inefficiencies at both the state and federal levels, with multiple incompatible streams of surveillance data on the same or related conditions including double data entry required, often by the same personnel (Figure 12–2). Recently, efforts have been initiated to integrate these systems at the federal level through the Health Information and Surveillance Systems Board (HISSB) at CDC. Such efforts will aid in integration at the state and local levels as well.

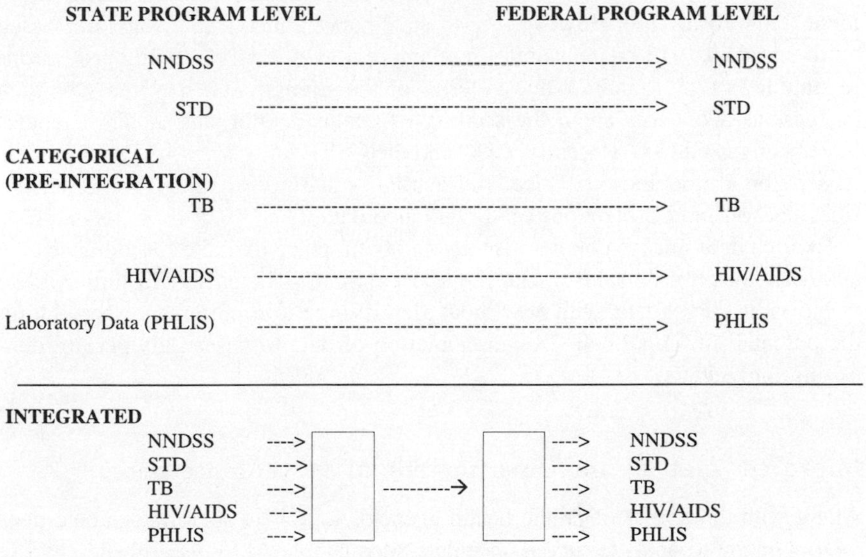

STATE PROGRAM LEVEL		FEDERAL PROGRAM LEVEL
NNDSS	--->	NNDSS
STD	--->	STD
CATEGORICAL (PRE-INTEGRATION)		
TB	--->	TB
HIV/AIDS	--->	HIV/AIDS
Laboratory Data (PHLIS)	--->	PHLIS

INTEGRATED

NNDSS	---->		---->	NNDSS
STD	---->		---->	STD
TB	---->	----------->	---->	TB
HIV/AIDS	---->		---->	HIV/AIDS
PHLIS	---->		---->	PHLIS

NNDSS = National Notifiable Disease Surveillance System
STD = Sexually Transmitted Disease
TB = Tuberculosis
HIV/AIDS = Human Immunodeficiency Virus/Acquired Immunodeficiency Syndrome
PHLIS = Public Health Laboratory Information Systems

Figure 12–2 Benefits of integrating infectious disease surveillance systems.

Protection of Confidentiality and Data Security

Protection of the confidentiality of surveillance data is key to public health surveillance. Legal assurances of confidentiality are necessary to balance the public good that comes from surveillance with the privacy of individuals from whom data are collected. In addition, even though surveillance is often legally required at the state level, successful surveillance still requires the cooperation of physicians, other data providers, and the community. Their cooperation will be more readily obtained if they are assured that the data they provide will be protected. Electronic systems to collect and store surveillance data, and to disseminate surveillance findings are not only a potential means to protect confidentiality but also a potential risk to confidentiality. Computer hardware, software, firewalls, and use of password and encryption technologies should be utilized to the fullest extent in surveillance system design.

To optimally balance the competing goods of public health benefits with individual privacy, state laws should *a*) specify the purposes of data gathering; *b*) inform the public of the uses of data; *c*) maintain strict confidentiality and data security, and other steps to prevent misuse of data; *d*) disclose data only when consistent with the public health purposes of surveillance; and *e*) obtain informed consent for secondary uses of surveillance data (e.g., for research purposes) in identifiable form (*17*). However, many state surveillance statutes are still based on the original 1913 model statute. A recent review of confidentiality protections in state laws (*16*) found a range in terms of the strength and specificity of such protections. Concerns about the security of health data at state health agencies have been raised (*63*). Recently, CDC and the CSTE have embarked on a process to develop a model surveillance confidentiality statute for states that better defines the uses and protections of surveillance data.

Explicit data release policies also need to be in place to make surveillance data available for public health research purposes. Such policies should limit release of individual level data, with or without identifying information, and should limit the potential for small cell sizes in tabulation of data to potentially permit identifying individuals.

Improved Analysis and Dissemination of Surveillance Data

Along with the ability of public health agencies to collect surveillance data goes the obligation to analyze surveillance data adequately and to disseminate and use surveillance findings for public health purposes. This may be a particular problem at state and local levels because of the resource limitations noted above and because of the lack of technical knowledge resources. Here again, the availability of rapidly advancing computer technology, statistical and mapping software, and Web-based systems to disseminate surveillance findings presents a great opportunity for state and local surveillance to realize its potential. Surveillance practitioners should make best use of these and other innovative mechanisms, including the media, to disseminate the key findings of surveillance, to encourage their use for local public health program design and evaluation, and to educate policy makers and the public. The limitations of surveillance data in terms of completeness, predictive value, timeliness, and its observational nature, which does not permit conclusions of causality, need to be adequately communicated in this process. Safeguarding the confidentiality of individuals in disseminating surveillance findings, particularly for local areas, is also a critical component of this process.

THE FUTURE OF STATE AND LOCAL PUBLIC HEALTH SURVEILLANCE

State and local public health surveillance practitioners have been actively involved in discussions of the future course of national public health surveillance. At the 1994 National Surveillance Conference, held in Atlanta and hosted jointly by the CSTE and CDC, attendees considered a blueprint for the future of national public health surveillance in the United States (9). The resulting document was endorsed by the CSTE membership in 1995. The blueprint proposes a National Public Health Surveillance System (NPHSS), which is described as a collaborative process among federal, state, and local levels to agree on what conditions should be under national surveillance. The blueprint describes the purposes and methods of surveillance, the case definitions to be used, data to be collected, the information systems to be utilized to collect and transmit the data, and defines the federal, state and local roles. By cataloging all surveillance efforts in one "virtual" national surveillance system, the blueprint forms a unifying framework to classify all surveillance efforts across the spectrum of public health. It provides visibility for surveillance as a non-categorical, core public health function, encourages collaboration and integration of surveillance efforts for efficiency and access to new data sources, and seeks to foster improved data quality through coordinated evaluation, training, and development of new surveillance methods. Importantly, it seeks to provide a single point to access and analyze surveillance data across public health disciplines. The NPHSS is not a proposal to combine all surveillance systems into one, but can be viewed as a conceptual (virtual) system to encompass all surveillance activities. Implementing the NPHSS will require engaging federal, state, and local public health partners, including CDC and other Public Health Service agencies, Association of State and Territorial Health Officers (ASTHO), CSTE, Association of Public Health Laboratories (APHL), National Association for Public Health Statistics and Information Systems (NAPHSIS), National Association of County and City Health Officers (NACCHO), State and Territorial Injury Prevention Directors' Association (STIPDA), and other state and national professional and public health organizations in an ongoing process. The NPHSS will provide a framework to address the issues identified in this chapter as state and local public health surveillance begins the next millenium.

REFERENCES

1. Langmuir AD. The surveillance of communicable diseases of national importance. *New Engl J Med* 1963;268:182–92.
2. Osterholm MT, Birkhead GS, Meriwether RA. Impediments to public health sur-

veillance in the 1990s: the lack of resources and the need for priorities. *J Public Health Management Practice* 1996;2:11–5.

3. Morris G, Snider D, Katz M. Integrating public health information and surveillance systems. *J Public Health Management Practice* 1996;2:24–7.
4. Institute of Medicine. The future of public health. Washington, D.C.: National Academy Press, 1988.
5. Hinman AR. Surveillance of communicable diseases. Presented at the 100th annual meeting of the American Public Health Association, November 15, 1972, Atlantic City, New Jersey.
6. Koo D, Wetterhall SF. History and current status of the National Notifiable Diseases Surveillance System. *J Public Health Management Practice* 1996;2:4–10.
7. Etheridge EW. Sentinel for health: a history of the Centers for Disease Control. Berkeley: University of California Press, 1992.
8. Birkhead GS. Recognizing and supporting the role of public health surveillance: intensive care for a core public health function. *J Public Health Management and Practice* 1996;2(4):vii–ix.
9. Meriwether RA. Blueprint for a national public health surveillance system for the 21st Century. *J Public Health Management Practice,* 1996;2(4):16–23.
10. Centers for Disease Control. Case definitions for public health surveillance. *MMWR* 1990;39(RR-13).
11. Centers for Disease Control and Prevention. Case definitions for infectious conditions under public health surveillance. *MMWR* 1997;46(RR-10).
12. Comprehensive plan for epidemiologic surveillance. Atlanta: Public Health Service, 1986.
13. Klaucke DN, Buehler JW, Thacker SB *et al.* Guidelines for evaluating surveillance systems. *MMWR* 1988;37(S-5).
14. Centers for Disease Control. Mandatory reporting of infectious diseases by clinicians and mandatory reporting of occupational diseases by clinicians. *MMWR* 1990:39 (RR-9).
15. Integrating public health information and surveillance systems. Atlanta: Public Health Service, 1995.
16. Gostin LO. Public health law: a review. *Current Issues in Public Health* 1996;2:205–14.
17. Gostin LO, Lazzarini Z, Neslund VS, Osterholm MT. The public health information infrastructure. *JAMA* 1996;275:1921–7.
18. Gostin LO. Health care information and the protection of personal privacy: ethical and legal considerations. *Ann Int Med* 1997;127:683–90.
19. Gostin LO, Ward JW, Baker AC. National HIV case reporting for the United States— a defining moment in the history of the epidemic. *New Engl J Med* 1997;337:1162–7.
20. Istre GR. Disease surveillance at the state and local levels. In: Public health surveillance. Halperin W, Baker EL (eds.). New York: Van Nostrand Reinhold, 1992.
21. Benenson AS (ed.). Control of communicable diseases manual. Sixteenth edition. Washington D.C.: American Public Health Association, 1995.
22. Centers for Disease Control and Prevention. 1998 sexually transmitted diseases treatment guidelines. *MMWR* 1998;47:1–111.
23. Centers for Disease Control and Prevention. Control and prevention of meningococcal disease and control and prevention of serogroup C meningococcal disease: Evaluation and management of suspected outbreaks. Recommendations of the Advisory Committee on Immunization Practices. *MMWR* 1997;46(RR-5):1–21.
24. Centers for Disease Control and Prevention. Injuries associated with self-unloading forage wagons–New York, 1991–1994. *MMWR* 1995;44:595–603.
25. Birkhead GS, Galvin VG, Meehan PJ, O'Carroll PW, Mercy JA. The emergency de-

partment in surveillance of attempted suicide: findings and methodologic considerations. *Public Health Rep* 1993;108:323–31.

26. Centers for Disease Control and Prevention. Decline in cigarette consumption following implementation of a comprehensive tobacco prevention and education program—Oregon, 1996–1998. *MMWR* 1999;48:140–2.

27. Tyler CW, Last JM. Epidemiology. In: Public health and preventive medicine. Fourteenth edition. Wallace RB (ed.). Stanford, Conn.: Appleton & Lange, 1998.

28. Snider DE, Stroup DF. Defining research when it comes to public health. *Public Health Rep* 1997;112:29–32.

29. Mariner WK. Public confidence in public health research ethics. *Public Health Rep* 1997;112:33–6.

30. 45 Code of Federal Relations (CFR) 46.

31. Cheadle A, Wagner E, Koepsell T, Kristal A, Patrick D. Environmental indicators: a tool for evaluating community-based health-promotion program. *Am J Prev Med* 1992;8(6):345.

32. Assessment of performance measures for public health, substance abuse and mental health. Perrin EB, Koshel, JJ (eds.). Panel on performance measures and data for public health performance partnership grants. Committee on National Statistics. Washington, D.C.: National Academy Press, 1997.

33. Health performance measurement in the public sector: principles and policies for implementing an information network. Perrin EB, Dorch JS, Skillman SM (eds.). Panel on performance measurements and data for public health partnership grants. Committee on National Statistics, Commission on Behavioral and Social Sciences and Education. Washington, D.C.: National Research Council, 1999.

34. Torrance GW, Feeny D. Utilities and quality-adjusted life years. *Int J Technol Assess Health Care* 1989;5:559–75.

35. Rousch S, Birkhead GS, Koo D, Cobb A, Fleming D. Mandatory reporting of diseases and conditions by health care professionals and laboratories. *JAMA* 1999; 282:164–70.

36. Centers for Disease Control and Prevention. Summary of notifiable diseases, United States, 1997. *MMWR* 1998;46:1–87.

37. Disease reporting: a health professional's responsibility. Public Health Letter (Los Angeles County Department of Health Services) 2;ob10;cb. September 1980.

38. Isaacman SH. Significance of disease reporting requirements. *Infectious Disease News* 1990; 3(10):23.

39. Centers for Disease Control. National Electronic Telecommunications System for Surveillance, United States, 1990–1991. *MMWR* 1991:40;502–3.

40. Devine O, Parrish RG. Monitoring the health of a population. Statistics in public health: quantitative approaches to public health problems. Stroup DF, Teutsch SM (eds.). New York: Oxford University Press, 1998.

41. Menck E, Smart C (eds.). Central cancer registries: design, management and use. Harwood Academic Publishers, 1994.

42. Jenson OM, Parkin DM *et al.* (eds.). Cancer registration: principles and methods. *IARC Scientific Publications,* number 95. Lyons, France, 1991.

43. Centers for Disease Control and Prevention. Prevention and control of influenza: recommendations of the advisory committee on immunization practices (ACIP). *MMWR* 1999:48(RR-4).

44. Baron RC, Dicker RC, Bussell KE, Herndon JL. Assessing trends in mortality in 121 U.S. cities, 1970–79, from all causes and from pneumonia and influenza. *Public Health Rep* 1988;103:120–8.

45. Centers for Disease Control and Prevention. Update: Influenza activity B United States, 1998–99 season. *MMWR* 1999;48.
46. Rosenberg ML, Hammond WR. Surveillance: the key to firearm injury prevention. *Am J Prev Med* 1998;15:1.
47. Berkelman RL, Bryan RT, Osterholm MT, LeDuc JW, Hughes JM. Infectious disease surveillance: a crumbling foundation. *Science* 1994;264:368–70.
48. Developing state-based chronic disease epidemiology capacity nationwide. Atlanta: Public Health Service, 1997.
49. Centers for Disease Control and Prevention. Monitoring Environmental Disease—United States, 1997. *MMWR* 1998;47.
50. Brown CM, Anderson HA, Etzel RA. Asthma: the state's challenge. *Public Health Rep* 1997;112:198–205.
51. Finelli L, St. Louis ME, Gunn RA, Crissman CE. Field epidemiology network for STDs (FENS). Epidemiologic support to state and local sexually transmitted disease control programs. *Sexually Transmitted Diseases* 1998;25:132–6.
52. Shramm M, Vogt RL, Mamolen J. Disease surveillance in Vermont: Who reports? *Pub Health Rep* 1991;106:95–7.
53. Harkess JR, Gildon BA, Archer PW, Istre GR. Is passive surveillance always insensitive? An evaluation of shigellosis surveillance in Oklahoma. *Am J Pub Health* 1988;128:878–81.
54. Konowitz PM, Petrossian GA, Rose DN. The underreporting of disease and physicians' knowledge of reporting requirements. *Pub Health Rep* 1984;99:31–5.
55. Do physicians report diseases? *Louisiana Morbidity Report* 1990;1(4):1–2.
56. Jones JL, Meyer P, Garrison C *et al.* Physician and infection control practitioner HIV/AIDS reporting characteristics. *Am J Pub Health* 1992;82:889–91.
57. Brachott D, Mosley JW. Viral hepatitis in Israel: the effect of canvassing physicians on notifications and the apparent epidemiological pattern. *Bull Wld Health Org* 1972; 6:457–64.
58. Vogt RL, LaRue D, Klaucke DN, Jillson DA. Comparison of an active and passive surveillance system of primary care providers for hepatitis, measles, rubella, and salmonellosis in Vermont. *Am J Pub Health* 1983;73:795–7.
59. Thacker SB, Redmond S, Rothenberg RB *et al.* Physician reporting of adverse drug reactions: results of the Rhode Island Adverse Drug Reaction Reporting Project. *JAMA* 1990;263:1785–8.
60. McDonald CJ, Overhage JM, Dexter P, Takesue BY, Dwyer DM. A framework for capturing clinical data sets from computerized sources. *Annals of Internal Medicine* 1997;127:675–82.
61. White MD, Kolar CM, Steindel SS. Evaluation of vocabularies for electronic laboratory reporting to public health agencies. *J Am Med Informatics Assoc.* 1999;6: 185–94.
62. HIV treatment through early detection and treatment of other sexually transmitted diseases—United States. *MMWR* 1998;47(RR-12).
63. O'Brien DG, Yasnoff WA. Privacy, confidentiality and security in information systems of state health agencies. *Am J Prev Med* 1999;16:351–8.

13

Public Health Surveillance in Low- and Middle-Income Countries

MARK E. WHITE
SHARON M. McDONNELL

The health of the people is really the foundation upon which all their happiness and all their powers as a state depend.

Benjamin Disraeli

This chapter deals with public health surveillance in settings of limited resources (*1*). Other chapters have discussed surveillance system design and implementation largely from the perspective of developed countries or settings of relatively abundant resources. The steps of system design and the underlying principles of collecting information for action do not vary because of the amount of available resources; however, in situations with limited (or absent) resources, there are both unique needs and unique opportunities for innovation. We address both the similarities and differences in the design and implementation of surveillance systems in low- and middle-income settings and provide examples of how some of the problems have been overcome or mitigated.

Health programs seek to increase healthy behavior, increase access to health care, and decrease death and illness, thereby improving the overall health of the public. The most important information for targeting and measuring the effects of public health programs are health outcomes such as rates of morbidity and mortality, and health-related behavior such as diet, smoking, and use of seat belts. There are numerous reasons for collecting health-related information. Five major reasons for collecting health-related information are listed below and each will be discussed:

1. Assessing health and monitoring health status and health risks.
2. Following disease–specific events and trends
3. Planning, implementing, monitoring, and evaluating health programs.
4. Financial management and monitoring information
5. Research

Assessing Health and Monitoring Health Status and Health Risks

Most often health status and risk are estimated by measuring the leading causes
of disease and death in a population. These indicators may assist in following
the health status or identifying priority goals for population health (e.g., *Healthy
People 2010*) (2). Internationally, the use of health indicators is very common
and additional work with the data can allow calculation of disability-adjusted life
years (DALYs) or years of potential life lost (YPLL) (*3,4*). In addition, periodic
systematic surveys of behavioral risk factors tracking health determinants or types
of behavior that influence health can be useful in targeting and evaluating programs. For example, in developing countries in which smoking rates have increased exponentially, there will be important changes in the risk of developing
lung cancer and cardiovascular disease; HIV/AIDS programs often rely on behavioral risk factor surveys to establish program design and evaluation.

Following Disease-Specific Diseases Events and Trends

Tracking disease trends (particularly infectious diseases) has been the main reason surveillance systems have been instituted (*5*). For epidemic-prone diseases,
a single case (e.g., of cholera, plague, or viral hemorrhagic fever) may be reason for action. For endemic or less severe diseases, surveillance systems may involve setting thresholds for concern and action for selected diseases. For example, a given district may decide that twice the expected number of cases of malaria
in a month may be reason to initiate investigation and control. The analysis of
information from public health surveillance systems on an ongoing basis may
provide the first clues to identifying and quantifying epidemics. Programs to eradicate polio (and previously smallpox) make extensive use of surveillance to monitor the progress toward reaching their goals (*6*). Eradication programs must rely
on surveillance, which becomes more important (and expensive) as the target disease approaches eradication (*7*).

Planning, Implementing, Monitoring, and Evaluating Health Programs

In international health, *management information* refers to program management—not patient management. Public health programs such as directly observed
therapy for tuberculosis or maternal health programs are designed to reduce the
burden of disease from specific causes. Information systems for low-income settings are often designed to provide information about the inputs, processes, and
outcomes of health programs. *Input information* refers to such things as financial and human resources used in programs. *Process information* systems measure things such as stocks of supplies, numbers of people treated, staff time, and
costs that are useful to measure the processes of service delivery. Input and
process information is useful to track the processes involved in health programs
and measure efficiency. If it is not explicitly considered in project design, lack
of accurate and timely information on the processes and management of the pro-

gram may be the step that limits and prevents the project from meeting its goals (see also Chapters 5 and 8). *Outcome information* measures the status of the population, for example rates of disease or behaviors affecting health. This information is essential for public health staff and planners to target interventions where they will do the most good and to monitor program effectiveness (*8*).

Financial Management and Monitoring Information

Financial information may be a subset of management information systems or these systems may be designed and managed separately. Financial information is often given high priority in high-income settings as it is linked with the funding of health services. Increasingly methods for obtaining financial information are sought for low- and middle-income settings to assist in prioritization and resource allocation. This type of information may come from a system of patient records or from systematic population-based surveys (*9*).

Research

Research is an important use of information and a core public health activity, but it represents a secondary use of the surveillance information. Surveillance information is a useful tool for generating hypotheses on causes of disease or risk factors, and it can also be used to test hypotheses about the effects of interventions. However, the primary purpose of public health surveillance is to provide information needed to improve the public's health. Unfortunately, information systems too often attempt to add long-term research questions and objectives to surveillance systems; this practice can lead to inefficient systems that fail to meet either the needs of implementers or researchers. Research questions are better addressed directly by special studies or systems.

COSTS OF MANAGING HEALTH PROGRAMS WITHOUT RELIABLE INFORMATION ABOUT LOCAL OUTCOMES

All of these reasons to collect information are valid, and each has a place in national information needs. Unfortunately, however, too often collection of information is viewed not as a priority but as a luxury. Developing and implementing useful information systems is a particular challenge in the resource-constrained environment of low- and middle-income countries. Many health conditions—diarrhea, malaria, pneumonia, and malnutrition—occur in settings with only rudimentary health care and few public health staff. Information systems that are poorly designed and implemented are the rule, and in settings where health resources and programs are severely constrained, the collection of information may seem beside the point. Additionally, too often most of the information budget has been spent on traditional systems (e.g., passive disease notification) that have been dysfunctional for years and may be poorly suited for current objectives (*10*). Since these systems are not perceived as useful to either planners or program managers, they encourage the view that health information is a drain on and impediment to successful implementation of control programs. Thus, health ministry personnel may not see the utility of establishing or re-engineering their surveillance systems (see also Chapter 8).

The result is that in situations of limited resources, measurable health objectives often cannot be identified because high-quality, population-based data are often missing. Instead of local data, planners must rely on information from international and regional sources such as United Nations International Children's Emergency Fund (UNICEF), the WHO, international conferences, nongovernmental organizations, and population laboratories (e.g., International Center for Diarrheal Disease Research, Bangladesh). Although health problems are similar in many limited-resource settings, relying on data from other countries can create major problems. For example, programs may be put in place that are not needed or no program may exist despite significant local need. Geographic differences in the impact of conditions associated with hepatitis B, iodine deficiency, HIV, tobacco use, or malaria can be significant. As an example, the need for country-specific data is illustrated by the finding of World Bank analysts that oral-rehydration therapy (ORT) in low-mortality environments is much less cost-effective than passive case detection and short-course chemotherapy for tuberculosis, whereas ORT in high-mortality environments is very cost-effective (*11,12*).

PLANNING THE PUBLIC HEALTH INFORMATION SYSTEM IN SETTINGS OF LIMITED RESOURCES

Before the specific information system is designed, it is important to review what is known and undertake a thorough priority-setting process that first characterizes the health status of the population and leads to the design and evaluation of effective public health programs. The activities and the information to support them must be connected logically; otherwise, the system designed may be piecemeal. Although this process appears linear, in reality it is far more fluid and less orderly (Table 13–1).

The form of a surveillance system should depend on the function and objectives for collecting the data. Throughout the world, surveillance objectives should be based on health impact, feasibility and acceptability of the proposed intervention, and the cost-effectiveness of the intervention (see chapter 8). When well-designed, public health surveillance systems directly measure outcomes accurately and systematically, and they become valuable tools for monitoring health programs (*13*). The selection of those diseases that should be maintained under local surveillance involves balancing resources and costs (*14*).

Decentralization of health systems and health sector reform are happening in nearly every country of the world (*15*). The process of decentralization may range from complete transfer of decision making and fiscal authority to almost no authority at local levels. These design decisions have enormous implications for health information and surveillance systems. Systems designed for centralized systems do not work well in the context of decentralization because the users

Table 13–1 Activities Needed to Establish and Manage a Country's Health and Types and Sources of Information Needed to Support These Activities

Activities Needed to Establish and Manage Health Services	Types and Sources of Information Needed to Support These Activities
1. Characterize overall health status of population (age distribution, major causes of mortality and morbidity)	Population-wide census and causes of mortality and morbidity i. Periodic community-level verbal mortality and surveys ii. Periodic health facility register or record review by agents iii. Regular reporting by health facilities and providers (complete vital record registration)
2. Determine health risks	Review of causes of morbidity and mortality for common risk factors Risk factor surveys
3. Rank health problems by health impact (severity, prevalence) to determine what health problems need to be addressed	Priority-setting exercises
4. Characterize high priority health problems and disease determinants	Targeted surveys of health providers, survey of health registers of other records, population surveys of risk factors; direct observational surveys of high-risk populations and geographic areas
5. Based on scientific knowledge, identify effective interventions for health problems and local situation	Scientific literature and health experts Local studies and field trials
6. Determine resources needed to implement interventions	Survey of health-care resources (facilities, supplies, trained staff, communications, transport) Survey of community resources, activities, and potential Evaluation of health budget
7. Prioritize activities based on previous steps	Decision analysis Expert opinion Political consideration and organizational capacity
8. Based on priorities (step 7) develop plans to prevent, control, and treat high-priority health problems	Health management literature Expert opinion Organizational capacity
9. Develop systems to manage and monitor delivery of prevention, control, or treatment programs	Individual and family health records Modules for i. Inventory of supplies ii. Tracking staff iii. Financial accounting

and their needs are different. Unfortunately, the health system may be decentralized without planning for the new information needs. Outmoded systems persist and new needs remain unmet (*16*).

Once there is agreement about the objectives of a system, the system should be planned specifically to meet that objective efficiently and effectively. Simple systems are most successful, especially in low- and middle-income countries where financial and human resources are often severely limited. It is easy to overwhelm the capacity of the system to provide accurate information by creating a system too complex to be implemented by people who have many other tasks. Trying to attain too many objectives often leads to confusion and failure. Actual integration of information systems is covered later in this chapter (as well as in Chapters 4 and 5), and is a priority for many countries.

Identifying measurable health objectives, assigning them priority, and then linking surveillance to those objectives is a priority both for the surveillance system and for health-system development in general (*11,12,17*). Linking surveillance to these ordered health objectives alleviates the pitfall of thinking of surveillance as just the reporting of disease. In fact, effective surveillance systems use information from multiple sources (such as sentinel sites, exit interviews, and regular surveys). Linking surveillance to objectives will help planners of the surveillance system to think creatively in efforts to build a surveillance system to measure all priority health objectives. Chapter 3 describes data sources that can be used in building surveillance systems. When resources are constrained there may have to be increased use of alternative sources such as case reports, sentinel sites, exit interviews, and surveys rather than more costly comprehensive methods available in situations with greater resources. It is noteworthy that using these data sources does not necessarily compromise the representativeness or utility of the information—if the system is well-designed and effectively implemented.

It is important to remember that public health surveillance systems exist only in the context of a functioning public health system. Surveillance should be put in place only when there is a planned or existing control program directed toward the health problem. The most important measure of a successful surveillance system is whether the information it provides is used by program managers to direct their work and improve public health. One way of considering the focus of information needs and objectives for a particular health problem is by looking at which cell of a two-by-two table best describes the situation (Table 13–2).

Surveillance through conventional disease reporting is most likely to be useful in those situations where the disease is described (etiology and transmission known) and there is some plan for taking action based on the information. Whereas the information or surveillance focus shifts more towards research and descriptive surveys when the disease is poorly described or control measures are unknown or not planned.

For each health objective, the method for tracking and evaluating that objective and its sub-objectives should be listed (Table 13–3). Once such a list is made, a grid can be constructed to show which method or approach will best measure the objective (Table 13–4). Completing a surveillance grid helps one visualize the overall structure and function of the surveillance system and think creatively about methods to obtain information.

The process of defining objectives, linking these objectives to indicators and then data sources and approaches will highlight surveillance needs. The process provides a basis for strengthening existing components, for identifying existing information that could measure objectives, and to develop innovative new in-

Table 13–2 Two-by-Two Table for Decision Making on the Focus of Planned Information Systems for Particular Health Problems, with Examples

	Disease well-understood	*Disease not well-understood*
Effective Control Available or in Place	**Information focus:** Monitor disease trends. Monitor the management of health programs and resources. **Examples:** Vaccination programs such as polio. Cervical cancer screening, early detection and treatment.	**Information focus:** Maintain and monitor control program. Conduct research to answer issues of risk factors and etiology through specific studies. **Examples:** The early days of HIV infection
No Effective Control Program Available or in Place	**Information focus:** Monitor trends of disease. Conduct research on effective disease control or ways to deliver control program to target population. **Examples:** Dengue hemorrhagic fever. Prenatal HIV transmission in low resource settings where cost of full treatment is prohibitive. Lung cancer prevention through behavioral modification to prevent teenage smoking initiation.	**Information focus:** Conduct research to establish etiology and investigate effective control measures. Registry and other targeted information sources may be helpful. **Examples:** Buruli Ulcer, pancreatic cancer, Creutzfeld-Jacob disease

formation system components. For example, in many countries, the process of linking surveillance to objectives highlights the need for mortality data and the absence of vital registration. In Table 13–4, the numerous potential uses of surveys as information sources are highlighted.

DATA SOURCES IN INTERNATIONAL HEALTH

Chapter 3 describes specific sources of data for public health information and surveillance systems. There are certain additional sources specific to low- and middle-income settings that deserve mention.

Vital-Event Registration

The measurement of vital events is the single most important addition that developing countries can make to their existing surveillance system. Death and birth rates—along with cause-specific, age-specific, and gender-specific rates—are very useful. In the United States, for example, 13 of the 18 health status indicators chosen to measure the health status of the population as part of the health objectives for the nation will be measured using vital records (2). At the very least a methodology for tracking important causes of mortality, and using these data to infer important sources of morbidity and disability-adjusted life years (DALYs) is fundamental.

Table 13–3 Examples of Objectives Linked to Surveillance Components That Will Measure Objectives

Surveillance-Linked Objectives	
Objective or Indicator	*Example of Methods To Obtain Information That Measures Objective*
Priority area #1—reduce diarrhea morbidity and mortality	
• Health status—reduce diarrhea mortality by 25% by 2010	• Vital-event registration in country or five sentinel areas
• Risk factor—increase female literacy of 10- to 14-year-olds to 80% by 2010	• Regularly conducted community survey
• Risk factor—Current drug-resistant diarrheal disease at 2%. No increase in drug resistant infections	• Monitor laboratory susceptibility for selected stool samples
• Health activity—Increase to 90% the proportion of 0- to 4-year- olds given appropriate home fluids by 2010	• Regularly conducted health survey or exit interviews
Priority area #2—Maternal morbidity and mortality	
• Health status—reduce maternal mortality by 25% by 2010	• Vital-event registration in country or five sentinel areas
• Health status—reduce cases of maternal morbidity by 50% by 2010 compared with 2000	• Sentinel health facility system or targeted survey
• Health activity—increase percentage of pregnant women receiving prenatal care to to 60% nationwide	• Regularly conducted community health survey
• Risk factor—increase female literacy of 10- to 14-year-olds to 80% by 2010	• Regularly conducted community survey or national data
• Health activity—Increase to 70% the percentage of women giving birth with trained assistants	• Community survey or exit interviews of women at all health facilities in district twice per year
Priority area #3—unintentional injury prevention. Reduce morbidity and mortality and better characterize injury risk by 2010	
• Health status—reduce morbidity and mortality from unintentional injury	• Vital records with detailed cause of death reporting. Facility-based records, sentinel health facilities, emergency room surveys
• Risk factor—describe major risk factors for unintentional injuries	• Review of records, community surveys, sentinel sites. Review of media reporting
• Health activity—increase and improve the quality of injury reporting	• Sentinel sites. Review of records
• Health activity—increase the use of motorcycle helmets to 60%	• Exit interviews in affected areas. Regularly conducted health survey. Exit interviews in selected areas. Observation

Developing countries and donors have placed too little emphasis on establishing or strengthening vital-event registration. In part these systems seem less exciting to outside donors or implementing agencies; in part they are perceived as too large and cumbersome. Vital registration could begin in small sentinel areas and expanded as it was evaluated and improved. The vital-registration system in the United States started in 1900 in 10 sentinel states, and it took 23 years

Table 13–4 Surveillance Components for Measuring Health Objectives in a Hypothetical Developing Country

Objectives	Population Based			Non-Population Based			
	Vital Registration	Disease Reporting	Surveys	Surveys	Sentinel Sites (either facility, laboratory, or health workers)	Laboratories	Special Studies (i.e. exit interviews or others)
Priority area #1—reduce diarrhea morbidity and mortality							
Reduce diarrhea mortality by 25% by 2010	x	x	x	x	x		
Increase female literacy of 10- to 14-year-olds to 80% by 1995			x			x	
No increase in drug-resistant diarrheal disease				x	x	x	
Increase percentage of 0- to 4-year-olds given appropriate home fluids to 90% by 2010			x	x			x
Priority area #2—reduce maternal mortality and morbidity							
Reduce maternal mortality by 25% by 2010.	x		x	x	x		
Reduce maternal morbidity cases by 50% by 2000		x	x	x	x		

Community surveys may be population-based depending on the sampling technique. Special surveys may target specific topics, sites, or populations. For example, emergency rooms, observational studies of seatbelt use.

(continued)

Table 13–4 Surveillance Components for Measuring Health Objectives in a Hypothetical Developing Country (Continued)

Objectives	Population Based			Non-Population Based			
	Vital Registration	Disease Reporting	Surveys	Surveys	Sentinel Sites (either facility, laboratory, or health workers)	Laboratories	Special Studies (i.e. exit interviews or others)
Increase percentage of pregnant women receiving prenatal care to 60% nationwide			x	x			
Increase to 70% the percentage of women giving birth with trained assistants			x	x	x		x
Priority area #3—unintentional injury prevention. Reduce morbidity and mortality and better characterize injury risk by 2010.							
Reduce morbidity and mortality from unintentional injury	x		x	x			
Describe major risk factors for unintentional injuries			x	x	x		x
Increase and improve the quality of injury reporting	x				x		
Increase the use of motorcycle helmets to 60%			x	x			x

Community surveys may be population-based depending on the sampling technique. Special surveys may target specific topics, sites, or populations. For example, emergency rooms, observational studies of seatbelt use.

for all states to be admitted into the system (18). Obviously, in the early stages of setting up a registry, some births and deaths would be missed. As late as 1974–1977, 21% of neonatal deaths were not registered in Georgia (19). Despite this underregistration, vital data are extremely useful. Once there is a system for collecting this information, the emphasis changes to slow, steady improvements in quality, completeness, and representativeness.

In areas in which routine mortality data are not available, the verbal autopsy (in which trained or untrained workers take histories from family members to classify deaths by cause) is a useful technique (20). In 1978, WHO detailed a list of approximately 150 causes of death that could be used by non-physicians to classify deaths by cause (21).

Included in vital registration are birth certificates. Reporting of births is directly linked to the extent to which births are attended, whether personnel are available to record these events, and whether reporting is linked with benefit. For example, if births are associated with receiving food supplements or any other positive outcome they are more likely to be reported.

In establishing vital-event systems, consideration should be given to including the registration of pregnancy. This is needed to measure the number of neonatal deaths, which in turn is needed to allow accurate infant-mortality rates to be calculated. Registration of pregnancies also allows measurement of prenatal care, fetal death associated with syphilis, family planning, and other important health concerns.

Regular, Periodic Surveys

Regular, periodic surveys can be an important component of a surveillance system. Surveys tend to be of two types: focused, non-population-based surveys to address specific information needs for a topic or a geographic area, and larger, possibly population-based surveys. Non-population-based surveys might include periodic surveys of motorcycle helmet or automobile seat-belt use to assist planning and managing injury control programs, or the laboratory surveillance for antibiotic resistance in hospitals (22). The most common source of population-based information in limited-resource settings are cluster surveys—multi-stage surveys with primary sampling units (23,24).

Surveys generally are single-purpose and are conducted intermittently on an as-needed basis, often at the request of international organizations. However, because the survey is the only method of gathering population-based information in many countries and surveys can be used to collect information on a variety of health topics, regularly scheduled surveys can constitute an excellent surveillance tool for health outcomes as well as determinants.

Previously conducted international or national surveys can serve as models for adaptation to local situations. Using questions and tools that have already been field tested may increase the quality of data collected and may allow for comparisons with other surveys. For example, WHO has useful questionnaires for diarrhea; acute respiratory-tract infections; immunization; and knowledge, attitude, and behavior associated with HIV infection. The CDC has questionnaires that cover child mortality, health-station practices, nutrition, morbidity of all types, HIV risk behavior among youths, and others. Once questionnaire modules have been developed, each module should be field-tested for readiness for implementation. Advance preparation and testing are very important. It is difficult and time-consuming, and therefore expensive to develop an effective questionnaire. Unfortunately, too often many of these steps are skipped. This leads to large, impractical survey designs with poor quality assurance, questionnaires that are difficult to administer, questionable data that is often impossible to analyze, and useless results. A large sample size does not provide control for bias, poor quality assurance, and design. The only significant difference between a large biased survey and a small biased survey is that the large survey costs more. Small, well-designed and executed surveys are much more valuable for managers and do not divert resources from the implementations they are meant to support. Stories abound of large resources being spent on poorly translated data-collection tools that are culturally inappropriate, and that do not answer the information needs for which they were designed.

In the data–collection tool (and the training to use it), it is advisable to reserve space for a small set (10 or so) of core questions that measure the highest-priority objectives for information desired by high-level policy makers. Not only will this demonstrate the timeliness of this surveillance component, it might also facilitate political and financial support for its continuation. Finally, when the time comes for a survey, the survey coordinator puts together the core questions, the last-minute questions from the policy makers, and the appropriate survey modules.

Data collection desired by international organizations (donors and non-governmental organizations) can be integrated into the ministry of health's schedule of surveys. Coordination of the survey should include steps that integrate desired input (proposed modules or questions) to be used by multiple stakeholders. The two groups can then collaborate to determine how the needs of both groups could be met. The international group can help train survey-unit staff and can help maintain a training manual on designing and conducting a survey, including interviewing techniques. This method is a cost-effective way to build local capacity and facilitate sustainability.

Sentinel Surveillance

Surveillance that uses sentinel sites or providers can play a critical role in limited-resource settings. At sentinel sites, more resources and more experienced and dedicated personnel can be used to collect information on more diseases, more detailed information about each case, and more difficult-to-collect information such as sexual behavior. Also, sentinel sites can often serve as sources of information about new conditions and can be used to determine the most effective methods for obtaining new data for the routine collection system.

There are several potential problems in interpreting data from sentinel sites. Sentinel sites are not designed to be representative of the population. Often sentinel sites may be selected from hospitals or other sophisticated facilities and tend to serve urban patients. Such data will not reflect rural, small, non-urban health stations where the majority of the population may live. Consequently, as sentinel systems are piloted, rural and small health stations should be included in the sentinel-site system.

Despite the lack of representativeness, sentinel sites can yield important information in a timely manner at a relatively low cost for several reasons: first, cause-of-death data are available, permitting timely data collection and analysis; second, because the number of visits and deaths is large (as in large urban centers), they yield more precise estimates and allow subgroup analysis by age, gender, or other important variables. Also, data are currently available, whereas systems of vital events and regular, periodic surveys are not generally established. For example, in Kinshasa, the Congo Ministry of Health used a hospital-based sentinel surveillance system to establish that measles remained an important cause of death for children <9 months old. The spread of clinically important resistance to chloroquine was detected because of increasing mortality from malaria in sentinel hospitals in numerous African countries (25).

At local levels resource constraints limit the number of sentinel sites. However, both health stations and districts can conduct a form of sentinel surveillance by limiting data collection on some health problems to a small sample of sites at infrequent intervals. For example, although children have their growth monitored throughout the year, the percentage with weight-for-age of <80% of standard might be calculated only once every 3 months on a consecutive sample of 30 children.

Exit Interviews

Interviews of patients who have finished their visits at health facilities, which can be called *exit interviews,* can be a flexible, easy, and cost-effective method of collecting information. Exit interviews are ideal for measuring progress toward local health objectives. They can be used to collect data for emergent problems or for routine surveillance, as well as to evaluate the performance of health workers and the management of the health services. For surveillance purposes, exit interviews can be used to collect information about the process indicators, health risks, health behavior, and health interventions (26). Unlike surveys, exit interviews can be conducted frequently.

Focus Groups and Case-Control Studies

Focus groups can make important contributions to the design of a surveillance system and to the understanding of the information within the system (27). As complex issues such as changes in behavior are assigned higher health priorities (e.g., HIV-related behavior, diet, home fluids, treatment practices, and reasons for not being vaccinated), focus groups are often used to gain new information.

Focus groups often provide an appropriate first step in generating ideas about why events and behavior occur. After ideas or hypotheses are available, surveys, exit interviews, and special studies (case-control studies) can be used to identify specific factors that should be incorporated into surveillance systems. Health-facility staff can use focus groups, along with exit interviews, to measure health objectives of local importance.

Through focus groups, health workers can obtain qualitative information from the community, which may be widely defined to include key informants such as school nurses, leaders, or groups of mothers. For example, a focus group may help determine, from groups of mothers, why children are not being vaccinated and what might be done to solve this problem. Information on access to and demand for health care requires qualitative information for decision making.

CHALLENGES FOR IMPLEMENTING SURVEILLANCE SYSTEMS IN LOW- AND MIDDLE-INCOME SETTINGS

The assessment of information systems in developing countries (settings of limited resources) reveals characteristics similar to but exaggerated from those in developed countries including: a plethora of vertical systems, low response capacity, little analytic capacity, political decision making and burdensome reporting requirements with no feedback (*10*).

In this situation the best solution is to work with decision makers and program managers to select and then carefully re-design and implement a surveillance system that directly improves the performance of a priority health program or activity. Actually seeing a useful surveillance system within their own setting is the most persuasive argument for surveillance for national health personnel.

The design of information systems for a specific purpose or objective must take the setting or situation into account. For example, the level of resources, security, geography, population dispersion and mobility, type of health system, literacy, centralization and privatization are examples. A complete description of the situation will help describe opportunities for information and constraints that must be considered (*28*). Increasingly, tools for assessing and evaluating information systems are being developed by WHO, CDC, and others to better describe both the health-care setting and the information systems in place and future needs for strengthening. In low- and middle-income settings an assessment of information systems most often reveals significant infrastructure and resource limitations that will affect the design and implementation of information systems. Typically, the categories of problems encountered, discussed in the sections that follow, are similar to high-resource settings but more exaggerated.

Limited Personnel Available for Public Health

Compared with high-income settings, lower- and middle-income settings must often rely on clinical personnel to carry out public health functions. Training and personnel systems for medical personnel reward and emphasize clinical specialties and advanced diplomas in academic research. Thus, there is little incentive or skill in public health program management or information systems. The lack of incentives for public health work or public health staff includes numerous management and infrastructure problems that are difficult to address. For example, in many countries salaries for workers in the public sector are insufficient so they must work a second or third job, further impinging on the time available for public health activities. The lack of competitive salary and a defined career ladder means that ambitious and well-qualified staff are not retained. This leads to rapid staff turnover and system inefficiencies. Additionally, public sector jobs may involve inflexible civil service regulations or political considerations that do not reward performance. Because health information is viewed as not useful, top managers may place less-effective managers or staff in the health information systems on the principle that they will do less harm. Finally, the lack of supervision and continuing education for public health workers leaves them isolated. This leads to a downward spiral of worsening information quality and decreasing use.

Solutions to address the lack of personnel for public health and prevention have included voluntary systems (using community health workers, traditional birth attendants, or village volunteers; e.g., UNICEF community surveillance). These voluntary systems deserve more attention but must be undertaken carefully. Health workers in the formal system may have little familiarity with these programs or workers. Thus, they neither use them well nor respect their constraints or skills. Nevertheless, there are exciting opportunities in this area that can link community and health system resources (29).

More familiar solutions are public health training programs designed to meet human resource gaps, either in numbers of personnel or in the types of skills they have (30). Typically this has been done either through short-term in-service training (particularly workshops) on public health surveillance or longer academic training programs. Short-term training has not shown significant benefit, considering the amount of expenditure in time and funds. Too often these are implemented in a piecemeal fashion with little regard for actual adult learning techniques and behavior change. Long-term training is commonly criticized for the lack of applicability of academic graduates to public health systems and the lack of sustainability of the programs. These concerns have resulted in programs targeting the specific needs of public health agencies such as the Field Epidemiology Training Programs or Public Health Schools without Walls (31,32). In countries such as Thailand, the Philippines, and Mexico, which have had these programs for 10 to 20 years, many top managers are either graduates of the programs or utilize information from graduates to make major decisions (33). These training program and the staff almost always work in re-forming surveillance systems to provide useful information systems leading to outbreak investigation and prevention and the production of health communication materials for various audiences.

One of the most important features differentiating successful from unsuccessful information systems is the presence of a supervision system. Technically credible supervision that occurs at regular intervals can make an enormous difference in the willingness and skill of health workers to participate in public health activities (10,34). There is much to be learned about addressing these problems; however it is quite likely that increased commitment to public health functions will be required both within ministries and the donor community.

Donor-Driven Development of Surveillance Systems

In resource-constrained systems, donors (multi-national, other governmental, private, or others) may provide significant levels of funds for the health and public health system. In addition to funding, donors are important sources for new ideas and innovative methods. However, besides additional funding, donors bring a subset of challenges that the country must confront.

Donor reporting and accountability systems can add an extra layer of top-level bureaucracy that may complicate implementation. Donors have needs for data to monitor their own projects and may require ministries to develop and implement surveillance systems to gather this information. While information needed by donors for reporting may be similar to that needed by ministries for implementation, the data or timing requirements may be different. This creates an additional reporting burden for the health systems and can impede health delivery. Such systems create friction between donors and ministries and are not sustainable.

In addition, donor funding may be contingent on meeting 1-year targets that are not possible considering the difficulties of field implementation (35). Short time frames do not allow ministries to make the major changes in bureaucracy and infrastructure. High-priority country programs may be put on hold to manage short-term projects.

Donors often require consultants to advise and assist ministry personnel in the design and implementation of projects. External consultants are expensive and may represent significant costs to the project. These costs are easily justified by good consultants who can catalyze the thinking and implementation of the project to help it move rapidly toward meeting its goals. Conversely, consultants with no experience may hinder implementation by insisting on impractical paradigms or, at best, must learn along with their counterparts. For surveillance, the ideal outside expert has successfully implemented a health information system in a ministry, has published or presented the results in a peer-reviewed context, and has a track record in successfully developing partnerships in low- and middle-income countries.

Non-governmental organizations (NGOs) have special benefits and risks. They can provide essential support to the delivery of clinical and public health services in a country. Unfortunately, too often the ministry of health or other governmental agency or the donor does not provide the guidance to these organizations. The result is competition for resources that undermines the humanitarian goals. For example, an NGO may be charged with strengthening a ministry of health. Because NGOs are typically able to pay much more than government agencies, the NGO may hire the best personnel away from the ministry it is trying to strengthen. Without careful planning for sustainability, these personnel may not be willing to re-enter the government at the end of the NGO project. If so, the ministry may actually be harmed.

Collaboration with the private sector and non-governmental agencies is essential in limited resource settings. Governments can use their expertise, their willingness to work in the most difficult and under-served areas, their human capacity, and their existing of bureaucracy to get necessary information and improve health services of all types.

Multiple Vertical ("Stovepipe") Systems in Place

Often an inventory of information systems reveals multiple systems that overlap but do not complement each other. What emerges are competing programs that mix objectives. For example, HIV/AIDS, polio, maternal and child health, sexually transmitted diseases, and the Expanded Programme for Immunisations (EPI), may each have independent surveillance systems that do not link centrally and do not integrate resources. In an eradication campaign, great resources must be spent to identify the last few cases of a disease to be internationally certified, which may leave fewer resources for programs that are more cost-effective in the short run (36). However, with careful design, such systems can be developed and supported in ways that strengthen the ongoing systems and programs of ministries (37).

Integrating information systems can increase efficiency of staff for public health and clinical functions, decrease the reporting burden, and allow sharing of resources such as staff, cars, and computers. There are several advantages to integration:

- surveillance information can be gathered with greater cost-efficiency
- requirements for health facility staff will be simplified and their training will be less duplicative

Integration is a significant challenge because the real and perceived needs of different programs often require collection of vast amounts of data from different parts of the health system (clinic logs, accounting systems, central records) or from the general populations (incidence rates, behaviors) in differing time frames. Therefore, it is difficult to meet all needs with one instrument (see Chapter 4) (38).

As an example, ministries in low- or middle-income settings often try to use one health–management information system to measure both management processes (such as stocks of vaccine in clinics) and public health outcomes (such as the incidence of cholera in the population.) Although the integration of systems appears logical and efficient, this combination is fraught with difficulties. A management process information system usually measures properties within health programs, while public health surveillance systems measure properties outside the health system and within the community (outcomes.) Both public health surveillance and management process information are needed by policy makers, implementers, media, and the population to make rational decisions about health. However, combining the two systems may lead to a complexity that seldom works well and does not enhance either objective, particularly when the persons collecting and managing the data do not understand the utility of and differences between the two types of information.

Integration usually occurs after the national system has struggled with multiple "independent" or vertical systems that have taxed resources and not effectively answered information needs. Therefore, the actual process involves bringing together existing systems with numerous stakeholders at all levels. This process is facilitated by identifying a group of credible experts at the top level who can work with program managers and local officials to coordinate activities and, where feasible, combine them. If users of the information, such as program managers or local officials, do not feel ownership of an integrated system, it is likely that they will either continue to use old vertical systems or develop new ones that they feel give them control and meet their needs. Most countries end up with a mix of integrated and vertical information systems supplemented by periodic surveys. The more these activities can be coordinated, the more efficient they will be.

Beyond routine reporting systems it is necessary to coordinate and integrate other sources of information. For example, to assure the development of a useful national surveillance system in a developing country, a survey unit or committee should be assigned the task of coordinating all national health surveys. The unit first works with program staff to develop surveillance questions in high-priority areas (e.g., diarrhea, vaccinations, HIV/AIDS, family planning, child survival, malaria, and tuberculosis). Two to five questions are often adequate for some conditions. The questions should be assigned priority so that the survey coordinator has some flexibility to shorten the overall questionnaire if needed.

More recently, in settings of limited resources planners are looking to the integration of vertical programs to increase the personnel and the incentives that might be available for high-priority diseases. For example, polio surveillance officers involved in the active surveillance of polio have begun to monitor other diseases, including cholera, measles, and meningitis (37). This increases local acceptability of these eradication programs and may lead to increased staff available for core public health functions in the lower and middle levels of the health system (health facilities and districts). The actual process of integration takes a high-level commitment by decision makers to allow sharing of resources (vehicles, staff time, and computers).

Lack of Laboratory Support for Confirmation of Outbreaks or for Management of Patients

In low-income settings laboratory services may be unavailable or non-standardized. Even the logistics of getting specimens to the laboratory may be difficult. Laboratory diagnosis increases the specificity of the surveillance system. The polio eradication program has done innovative work toward trying to overcome many of these problems all over the world. For example, they have used the private sector to help transport specimens to the laboratory and the laboratory results have been used to insure that the surveillance system results are supervised and accurate (39). Expanding the services of laboratory improvements built from vertical programs remains a significant challenge. Regional approaches, across national boundaries may be necessary to provide the laboratory services needed. Increasingly, national laboratories must provide guidance to laboratories within the country about core public health laboratory services.

Unsatisfactory Response Capability and System Not Held Accountable for Response

A culture of credibility for data or information must be combined with the belief that information is collected in order to take action. The design and implementation of surveillance systems needs to take into account the legal and administrative benefits and consequences of reporting. Countries may have elaborate regulations for reporting that are not practical to enforce. Physicians are often not trained about disease reporting. In addition, whether they work in public or private institutions, they often do not see that reporting disease has any benefit to themselves or anyone else and they rarely face consequences for not reporting. In the absence of action or at least feedback even when action is not possible, people lose interest in case notification. Lamden, in a study in the United Kingdom, a relatively resource-rich setting, found that notification of outbreak-prone diseases took on average 16 days to reach the person who could take action in controlling communicable disease, which significantly reduced the ability to respond effectively to outbreaks (16). The reporters suffered no consequences for this lack of timeliness.

In low-resource settings, outbreaks of infectious disease are seldom detected or responded to until late in the course of the outbreak—after media involvement and political consequences have occurred (see also Chapter 16). Health workers are rarely encouraged to report public health problems, and they seldom have the resources they believe are necessary to initiate action.

Integrated, well-thought-out surveillance at the health-station and health-center level warrants more focused attention—especially to data collection, analysis, and dissemination of results as a basis for public health action. Surveillance responsibilities should be specified in employee work plans and completion of surveillance duties used to assess health-worker performance.

Although WHO has surveillance and evaluation training modules for vertical programs such as EPI and Control of Diarrheal Diseases (CDD), there are few general surveillance training modules for district or health-station levels (40–43). Local surveillance is critical because major health problems in developing countries require innovative public health action at the local level. Local surveillance and public health action based on surveillance may be less urgent for programs with high effectiveness and ease of administration, (e.g., vaccinations), or for programs that depend solely on the formal health-care system (e.g., acute respiratory infections or tuberculosis). However, local surveillance and linked public health action will be essential for most of the priority diseases (e.g., diarrhea, malaria, and HIV) and related prevention activities (oral rehydration solutions, chloroquine for all cases of fever, and condoms). In general, these interventions require extensive behavior change on the part of clients and also require local problem solving, surveillance of objectives, strategy reformulation, and creative intervention by health workers.

To address the usefulness of data at local levels, data collected routinely by health stations should be limited to high-priority conditions. For example, mandatory reporting could be limited to 10 selected diseases on the basis of established priorities or reporting laws. In addition, the health facility should meet certain standards before reporting requirements are expanded: the health station staff should be *a*) reporting regularly, *b*) displaying information collected, *c*) able to describe the meaning of the data, *d*) using the data to solve health problems with national and community input, and *e*) using the data to evaluate programs targeted at certain health problems. If these are all being done, the staff is likely to see the usefulness of surveillance information in program management and will likely be more enthusiastic about the public health functions and able to initiate collecting more information.

Many health facilities are limited to just reporting the number of cases of disease (i.e., summary-count data) via simple patient registers. As they become more able and interested, additional case-patient data (e.g., age and date of onset of disease) can be collected for selected health problems, and additional diseases can be added on the basis of priority setting (e.g., AIDS or moderate and severe malnutrition). The practice of collecting data intermittently for special purposes can be expanded, and data items found to be useful at sentinel sites can be added to reportable conditions from all health stations or at least can be expanded to a larger number of sentinel sites.

Display and interpretation of surveillance data and planned action based on the interpretation can be integrated into assigned duties of health workers and into the duties of their supervisors. Each health worker should have a detailed task analysis or job description, with the task analysis linked to national and local health objectives. Public health surveillance systems require good managers who understand how to use surveillance skills, quality assurance, and communications to bring the system to life and maximize its effectiveness as a tool to improve the health of the public.

Infrastructure and Communications Constraints

Lack of transportation for health staff to do public health work—including the investigation of cases, contact tracing, control of disease, or transporting specimens to laboratories—is frequently named as a significant constraint. The lack of basic equipment and supplies represents another obstacle. In a recent survey in Tanzania many of the health facilities did not have reporting forms, and health personnel often had not been trained to use the forms for reporting diseases within the surveillance system (P. Nsubuga, personal communication).

Electrical power may be available only erratically and, in some settings, not at all. There may be surges of power on the line that disable equipment or create errors in data bases In some places, there simply is not the resource or education base, or both, to create a computer-based system. In such settings, health workers may still rely on a handwritten reporting system. When this happens, it becomes even more challenging than usual to maintain quality control during the collection and tabulation of data, as well as to stimulate review and use of the information created through analysis of the data collected. It may also be a challenge to convince officials higher up in the public health or governmental systems of the validity and value of information that appears on hand-lined paper in handwritten script.

Often computers are not available, and when they are, they may be old or inaccessible to those who need them. Frequently computers are viewed as status symbols, resulting in inappropriate placement with, for example, executives who neither need to nor know how to use them, while not available for data entry and analysis. More positively, the increasing availability of computers in developing countries allows health workers to analyze surveillance data and even to connect electronically at regional and international levels. As the prices of computer hardware decreased, computers have been moved to zonal, state, and provincial levels. In many countries surveillance data have been analyzed with computers at the national and district levels for several years. Increasingly countries are reporting data to WHO electronically. *Epi Info,* an epidemiology computer program designed to assist data management and analysis, is available free and over the Internet (*44*). This program is available in seven languages (English, French, Spanish, Arabic, Russian, Chinese, and Serbo-Croatian), and manuals are also available in Italian, Portuguese, German, Norwegian, Hungarian, Czech, Polish, Rumanian, Indonesian, and Farsi.

Mapping of surveillance data has increased because inexpensive mapping programs that can display maps by district, health station, and village and can be linked to surveillance data bases. A mapping program called *Epi Map* is compatible with *Epi Info* and can create maps of surveillance data automatically (see Chapter 11).

CASE STUDY: TWO SURVEILLANCE SYSTEMS IN THE PHILIPPINES

In 1989, the Philippine Department of Health (PDOH), concerned about epidemics that were reported via the media but were not identified by the health information system, reviewed reports and determined that fewer than 10 outbreaks were reported to the central level per year in a country of over 60 million people. The PDOH then developed a sentinel surveillance system to provide early warning of outbreaks of selected infectious diseases. In its first year of operation, the system identified several outbreaks. One of these was an outbreak of tetanus that was traced to fireworks injuries in the annual New Year's celebration. Review of the causes of this outbreak led to the development of an injury-control program that reduced the numbers of injuries and eliminated the unexpectedly high number of cases of tetanus (*45*). The surveillance system showed that a surprising number of children in the age range of 1 to 2 years were having measles. This discovery led to a change in policy that allowed children of this age to be vaccinated for measles. When Mount Pinatubo erupted in 1992, the National Epidemic Sentinel Surveillance System (NESSS) staff were mobilized to conduct daily surveillance on over 100,000 evacuees (*46*). The system was well established by 1995. In that year the NESSS detected 80 epidemics that subsequently were formally investigated (*47*). These included 25 outbreaks of bacteriologically confirmed typhoid fever; 15, of clinical dengue; 10, of clinical measles; seven, of food poisoning of unknown cause; five, of laboratory-confirmed cholera; four, of human rabies; three, of malaria; two, of mushroom poisoning; two, of meningitis; two, of paralytic shellfish poisoning; and one each, of unspecified viral encephalitis, diphtheria, laboratory-confirmed chickungunya fever, leptospirosis, and puffer fish poisoning. All these outbreaks were investigated and in most cases control measures were implemented as a result of reports by the investigators.

In 1990, in response to reports that many vertical health information systems were inefficient, the PDOH revised routine reporting by creating the Field Health Surveillance Information System (FHSIS), a centrally designed integrated information system, which aimed to integrate management information, vital statistics, and notifiable diseases information systems. Because this system had the broad objectives of combining public health surveillance and process management information for many programs, it was instituted in all health facilities run by the government. Data tables were designed at the central level to make it easy for local health personnel to analyze their own information as well as to pass it to the provincial level, where data were computerized, reanalyzed, and sent upward. After a short period of pretests, the system was instituted nationwide. Unfortunately, the FHSIS fared less well than the NESSS. In the mid-1990s, the PDOH decentralized and the central budget was decreased. The staff of FHSIS were not able to adapt the system to decentralization; it became increasingly difficult to get data from many independent health units, data quality was difficult to estimate, and reports to the central managers fell years behind. In early 1999, we assessed parts of the Philippine health system including the FHSIS. About half the units of local governments we visited reported that they found the FHSIS useful and said they were continuing to fill out the forms and analyze the information for program purposes at their level. The rest said they had abandoned the FHSIS altogether because it was an impractical system designed to meet the needs of central managers. At the central level, the most recent national report available covered the year 1995. Only 50 copies had been printed.

In contrast, throughout the 1990s, program managers and top PDOH management increasingly relied on the uninterrupted flow of sentinel surveillance data from the NESSS to estimate disease burden and to monitor program impact. The NESSS was gradually expanded to include surveillance for fireworks injuries (hospital-based), HIV infection (community-based), acute flaccid paralysis (AFP) and poliomyelitis (facility-based), and HIV behavioral risk factors (community-based). In 1999 the PDOH reorganized and merged all population-based health information systems (including FHSIS) under the managers of the NESSS in the hope that the quality and timeliness of the other systems would rise to meet the levels achieved with the NESSS.

As described above, the NESSS and allied surveillance systems successfully met the needs of leaders of the PDOH and other constituents, while the FHSIS struggled to meet its objectives. Why do some systems succeed and others do not? One can identify some of the lessons by reviewing the steps in the implementation of the systems.

The first step in designing a surveillance system is to identify the objectives. Too often, large integrated surveillance systems like the FHSIS have broad and ambitious objectives of integrating many process-management, vital-statistics, and population-outcome measurements into one system for an entire nation. These ambitious plans are seldom matched with sufficient resources, and the system struggles under unrealistic expectations and lack of focus. In contrast, the original objective of the Philippines NESSS was narrow—i.e., to identify large epidemics of acute infectious disease quickly enough that appropriate public health interventions could be applied promptly. It was much easier for the staff of the NESSS to focus their efforts on meeting their objective and thus to provide early successes that showed PDOH management and other constituents that the system was useful. It was then possible to build the NESSS into a more integrated system by adding tasks one at a time over the years, as it moved from a strictly facility-based system to include a community-based component. Gradual growth allowed constituents within PDOH to accept and mold the system to their needs. It should be noted that the transition to community-based sentinel surveillance allows the system to make better estimates of incidence and prevalence rates (which require population-based denominators) and increases the system's ability to promote equity (48).

The purpose of surveillance is to provide information needed by managers and other decision makers. Thus, it is essential to design the system to provide information in a format that they can readily understand and use. The NESSS system was designed by the staff of the Department of Health and Field Epidemiology Training Program trainees who worked closely with users of the information or were users themselves. In contrast, large integrated information systems are often designed by computer specialists and systems analysts who are unfamiliar with the needs of decision makers in the field. It is easy for system designers to focus entirely on hard issues of data collection, tabulation, analysis, and reporting without recognizing the need for ownship that is critical for sustainability. The problem is compounded if the designers are consultants from outside the system, which increases the chance that health personnel will assume the system is imposed on them from the outside. This makes it less likely that they will feel ownership and sustain the system after external funding is discontinued. Thus, it is very important to involve users in the design of an information system, especially in the definition of the data to be collected and the format in which the resulting information will be presented. This principle can be carried too far, however. Systems designed for the objectives of multiple users (researchers, program managers, donors) may end up collecting so much information that they fail to meet the needs of most of the users.

In middle- and low-income countries, donors often provide funding for projects, and those same donors are key consumers of surveillance and other health information. In the Philippines, donors were skeptical about the utility of the NESSS for PDOH and themselves, so they declined to provide funding for creating the sentinel surveillance system. Because NESSS was funded with limited local funds, it had to be small and focused. As the system demonstrated its utility, top PDOH managers and donors gradually added funds for activities (such as HIV behavioral risk factor surveillance). The system grew incrementally. On the other hand, those same donors felt the need for higher-quality national data to use in monitoring their many projects; this perceived need was shared by top PDOH management. Therefore, the FHSIS was well funded at the start, but was required to cover the entire nation in a short period. With the funding came the need to meet donor agendas and to keep to what was—in retrospect—an impossibly tight time schedule to provide the national data that donors and top managers needed acutely. In the end, these tight deadlines made implementation of the broad-based system a formidable challenge.

Frequency of reporting depends on how often users need information. The NESSS reports on epidemics had to be created and disseminated frequently to allow time to conduct investigations and to apply appropriate interventions in order to prevent future cases. In order to meet this need, the new system was designed to provide weekly reports. Because the FHSIS to be was a national system with many users, reports were planned for different levels at different times. This proved difficult in practice and reporting, especially at the national level and reports fell far behind schedule.

The larger the size of the population under surveillance, the slower the process of collection and analysis. This is a crucial trade-off in any surveillance activity. In order to provide weekly reports, the NESSS designers chose a sentinel design with 14 facilities. Because admissions to facilities may depend on changes in referral patterns or other factors in addition to rates of illness in the population, the NESSS data provide only very rough estimates of rates of illness in the population. The FHSIS mandate involved providing information on all health facilities so it covered all health units. Whereas the NESSS trade-off provided rapid reports while sacrificing geographic completeness, the FHSIS design required geographic completeness. However, this large scale made implementation and quality control difficult. For broad geographic coverage of many variables, it is often most practical to depend on periodic surveys rather than on ongoing information systems. In many cases, national surveys have proved to be more satisfactory sources of national estimates in the Philippines than has the FHSIS or the NESSS.

Designers of information systems are often faced with top managers or donors who demand information systems that are good, fast, and cheap. It is useful to draw these three attributes on a triangle and explain that it is practical to provide any two sides, such as good and cheap or fast and good, but that it is very difficult to build a system that is good, fast, and cheap. This involves the decision makers in the discussion about the trade-offs that inevitably have to be made in all information systems.

Important factors for the success of the NESSS included its focus on designing the entire system around customer needs, emphasis on building and maintaining human capacity, and quality assurance. As the NESSS developed, the staff designed each new system beginning with consideration of how the reports needed to be designed and delivered in order to meet the needs of the users and then worked backwards to design the system to produce these reports (Table 13–5).

System designers tend to focus on hard issues of data collection, flow, tabulation, analysis, and reporting. It is easy to forget that a surveillance system is made up of people. Its success and sustainability depend on the attitudes and competencies of the people running the system. High-quality ongoing training, supervision, and career paths for surveillance system staff are critical ingredients in successful information systems. As the NESSS was piloted, its managers realized the importance of a cadre of competent and dedicated people to run it. Too often, planners of surveillance systems focus on data and only realize the im-

Table 13–5 Steps in the Development of the Philippine National Epidemic Sentinel Surveillance System

Data Side	Human Capacity Side
1. Identify the health problems thought to cause burden of disease	Consult top managers, donors, international agencies, experts
2. Determine who will make interventions	Involve users in design
3. Determine information users need to make interventions	Involve users in design
4. Decide how often decision makers need reports	Involve users in design
5. Identify who collects, tabulates, analyzes, reports, disseminates information	Identify manager, staff to analyze, report, and enter data
6. Design report	Involve users and staff in design
7. Make shell tables	Involve staff in design
8. Design questionnaire	Involve staff in design
9. Pilot questionnaire	Involve staff in implementation and evaluation
10. Pilot data flow and analysis	Involve staff in implementation and evaluation
11. Pilot system	Train staff in system and involve them in evaluation
12. Run system	Involve staff in ongoing training and quality assurance monitoring
13. Evaluate system: Was information used? Is data and analysis of good quality?	Involve staff and users in design of external evaluation and in review of evaluator's report
14. Revise system	Involve staff and users

portance of good personnel after the system falters. NESSS built staff by developing competency-based training for the nurses, who supervised implementation of each site, and for data entry clerks. Analysis and reporting of surveillance data is not a trivial task. Successful surveillance systems provide training and quality assurance for analysis and reporting functions, which are typically done by professionals. The NESSS sponsors yearly meetings where surveillance staff meet and present successes and problems. The system also includes ongoing monitoring and periodic external evaluations. In contrast, the FHSIS was severely constrained by limited funding for staff training and development. To meet this need, an innovative computer program was written to automate data analysis (47). This program used the metaphor of "a black box" into which clerks could enter data. The program analyzed the data and produced a variety of useful reports without the need of human analysis. While this was a cost-effective way to provide reports, some health workers felt uneasy that they did not have access to their own data and they were unable to modify the analysis done by the program. Some seemed to feel that the program might replace rather than complement their own analyses. This decreased acceptance and use of the program.

Both NESSS and FHSIS successfully met many of their goals, but neither was able to meet all the information needs of the PDOH. Their experience illustrates several key points about successful surveillance systems:

- Objectives are realistic, clear, and focused on providing the information needed to implement programs to improve public health.
- Resources and expectations are realistic and balanced.
- Stakeholders understand that all surveillance systems involve compromise and gradual improvement based on monitoring and evaluation.
- Users are involved in the design of reports.
- Processes for data collection are appropriate to the data.
- Staff are involved in design of processes and monitoring.
- There is ongoing training and career development for staff at all levels (including those who analyze and report information, not just data entry clerks).
- Ongoing monitoring is used to improve processes.
- Periodic external evaluations are used to build the system and confirm its utility as a public health management tool.

SUMMARY

The vision for surveillance systems in developing countries involves systems that are linked to health objectives, ordered by priority, limited in scope, and not burdensome at the health facility level. These systems may involve not only innovative data sources and methods to deal with the resource constraints, but also the opportunities that come with increasing emphasis on decentralization. It is hoped that improvements will come in methods to obtain population-based data gathering from vital-event registration and surveys. Donors and international agencies can be instrumental in assisting countries to strengthen their own capacity at gathering this type of information rather than creating multiple vertical systems that do not connect.

In implementing surveillance and health systems, developing counties can avoid the mistakes that industrialized countries have already made. These include poorly planned and fragmented surveillance systems, surveillance systems that are not linked to objectives, health objectives that are not explicit and often politicized, large divisions between curative and preventive medicine, and differences in health care between rural and urban areas. Most important are the infrastructure and managerial supports that are necessary to motivate the personnel who run the system despite significant obstacles. Surveillance in developing countries is accompanied by numerous logistic problems but also presents unique opportunities. The careful setting of health priorities and the meticulous allocation of limited resources to the interests of the public's health can be the results of surveillance in such settings.

Surveillance data need to be collected based on the frequency of decision making. For certain types of information every 3–5 years may be sufficient for the program needs. Health objectives provide national politicians and health leaders a plan to ensure the public's health. With a surveillance system that is linked to these objectives, leaders will be able to monitor progress made toward meeting national objectives. With analysis and action at the district and health facility level, local health staff can take rapid and appropriate action.

The authors wish to acknowledge Manuel M. Dayrit, Felilia White, Edna Lopez, Maria Concepcion Roces, Maria Consorcia Lim-Quizon, and the many others who developed the Philippine National Epidemic Sentinel Surveillance System used as an example in this chapter.

REFERENCES

1. World Bank. World development report. London: Oxford University Press, 1997.
2. Centers for Disease Control. National Center for Health Statistics. Health status indicators for the year 2000. *Statistical Notes* 1991;1:1–4.
3. Murray JL, Lopez AD. Global burden of disease summary. Geneva: World Health Organization, 1996.
4. McDonnell S, Vossberg K, Hopkins RS, Mittan B. YPLL as a guide to county health planning. *Public Health Reports* 1998;113:55–61.
5. Langmuir AD. The surveillance of communicable diseases of national importance. *NEJM* 1963:268(4):182–92.
6. Centers for Disease Control and Prevention. Progress toward global poliomyelitis eradication—1997–1998. *MMWR* 1999:48(20):416–21.
7. Henderson DA. Eradication: Lessons learned from the past. *Bull WHO* 1998;76 (Suppl 2):17–21.
8. Starling CF, Couto BR, Pinheriro SM. Applying the Centers of Disease Control and Prevention and National Nosocomial Surveillance System methods in Brazilian hospitals. *Am J Infection Control* 1997;25:303–11.
9. Duran-Arenas L, Rivero CC, Canton SF, Rodreiguez RS, Franco F, Luna RW, Catino J. The development of a quality information system: a case study in Mexico. *Health Policy and Planning* 1998;13:446–58.
10. Sandiford P, Annett H, Cibulskis R. What can information systems do for primary health care? An international perspective. *Soc Sci Med* 1992:34(10):1077–87.
11. Jamison DT, Mosley WH. Disease control priorities in developing countries: health policy responses to epidemiological change. *Am J Public Health* 1991;81:15–22.
12. Jamison DT, Mosley WH (eds.). Disease control priorities in developing countries. Oxford and New York: Oxford University Press, 1993.
13. Thacker SB, Berkelman RL. Public health surveillance in the United States. *Epidemiol Rev* 1988;10:164–90.
14. Carter A. Setting priorities: the Canadian experience in communicable disease surveillance. In: Proceedings of the 1992 International Symposium on Public Health Surveillance. *MMWR* 1992;41(Suppl):79–84.
15. Creese AL, Martin JD, Visschedijk JHM. Health systems for the 21st century. *WHO World Health Statistics Quarterly* 1998;51:21–7.
16. Lamden K. Disease surveillance at district level [letter; comment]. *Lancet* 1998; 352(9134):1153–4.
17. Walsh JA, Warren KS. Selective primary health care: an interim strategy for disease control in developing countries. *N Engl J Med* 1979;301:967–74.
18. U.S. Bureau of the Census. Historical statistics of the United States, colonial times to 1970. Bicentennial edition, Part 1. Washington, D.C.: Government Printing Office, 1975.

19. McCarthy BJ, Terry J, Rochat R, Quave S, Tyler CW. The underregistration of neonatal deaths: Georgia 1974–1977. *Am J Public Health* 1980:977–82.
20. Kielmann AA, Taylor CE, DeSweemer C *et al.* Child and maternal health services in rural India: the Narangwal experiment. Baltimore: Johns Hopkins University Press, 1983.
21. World Health Organization. Lay reporting of health information. Geneva: World Health Organization, 1978.
22. Espitia VE. Intentional and unitentional fatal injuries—Cali, Colombia, 1993–1996. Bogota, Columbia: Ministry of Health, 1997.
23. Expanded Programme on Immunization. The EPI coverage survey. Training for mid-level managers. Geneva: World Health Organization, 1988.
24. Lemeshow S, Stroh G. Sampling techniques for evaluating health parameters in developing countries. Washington, D.C.: National Academy Press, 1988.
25. U.S. Agency for International Development and the Centers for Disease Control. African child survival initiative, 1989–1990. Bilingual annual report. Washington, D.C.: Government Printing Office, 1990.
26. Abramson JH, Abramson ZH (eds.). Survey methods in community medicine: epidemiological research, programme evaluation. Fifth edition. New York: Churchill Livingstone, 1999:166–70.
27. Scrimshaw NS, Gleason GR (eds.). Rapid assessment procedures. Boston: International Nutrition Foundation of Developing Countries (INFDC), 1992: 326–31.
28. Centers for Disease Control. Guidelines for evaluating surveillance systems. *MMWR* 1988(Suppl No S-5):1–20.
29. John TJ, Samuel R, Balraj V, John R. Disease surveillance at district level: a model for developing countries. *Lancet* 1998;352(9121):58–61.
30. Adams OB, Hirschfeld M. Human resources for health. *World Health Statistics Quarterly* 1998;51:28–32.
31. Music SI, Schultz MG. Field epidemiology and training programs: new international health resources. *JAMA* 1990;263(June 27):3309–11.
32. Cardenas V, Sanchez C, De la Hoz F *et al.* Colombia Field Epidemiology Training Program. *Am J Pub Health* 1998;88(9):1404–5.
33. Evaluation of the Field Epidemiology Training Program (FETP). Administrative Report for Contract No. 200-96-0599-03. Arlington, Va.: Batelle, 1998.
34. Henderson DA. Surveillance of smallpox. *Int J Epidemiol* 1976;5(1):19–28.
35. Morris S, Gray A, Noone A, Wiseman M, Sushil J. The costs and effectiveness of surveillance of communicable disease: a case study of HIV and AIDS in England and Wales. *J Pub Health Med* 1996;18:415–22.
36. Taylor C. Surveillance for equity in primary health care: policy implications from international experience. *Int J Epi* 1992;21:1043–9.
37. Sutter RW, Cocchi SL. Comment: ethical dilemmas in worldwide polio eradication programs [comment]. *Am J Pub Health* 1997;87(6):913–6.
38. Salisbury D. Report of the workgroup on disease elimination/eradication and sustainable health development. *Bull WHO* 1998;76(Suppl 2).
39. Centers for Disease Control and Prevention. Progress toward global poliomyelitis eradication—1997–1998. *MMWR* 1999;48(20):416–21.
40. Expanded Programme on Immunization. The EPI coverage survey: training for mid-level managers. Geneva: World Health Organization, 1988.
41. Galazka A, Stroh G. Guidelines on the community-based survey of neonatal tetanus mortality. Geneva: World Health Organization, WHO/EPI/GEN/86/8, 1986.

42. Programme for Control of Diarrhoeal Diseases. Household survey manual: diarrhea case management, morbidity, and mortality. Geneva: World Health Organization, CDD/SER/86.2/Rev.1, 1989.
43. McCusker J. Epidemiology in community health. Nairobi, Kenya: African Medical and Research Foundation, 1978.
44. Dean, AG, Dean JA, Coulombier D *et al. Epi Info.* Version 6. A word-processing, data-base, and statistics program for public health on IBM-compatible microcomputers. Atlanta: Centers for Disease Control and Prevention, 1995.
45. Annual National Epidemic Sentinel Surveillance Report, 1995. Department of Health, San Lazaro Compound, Santa Cruz Manila, 1995.
46. Centers for Disease Control and Prevention. Surveillance in eradication camps after the eruption of Mt. Pinatubo, Philippines. *MMWR* 1992;41:SS1:963.
47. Marte AB, Schwefel D. The Philippine management information system for public health programs, vital statistics, mortality, and other notifiable diseases. *International Journal of Bio-Medical Computing* 1995;40:107–14.
48. Taylor CE. Surveillance for equity in primary health care: policy implications from international experience. *Int J Epidemiol* 1992;21:1043–9.

14

Surveillance of Quality in Health Care

JAMES F. MURRAY

The needs of each and every individual are of equal importance, and those needs must be made the basis for the planning of societies. All resources must be used in such a way as to ensure that every individual has equal opportunities for participation.

1982 U.N. General Assembly

In recent years managed-care organizations (MCOs) in the United States have created surveillance systems with the capacity to acquire information about health-care processes and outcomes that were previously unavailable or prohibitively expensive and to take action based on that information. This chapter focuses on managed care's use of surveillance for assessing the quality of health care and will address the following issues.

- What conditions initiated an emphasis on quality surveillance?
- Why did quality surveillance become an issue and flourish under managed care?
- What are the traditional definitions and approaches for assessing the quality of health care?
- What resources, both data and other types, are available for quality surveillance?
- What are some examples of specific applications of quality surveillance?
- How have MCOs and others implemented quality surveillance?
- How have MCOs, government regulators, employers, and individual consumers received quality surveillance results and subsequently acted on this information?

The terms *managed care organization, MCO, managed care,* and *managed care health plan* are used interchangeably in this chapter to describe any organization that assumes responsibility for both the financing/insurance function and delivery of health care. Specific managed-care structures such as health maintenance organizations (HMOs) and preferred provider organization (PPOs) are used when those terms are most descriptive.

MANAGED CARE

MCO's focus on quality surveillance comes from their mission statement. MCOs have declared themselves responsible for both the financing and delivery of health care to a defined population. Success at this mission depends on access to information on population demographics, health-care utilization patterns, and associated medical costs. This responsibility and access to information is the cornerstone and catalyst for quality surveillance.

Close relationships between beneficiary and payer are found in government systems of health care (i.e., Medicare, Medicaid, and the Veterans Administration [VA] systems). With the exception of the VA, however these government insurance plans do not encompass the delivery of health care within their structure or processes; their mission is payment only but they have established important precedents. Many health-care data standards have their origins in government-sponsored systems. Quality and cost concerns initiated measurement and management efforts to balance both dimensions (1–3).

Within the traditional fee-for-service health-care system, however, the ability and incentive to comprehensively assess and improve quality on a *system-wide* basis did not exist. Traditional fee-for-service systems could not define a population for which insurers or providers could unambiguously be held accountable. Even if a population could be defined, accountability of insurers or providers was hampered by the cottage industry nature of health care. There was no system to facilitate communication and coordination between providers. Capturing all of the relevant information about the health services received by an individual, much less a population, was difficult if not impossible. Assessment of quality in our health-care system was therefore sporadic and fragmented. Quality measurement and improvement efforts were confined within delivery sites (e.g., hospitals) and did not take a population-based approach. This created a system where no single person was responsible for the care of an individual; no one could determine whether the overall care received by an individual was optimal. This situation changed with managed care. From what previously existed as a set of unconnected providers with no standardized processes and little incentive to optimize the cost and quality of health care, managed care created a system where both cost and quality of care had the potential to be better coordinated and comprehensively managed.

Concern about the rising cost of health care was a major catalyst and incentive for the growth of managed care. Managed care offered cost savings at a time when the traditional health-care system, with no incentive to control costs, was experiencing staggering medical cost inflation. Examples of how MCOs achieved success in cost containment will be explored in the next section. The cost advantage of managed care drove up payer demand for this type of system, causing a proliferation of MCOs to spring up. This resulted in a dramatic shift of the U.S. population into managed care (4–15).

In addition to financial management, managed care placed an emphasis on maintaining the health of its population. The original nomenclature and model of managed care was the HMO. HMOs were founded on the belief that a healthy population would have less need for catastrophic (i.e., reactive, intensive, and expensive) services. Regular visits and screening procedures (such as cancer screening and immunizations) took on great importance to provide early warnings or prevention of problems to come.

In recent times there has been an evolution of managed care beyond an HMO. There has been a proliferation of structures and philosophies that defy easy categorization or nomenclatures. What has stayed consistent is the dual mission that accepts responsibility for both the financing and delivery of care.

Managed Care and Cost Containment

MCOs achieved cost savings through successful efforts in cost containment. These efforts have had both a positive and a negative impact on their approach to and success in performing quality surveillance. A fundamental change under managed care was in provider selection and access to specialists and hospitals for beneficiaries. Traditional fee-for-service insurance allowed beneficiaries open access to the providers of their choice; managed care restricted beneficiaries to a pre-selected set of providers that were either employees of the MCO (the staff model) or had a contracted relationship with the MCO (the group or independent provider model). This restricted provider network allowed the MCO to exercise tighter controls on the delivery of care and associated costs/reimbursement policies and procedures. This arrangement facilitated the implementation of quality surveillance since policies and procedures for quality initiatives (e.g., data submission requirements and access to necessary information such as medical records) were included in the provider contracts. However, on the negative side, limitation of choice and restricted access to providers has adversely affected the perception of quality under managed care.

A second effort was utilization management (UM), a second level of review on medical decisions in which the MCO makes the final decision on the appropriateness and necessity for specific, usually expensive, medical services (16). For example, use of emergency room services and admission to a hospital requires the authorization of the MCO. Failure to obtain such authorization may result in the denial of payment for the service. Additionally, the amount and extent of usage is also closely monitored; the duration of inpatient stays, for example, requires the approval of the MCO. Any additional days in the hospital past the approved length of stay may not be covered. This type of management and data collection process is potentially a benefit to quality surveillance and improvement efforts. However, the entire process has had a negative impact on the perception of quality in MCOs. Because it sometimes denied requested services and initiated disagreements on what was necessary and appropriate UM was not well received by providers and patients. In conjunction with limited provider access, UM contributes to the attitude that managed care withholds necessary services.

An innovation under managed care was capitation. Capitation is a fixed prepayment to a provider (such as a physician) to supply a set of services for a defined population (17–19). For example, under capitation a primary care physician (PCP) receives a fixed payment for each MCO member in his practice. The PCP is subsequently responsible for all acute, preventive, and chronic primary care services delivered at his or her primary care office. A variant of a capitated arrangement is a "carved-out" service. This is a packaged set of related services for which a fixed reimbursement is paid to the provider. Both capitation and carved-out services have risks and benefits for the provider and health plan. On the benefit side, the provider gains a certain amount of autonomy in the delivery of care. However, the provider now has a financial risk that creates an incentive to carefully manage the resources consumed. This incentive is often described as a perverse incentive because it creates an environment where withholding services may result in greater financial reward for the provider. This type of environment is the opposite of the traditional fee-for-service system that rewarded the provider for doing more—which has a different type of risk of providing unnecessary and potentially harmful services.

The benefit of capitation to the MCO is bounded financial risk for delivering required services to its members. The downside for the MCO is further concern that managed care promulgates and supports an environment that may withhold necessary services. Capitation and carve-outs have had mostly a negative impact on the quality of surveillance. These strategies can adversely affect access to accurate and comprehensive data. This issue will be explored more fully below.

These innovations and cost management techniques created savings for both employers and employees and profits for the health plans. However, the success in cost containment, coupled with the increasing numbers of beneficiaries being driven into managed health care, fueled a mounting concern that the emphasis on costs adversely affected the quality of health care under managed care. In reaction to this concern, the concept of accountability was introduced. Accountability, in its simplest definition, is the quality surveillance holding a specified entity responsible for the quality of care delivered.

ACCOUNTABILITY AND QUALITY IN HEALTH CARE

This section will provide a brief overview of the foundations of quality measurement. Ernest Codman is credited with introducing a concern for health-care quality by an introspective assessment of surgical practice at Massachusetts General Hospital in the early 1900s (20,21). Various definitions and measurements of quality were proposed in the ensuing years. Drawing on all of the work since Codman, Donabedian produced a definitive taxonomy of quality in health care (22–24). Donabedian institutionalized what has become known as the triad of quality: structure, process, and outcomes.

By the mid-1980s, concern about health-care costs had generated interest in total quality management (TQM) and continuous quality improvement (CQI) (25–30). These concepts and related tools had previously proven quite successful in the service and manufacturing industries. Their use in the health-care industry began in hospital settings where complex systems provide a broad range of services to their admitted populations that were amenable to the adaptation and implementation of TQM and CQI. Quality-improvement programs were initially targeted at service-related issues (such as improving the admission process) or optimizing the use of scarce resources (e.g., scheduling operating rooms).

For the reasons previously discussed, managed care had the potential to measure quality using Donabedian's framework and implement improvement efforts using the TQM/CQI paradigm. This ability, combined with the growing concern about cost containment and the perception of poor quality within managed care, created an environment that began demanding objective evidence of acceptable quality.

SOURCES OF DATA AND INFORMATION SYSTEMS

One of the fundamental principles in the quality paradigm is "You can't manage what you can't measure" (*31*). Given the marketplace demand to measure, report, and manage quality, health plans needed to develop and implement quality surveillance systems. Initial efforts by health plans were directed at mining their readily available sources of data. The most prominent source was their administrative claims data. Although these administrative claims systems were developed for reimbursement and financial management, they have significant potential to assess, inform decisions and initiate action on the quality of care being provided to MCO members. Managed-care data systems contain complete demographic information along with medical and pharmacy claims for health-care services received by beneficiaries. There are many examples of how administrative data can be used effectively for quality surveillance. Among these examples are the identification and tracking of patients with specific diseases (e.g., targeted chronic diseases) or who are receiving specialized types of care (e.g., pre-natal care registries), or the tracking of needed services (e.g., vaccinations, and mammograms) incontrovertibly linked to health outcomes (*32*). Applications are described more fully below. When administrative data are necessary but not sufficient they can be complemented with primary data-collection efforts from other data sources. This hybrid of data sources allows optimization of the data and emulates other public health data surveillance (see also Chapter 3). In summary, access to this kind of information is an enabler of quality surveillance on the structure, process, and outcomes of care provided by an MCO. In the sections below, the structure and content of these administrative data systems are discussed.

MCO Administrative Claims Data

No two managed-care administrative claims data sets are identical. They have not developed in a systematic and consistent fashion with well-defined standards. However, largely due to the data requirements from the Health Care Financing Agency (HCFA) for Medicare reimbursement, standards do exist. These standards have been generally adopted intact though they are frequently modified and enhanced by the health plans to suit their own needs. In spite of customizing, the overall result has been common structures and data elements at the core of most managed-care data sets.

In general, there are four basic types of MCO administrative data. Three types of data coincide with the three major sites of health-care services. These types are *a*) hospitalizations and outpatient procedures; *b*) outpatient physician, specialist, and ancillary services (e.g., laboratory and radiology); and *c*) pharmacy services. The fourth data type describes the population (i.e., members/beneficiaries). It includes information on the following: *a*) demographics, *b*) family composition as defined by insured individuals on the same policy, *c*) benefit design, and *d*) enrollment time frames and current status for the covered population. We will examine the potential issues and concerns for quality surveillance then examine each of these data sets and the common elements within them.

The first issue is the limited clinical validity and completeness of MCO administrative data. The primary purpose and rationale of the data was for financial reimbursement and management. Although the data sets contain "clinical" information, they are not a comprehensive clinical data set that adequately captures and/or describes all of the clinical issues in a member's health-care visit. For example, there is no information on key clinical findings or measurements (e.g., blood pressure, laboratory results, radiologic findings). The lack of complete clinical information limits the quality surveillance that can be accomplished with the data.

The clinical information that is present comes from several accepted coding standards. Diagnostic information is coded using the *International Classification of Disease, Version 9 (ICD-9)*. The *ICD-9* coding system is large, containing over 15,000 codes. However, despite its volume of codes, it has clinical limitations. Its size and the way in which it is used in practice can introduce unwanted coding variation. Clinical variation in coding occurs due to inherent uncertainty in the diagnostic process and the recording of working diagnoses until a definitive diagnosis can be made. Administrative variation occurs from the way in which different providers can and will code similar conditions. This variation affects the issues of data validity and reliability and will be examined later in this chapter.

Information on clinical procedures is important for determining the appropriate amount of reimbursement. There are several accepted methods for coding procedures performed during a health-care encounter. The standardized coding methods are *a*) *Common Procedure Terminology Version 4 (CPT-4)*, *b*) *ICD-9,* and *c*) the *Health Care Procedure Classification System (HCPCS)*. The procedural information is subject to similar concerns on validity (i.e., coding error) and reliability (i.e., variation) as the *ICD-9* diagnostic codes but to a lesser degree. Procedure codes are closely tied to reimbursement, and more likely to be audited. However, since procedure codes are linked to reimbursement, a phenomenon occurs known as *up-coding* which is the selection of a procedure code that can be justified for clinical appropriateness while maximizing the reimbursement amount for the provider.

Data Formats

Inevitably, the ability and utility of quality surveillance using administrative data comes down to what data are available, what they represent, and how they are interpreted. This section will briefly describe the four unique data formats for each of the four different types of data. This section will briefly outline the common data elements for each data type found in managed-care administrative data sets.

Inpatient Data

The HCFA data format for reimbursement to hospitals and outpatient surgical facilities is the HCFA 1450 (also known as the UB-92). This format is used by facilities for reimbursement (e.g., room and board charges). It is not used for reimbursement to a physician (see HCFA 1500 below). Because of the complex nature of institutionalized care, the form is quite long and complicated. Table 14–1 shows the most common data elements used by MCOs unique to the HCFA 1450.

Outpatient Data

The HCFA data format for reporting physician and ancillary services is the HCFA 1500. Table 14–2 contains the most common data elements of the HCFA 1500 used by MCOs.

Table 14–1 Data Elements in the HCFA 1450 or UB-92

Data Element	Description
Member ID	Unique member identification number
Facility ID	Unique code that identifies the facility requesting reimbursement for the inpatient, emergency room, or outpatient services provided
Facility location	Data on the address, city, state, zip code of the facility
Admission date	Date on which the patient was admitted
Discharge date	Date on which the patient was discharged
Type of admission	Emergency, urgent, elective, not available
Diagnosis-related group (DRG)	Clinical classification system used to group hospital inpatients according to the major reason for admission (i.e., principal diagnosis and procedure codes)
Length of stay	The number of days the beneficiary was in the institution
Total charge	Total charges for the event
Principal diagnosis	The condition considered primarily responsible for the admission or outpatient event
Secondary diagnoses (up to 8 additional)	Additional diagnoses that co-existed at the time of admission or developed subsequently
Admitting diagnoses	The condition identified at the time of admission requiring hospitalization
Principal procedure Code and date performed	The principal inpatient procedure and its date. The principal procedure is for definitive treatment rather than diagnostic or exploratory purposes
Secondary procedures and dates	Up to 5 additional procedures and dates on which they were performed during the stay
Patient discharge status	Identifies whether patient was alive or dead; if alive, the location to where the patient was discharged (e.g., home)

Table 14-2 Data Elements in the HCFA 1500

Data Element	Description
Member ID	Unique member identification number
Physician ID	Unique physician identifier
Physician location	Data on the address, city, state, zip code of the physician
Date of service	Date on which the service was performed
Date episode started	If this is continuation of care for a particular condition, indicate date on which care was initiated
Referring physician ID	Unique ID for the referring physician
Diagnosis 1 through diagnosis 4	The conditions treated during the visit. Each diagnosis is linked to one or more of the procedures performed during the visit
Procedure 1 through procedure 6	The procedures performed during the visit. The are coded using either CPT-4 or HCPCS coding standard
Charges 1 through charges 6	The charges for each of the procedures performed during the visit
Total charges	Summation of all individual charges

Pharmacy Data

The next data format is for the reimbursement of pharmacy claims. It is not a HCFA-originated format but was created and institutionalized by the National Council of Prescription Drug Programs (NCPDP). Specific drugs are identified using the National Drug Code assigned to every pharmaceutical product by the Food and Drug Administration (Table 14-3).

Member Data

The remaining data set is the member enrollment and eligibility file (Table 14-4). This data set contains the demographic and benefit coverage information for the members of the MCO. There is no precedent or industry standard for this data.

Table 14-3 Data Elements in the NCPDP Data Set

Data Element	Description
Member ID	Unique member identification number
Pharmacy ID	Unique pharmacy ID
Pharmacy location	Data on the address, city, state, zip code of the pharmacy
Date of service	The date on which the prescription was filled
Product NDC code	Unique national drug code (NDC) number for the medication
Quantity	The amount of medication given to the patient
Supply	The anticipated amount of time that the medication will last if taken as directed
Prescribed ID	The unique ID of the provider prescribing the medication
Total cost	Total cost of the prescription considering dispensing fees, copayment amounts, medication cost
Dispensing fee	Amount paid to the pharmacy for dispensing the medication
Paid amount	The cost of the medication
Copayment	The amount paid by the member for the medication

Table 14–4 Standard Data Elements for Population Demographics and Benefit Design

Data Element	Description
Member ID	Unique member identification number
Member location	Data on the address, city, state, zip code of the member
Date of birth	Patient birth year—used to calculate age
Sex	Sex of the member
Race	Race/ethnic origin of the member—not commonly found due to confidentiality concerns
Enrollment start	The date that the member was enrolled in the health plan under their current coverage
Enrollment end	The date that enrollment ended for a member. This field is blank for active members
Guarantor/dependent status	This field indicates who in the family is the responsible party for payment and/or carries the insurance coverage
Zip code	Member ZIP code
MSA	Metropolitan Statistical Area—geographical regions designated by the census bureau
Benefit information	Each plan and insurance product will have different benefit designs relative to the set of covered services, copayment amounts, deductibles, and coverage limits
Other demographics	Many fields contain personal identifying information that are generally held confidential by the plan. These items include family composition and relationships, employer, covered benefits to include copayment amounts

The data contains many sensitive data elements subject to confidentiality concerns. The issues of privacy, confidentiality, and legal concerns on access and use of such information have been discussed elsewhere (see also Chapter 10).

The discussion above does not represent a comprehensive review or inventory of all data elements collected by an MCO. It is presented as a minimum data set for the examples and application of quality surveillance to be presented later in the chapter.

Data Issues

A common concern on the use of administrative data for any purpose is the quality and validity of the data. There are important issues to understand about MCO administrative claim data before they can be effectively used for quality surveillance.

Data Quality Checks

As with any data set there are standardized checks to determine the validity of the data for the intended analysis. The following list is not comprehensive but provides a minimum set of data checks that should be performed.

- Extent of data missing—Do any data fields contain significant amounts of missing data?

- Data validity—Do the data within each field contain valid responses consistent with the meaning and content of that specific data field and data type? An example of a data field validity check is to determine if all *ICD-9* codes are found in the standard *ICD-9* dictionary. An example of a data type validity check would be to ensure that data fields represent valid and meaningful dates.
- Clinical validity—Are diagnostic information and procedural information consistent with each other and with the demographics of the population? Common problems include gender mismatch (e.g., males having a baby) and age mismatch (e.g., elderly women having a baby).
- Concurrent validity checks—One approach to assess concurrent validity is to check results against a national standard (e.g., compare prevalence rates of disease against published statistics). If widely divergent findings are found, then the user must determine if there is a plausible explanation for such a difference. If large, unexplained discrepancies are found they may invalidate the data for the intended analysis.

Validity of Diagnosis and Procedure Codes

Because of the complexity of the different coding systems, coding inaccuracies may occur. Ultimately, the validity of the clinical diagnosis and procedure recorded in the administrative data depends on how well they match a "gold standard." While medical records are far from an ideal gold standard, they are often considered as the definitive source of patient information. In two independent studies comparing the use of managed-care claims versus data obtained from review of the medical records, the level of agreement between administrative data and the medical record is acceptable for clinical information contained in the diagnostic and procedural codes (*33,34*). Although the level of agreement between automated claims and medical records is often quite high, the ideal strategy for determining clinical information most accurately is a combination of automated claims and medical record data. However, when only administrative data are available, the user should not allow the perfect to get in the way of the good enough.

Convenience Sample

Any MCO population and the related administrative data are inherently a convenience sample. Unlike a random or stratified sample of a population, a nonrandom sample raises issues about the generalizability of observed results. There may exist unobserved biases or confounding factors in the data. Selection bias is a specific form of bias in which members in the MCO have entered the health plans due to some unobserved yet systematic factor that introduces a bias into the observed results. An example of selection bias is "adverse selection," where a health plan may attract a population with higher levels of comorbidities or health risks. If bias exists, quantification and correction of the bias is critical before making inferences from the data. However, selection bias and its underlying causes are easily recognized. Some creative bias identification and quantification techniques have been developed (*35–37*). These techniques can not only assist in identifying selection bias, but also quantify the magnitude and/or control for selection bias. The surveyor can then determine if the presence, direction, and magnitude of the bias will adversely affect the outcomes of interest and the conclusions that can be drawn from the data. If selection bias exists, valuable information and valid conclusions may, under the right circumstances, still be extracted from the data. Correction of selection bias requires that a case mix or risk adjustment be performed to control for known confounding factors.

Enrollment Time Frames and Population Counts

Members who enroll and disenroll from a health plan at different points in time adversely affects both cross-sectional and longitudinal analyses. The method for counting the population requires adjusting for the differing time frames of enrollment. There are several methods for counting a population.

The first method uses a prespecified time requirement for enrollment. The specific details for an acceptable time frame and other enrollment criteria depend on the analysis being performed. The enrollment criteria may range from requiring absolute continuous enrollment over a specified time frame to allowing one or more breaks in enrollment that do not exceed a specific amount of time. For example, when assessing the immunization rate of children at 2 years of age, the inclusion criteria may require that all children be continuously enrolled from birth to 2 years of age. The continuous enrollment criteria may be slightly relaxed to allow a single break not to exceed a certain limit (e.g., 45 days). There are several reasons why allowing a break is reasonable and acceptable. Possibilities are *a*) a small lag time in communicating enrollment or benefit change information may occur between the employer and the health plan, or *b*) it is not uncommon that a Medicaid beneficiary may incur a single 30-day break in coverage during a calendar year.

The second method of counting a population is the effective membership approach. Effective membership is commonly used in determining the denominator of a rate or proportion for a particular event or outcome of interest. A time period of interest is determined (e.g., 1 year). Members are counted in the denominator and reflect the proportion of the time they were enrolled in the plan over the time period of interest. For example, if analyzing the admission rate for ischemic heart disease in a population over the course of 1 year then a member will be counted in the denominator based on that proportion of time enrolled during the year. A member enrolled for the entire year would count as 1; a member enrolled for only half of the year would have an effective membership of one-half and be counted as half a person in the denominator of the rate.

Different Contracting Strategies and Payment Mechanisms

Managed-care organizations may introduce variation into their data if they use different contracting and payment mechanisms for the providers in their networks. This may or may not adversely affect the validity of the data. As discussed, one of the innovations of managed care was capitation and carve-outs. Capitation and carve-outs are common causes of missing data. First, there is less incentive on the part of the provider to submit comprehensive data since detail on the services performed may not be required for payment. Second, any data that is submitted may be less reliable since there is no financial auditing of the data. If capitated or carved-out services are part of the health plan's contracting strategy then the user must determine the extent to which this practice adversely affects quality surveillance data for valid measurement of the specific processes or outcomes of interest.

Another payment mechanism that affects data completeness and validity is benefit design (e.g., the use of copayments). Benefit designs that do not cover certain goods or services will result in missing data since reimbursement claims are not submitted. For example, pharmaceutical coverage does not commonly pay for over-the-counter medications. Therefore, information on use of these medications is not available. Copayments can also adversely affect the data quality. In some circumstances the copayment required by the member equals or exceeds the costs of the medication or service. Again, missing data can be missed because a reimbursement claim is not submitted to the health plan.

Different Providers for Different Sets of Covered Services

In addition to payment mechanisms, there may be missing data due to services not covered by the health plan's contract. For example, an MCO may receive a contract for medical services but the pharmacy benefit administration is given to another organization. This creates an incomplete picture for both organizations since the medical and pharmacy experiences of the member cannot be linked. There is no simple solution to this problem other than the exclusion of members from the analysis for which complete data are not available.

Administrative claims data, while not perfect, have several advantages over primary data collection and other surveillance methods (38). The acquisition of the data is attractive from a cost perspective since it comes as a by-product of the claims payment process. Claims data can easily cover large numbers of patients with less inconvenience to health plan providers and members. Administrative claims data will provide valid cost and resource data from the perspective of the payer.

Administrative claims data may be used to construct individual episodes of care for selected conditions at the level of the individual member. Episodes of care are temporal analyses that link the longitudinal experience of a member across all places of service for all services related to a particular condition. Episodes of care can be used to determine access and coordination of care for the targeted condition. In addition to the clinical diagnostic and procedural information, episodes will capture all relevant charge data, enabling more robust economic analyses to be performed (39–41).

While there are many potential pitfalls in the use of administrative data sets, successful navigation through these data issues yields a powerful resource for surveillance. A recent study by Fink concluded that "HMO data sets are significant improvements over indemnity plan data, and where available, their accuracy in measuring health services utilization is superior to surveys" (42). If the weakness of the data is recognized and proper analysis is done to assess the quality of the data, administrative claims data are a powerful resource for quality surveillance.

SURVEILLANCE EXAMPLES

Quality surveillance will be presented in the context of accountability (i.e., quality surveillance with the goal of holding a health plan or provider responsible for the quality of care delivered) and with an emphasis on the population-based measurement and improvement of health outcomes. Two examples of quality surveillance using managed-care data will be explored: *a*) identifying a population with a chronic disease from administrative data bases and *b*) using quality and accountability measures in surveillance systems.

Identifying a Chronic Disease Population from Administrative Data Sources

A first step in quality surveillance is the development, validation, and implementation of administrative data algorithms for identifying members with targeted conditions (e.g., chronic diseases). Health-plan members with chronic disease need continuing medical care and management of their condition to optimize their health outcomes. The identification and tracking of these members are critical to both the quality and the financial concerns of the MCO.

The administrative data sets of MCOs are good for identifying and tracking members with chronic disease (*43,44*). Once the members are identified then additional analyses can assess other measures of interest. Examples of such measures are *a*) the prevalence of disease, *b*) prevalence by patient demographics and provider characteristics, and *c*) the relationship between treatment patterns and patient outcomes.

The methodology for identifying members with a chronic disease uses the relevant diagnosis (i.e., *ICD-9*), procedure (i.e., *CPT-4, HCPCS,* or *ICD-9*), or pharmacy codes (i.e., *NDC codes*) that are indicative of the targeted condition. The first example comes from the Healthplan Employer Data Information Set (HEDIS), which is a quality surveillance and accountability system based in part on managed-care administrative data. The background and purpose of the HEDIS are discussed in a later section. The following administrative data algorithm is used by the HEDIS for the identification of hypertensive members for its "Control of High Blood Pressure" performance measure (*45*). A health-plan member is considered to have hypertension if

- there is at least one outpatient encounter with an *ICD-9* diagnosis code of 401 or 401.x in the last 6 months,
- AND the diagnosis of hypertension during that time period is confirmed by chart review. The documentation in the medical record must consist of one or more of the following words or phrases: *hypertension; HTN; high blood pressure; HBP; or ↑ BP*).

The HEDIS hypertension algorithm starts with the administrative data but requires validation of hypertension in the associated medical record. However, some algorithms rely solely on administrative data without medical record validation. For example, Quam developed a different approach for the identification of hypertensive members (*46*). A member can be flagged as hypertensive based on the following criteria:

1. At least one claim with an *ICD-9* code (primary, secondary, or otherwise) of one of the following codes:
   - 401.xx—essential hypertension
   - 402.xx—hypertensive heart disease
   - 403.xx—hypertensive renal disease
   - 404.xx—hypertensive heart and renal disease
   - 362.11—hypertensive retinopathy
   - 437.2—hypertensive encephalopathy

   Two separate claims on two different dates of services with any of the above diagnosis codes improve the ability to identify accurately a member as being hypertensive. However, the claims may not have come from a pathologist, radiologist, or independent laboratory.

2. Optimal identification occurs when medical claims are combined with pharmacy scripts. If only one medical claim is found with the appropriate diagnostic information, the member may still be flagged as hypertensive if at least one pharmacy claim is found during the relevant time period for a drug in one of the following therapeutic classes:
   - calcium antagonist
   - loop diuretics
   - thiazide and related diuretics
   - potassium-sparing diuretics
   - beta-adrenergic blocking drugs
   - peripherally acting anti-adrenergic drugs
   - centrally-acting anti-hypertensives
   - vasodilating anti-hypertensives
   - angiotensin-converting enzyme (ACE) inhibitors
   - angiotensin II receptor blocking drugs
   - other anti-hypertensive drugs

Consider the differences in these two algorithms. The HEDIS algorithm, due to the medical record validation component, ensures that all members being assessed are hypertensive (i.e., it maximizes positive predictive value). However, if an error rate of less than 5% in the positive predictive value is acceptable, then the Quam algorithm performs well without the medical record validation. The Quam algorithm using both administrative medical and pharmacy claims had a 96% agreement with the medical record yielding an error rate in the positive predictive value of only 4% (*46*).

A key point in these examples is that the development of any administrative data algorithm should include the validation of the algorithm and determination of its operating characteristics (i.e., the sensitivity, specificity, and positive predictive value of the identification algorithms). The appropriateness of the algorithm for its intended usage requires careful assessment by the analyst on the cost and complexity of the methodology versus maximizing these operating characteristics. For example, an administrative data approach to finding individuals with chronic disease uses readily available data and therefore will be less expensive to implement. However, sole reliance on an administrative-claims-data approach will have a higher level of sensitivity (i.e., ability to detect all of the individuals with the disease). Administrative data sources are inherently biased because all individuals with a condition may not see a physician in the analytical time frame selected or the individual may see a physician but the physician does not record it on the medical claim. Validation of an algorithm is necessary to fully understand any bias and determine the operating characteristics of the algorithm and determine its appropriateness for the intended use. Validation of an administrative data algorithm can be accomplished by selecting a sample of members with and without the disease from the population. The administrative data sample is compared to a "gold standard" source, often the medical record. The information from the medical record is used to confirm or refute the diagnosis of the chronic disease for those members. This was the type of validation performed for the HEDIS hypertension algorithm. The HEDIS hypertension algorithm using only administrative data has a sensitivity of 54%, a specificity of 95%, and a positive predictive value of 88% (45). Since the goal of the HEDIS measure is to assess performance in a sample of the hypertensive population, the critical parameter was the positive predictive value. The positive predictive value was improved from 88% to 100% by the requirement of medical record validation.

Quality and Accountability Measures

Accountability is the measurement of health-care delivery systems on quality (i.e., their structures, process, and outcomes) with a specific focus on a particular individual or organization that is held responsible for a particular aspect of quality. For example, a physician (i.e., the unit of interest or accountability) may be measured on the percentage of children who have received all of their required immunizations (i.e., the process of interest) in the past year. On the basis of these results, decisions may be made (e.g., selection of the physician by a health-plan member) or certain actions may be taken (e.g., initiation of an immunization quality improvement program).

The first concern in accountability and therefore in quality surveillance is that the quality measures are relevant, scientifically sound, and feasible (47–49). Since the end result of accountability is either a) decision making by the MCO, payer, or consumer; or b) quality improvement, quality measures must meet all three of these characteristics to function adequately and appropriately as accountability measures.

Quality and accountability measures must be relevant to the evaluation and decision-making purposes for which they are intended. Quality measures are relevant to the extent that they achieve one or more the following:

- The measure addresses issues that are important and meaningful to the intended audience (i.e., consumers, employers and other payers and providers). Health outcome measures are generally preferred but not yet the dominant type of measure. Structure and process measures are more often selected due to their ready availability, their relative ease of implementation, and the incontrovertible link they have to outcomes.

- The measure has a clear unit of accountability (i.e., a physician, health-care system, or other entity) that is held responsible for the measured results.
- The measure should be actionable and have a potential for improvement. For a measure to be actionable there must be clear interventions that can be made to improve performance. The opportunity for improvement exists when *a*) there is a large gap between current practice and ideal practice or *b*) significant variability exists between health plans (i.e., there are meaningful differences in the results achieved by health plans on the measure).
- The structure, process, or outcome being measured is controllable or can be influenced by the unit of accountability. Related to controllability is the previous criterion on a measure being actionable and relevant to quality improvement.
- The measure is useful in decision making (e.g., identifying opportunities for quality improvement, aid in selecting a health plan or physician by a consumer).
- The measure has significant financial impact. The emphasis should not be solely on cost reduction but more driven by value (i.e., cost considering effectiveness and quality). The concept of value may be measured by concepts such as cost-effectiveness (*50*).

No measure will meet all of these criteria; however, given the complexity and cost of collecting the information, measures that meet multiple criteria for relevance are desirable.

Quality and accountability measures must have a strong rationale and evidence base. As Deming said, "That which gets measured gets done" (*31*). For this reason, any accountability measure will have the effect of stimulating and encouraging a particular medical or administrative practice and must be scientifically sound. Scientific soundness is the combination of a solid evidence base combined with acceptable measurement characteristics. The following criteria describe this complex construct.

- Defensibility: The measure is based on solid evidence that comes from the clinical literature of ideally nationally accepted guidelines or review panels. Examples are the U.S. Preventive Services Task Force (USPSTF) and guidelines from the National Heart Lung and Blood Institute (NHLBI) of the NIH.
- Reproducibility: Repeated usage of the measure will produce the same results in the same or similar populations and settings.
- Validity: The measure makes sense logically and correlates with other measures assessing the same aspect of care.
- Accuracy: The measure is a valid representation of what is actually observed.
- Appropriateness of statistical sampling: Random samples are preferable to avoid issues of confounding and bias. The sample of members must be sufficiently large enough to have either acceptable reliability, statistical

power to detect meaningful differences, or a specified threshold of acceptable performance (51,53).

- Appropriateness of statistical analysis: The proposed statistical analysis and inferences must follow accepted statistical methods (54,55). This may include case mix and risk adjustment, if necessary (56).
- Comparability of data sources: The sources of data for calculating results must be well understood and clearly specified (55). It is important that any variability observed in the results is largely attributable to the unit of accountability (e.g., health plans) and not due to variability in the underlying data sources.

Well-defined quality and accountability measures will satisfy all of these criteria.

The final construct required of quality and accountability measures is that of feasibility, and one of the largest components of feasibility is data access. For this reason, quality and accountability performance measures often rely on information contained in MCO administrative data sets. An explicit objective of the HEDIS measurement set is to rely on readily available data and simultaneously foster improvements in managed-care information systems. In addition to data availability and ease of access, the other feasibility criteria are

- The measure must be precisely defined to insure consistency in both the data collection process and calculation of the results.
- The specifications of the measure must be efficient (i.e., it has to be possible to produce the results of the measure at a reasonable cost).
- Patient confidentiality must be preserved at all times. Patient confidentiality must be considered during both the collection of data and the public reporting of the results.

An Example of a Quality and Accountability Measurement System

There are many examples of quality and accountability measurement systems (57). As previously cited, a leading example is HEDIS from the National Committee for Quality Assurance (NCQA), a not-for-profit organization with the mission of evaluating and publicly reporting on the quality provided by a variety of health-care providers. These providers include: a) managed-care plans (i.e., employer-sponsored HMOs, Medicare, and Medicaid), b) PPOs, and quite recently, c) large groups of physicians accepting responsibility for financial risk and delivery of health-care services. The HEDIS is a set of standardized performance measures that assess various aspects of the structure, process, and outcomes of care (58,59). The current consumers of HEDIS information are a) purchasers, both private and public (i.e., Medicare and Medicaid), b) consumers, c) organized labor, d) medical providers, e) public health officials, and, f) the health plans themselves.

At the time of publication, the HEDIS 2000, the most current version of the accountability measurement set, was divided into eight domains (45):

- *Effectiveness of care.* This HEDIS domain assess how acute, chronic, and preventive care is delivered by a health plan. The goal is to determine how well the plan does on implementing clinical processes and achieving good outcomes. The domain comprises process and outcome measures.

- *Access/availability of care.* This HEDIS domain assesses whether care is available to members when and where they need it and whether it can be obtained in a timely and convenient manner. It comprises process measures.
- *Satisfaction with the experience of care.* This HEDIS domain provides information about whether a health plan is able to satisfy the diverse needs of its members. It comprises process and outcome measures.
- *Cost of care.* This HEDIS domain compares health plans based on the "cost" of the services they deliver. Cost is a measurement dimension separate from quality achieved.
- *Stability of the health plan.* This HEDIS domain comprises indicators on the fiscal and operating soundness of a health plan. Health plan stability is important, because consumers make enrollment decisions that generally bind them for a one-year period. The domain comprises structure and process measures.
- *Use of services.* This domain reports how a health plan uses its resources. Use of services indicates how efficiently care is managed and whether needed services are being delivered. It comprises process measures.
- *Informed health-care choices.* Health plans should assist members in being active partners in their health-care decisions. The objective of this domain is to develop and report measures that assess how effectively health plans accomplished this result. As of the HEDIS 2000, this domain consisted of a single-process measure; development efforts were under way to expand it.
- *Health plan descriptive information.* This HEDIS domain reports the attributes and operating characteristics of the health plan itself; in particular, in a variety of elements of plan management (including a description of selected network, clinical, utilization, and risk management activities). This domain comprises structure measures.

The HEDIS measurement set contains many of the traditional public health surveillance concerns mostly found in the HEDIS 2000 Effectiveness of Care domain. Notable examples include

- vaccination status of adolescents
- advising smokers to quit
- antidepressant medication management
- appropriate use of medications for people with asthma
- beta blocker treatment after a heart attack
- breast cancer screening
- cervical cancer screening
- check ups after delivery
- childhood immunization status
- *Chlamydia* screening
- cholesterol management after acute cardiovascular events (i.e., screening and control of LDL cholesterol)

- comprehensive diabetes care (i.e., screening and control of HbA1C, screening and control of LDL cholesterol, diabetic retinopathy exams, diabetic nephropathy screening)
- controlling high blood pressure
- influenza shots for older adults
- follow-up after hospitalization for mental illness
- management of menopause (informed health-care choices domain)
- prenatal care in the first trimester
- health of seniors (i.e., health measurements status) (60)

The full specifications for these measures are available from the National Committee for Quality Assurance (45).

The HEDIS relies on managed-care data sets to construct its performance measures. Given the potential constraints and limitations of these data sets, the HEDIS has defined two approaches for implementing a measure. One approach relies solely on administrative data when the data is sufficiently comprehensive and valid. The second approach, known as the hybrid method, uses a combination of administrative data and medical chart review on a sample of the population. The following is an example of how childhood immunization rates can be assessed for an entire population using the administrative data method (45,47). The first step is to identify the targeted population for the denominator of the rate. For the HEDIS immunization measure, the specifications of the population and denominator are

- The specification is that all members whose second birthday occurred during the evaluation year and who were members of the plan as of their second birthday, and
- The denominator is that all must be continuously enrolled as a member of the health plan for the 12 months before his or her second birthday. Members who have had no more than one break in enrollment of up to 45 days during this time period are considered continuously enrolled.

Members who meet the inclusion criteria will be evaluated for which immunizations they have received. The required immunizations define the numerators of the immunization rates. There are six numerators, one for each of the required immunizations. The calculations of the six numerators are described below:

- *DTP*. A member must receive at least four DTP or DTaP vaccinations (*CPT-4* code 90700, 90701 or 90711, 90720 or 90721) with different dates of service by the child's second birthday, or an initial DTP or DTaP followed by at least three DTP, DTaP, and/or DT (*CPT-4* code 90702).
- *Polio*. A member must receive at least three polio vaccinations (OPV or IPV) (*CPT-4* code 90711 or 90712 or 90713) with different dates of service by the child's second birthday.
- *MMR*. A member must receive at least one MMR vaccination (*CPT-4* codes 90705 or 90707 or 90708 or 90710 for measles; 90704 or 90707 or 90709 or 90710 for mumps; or 90706 or 90707 or 90708 or 90709 or 90710 for rubella) with a date of service falling between the child's first and second birthdays.

- *HIB.* A member must receive two H influenza type B vaccinations (*CPT-4* code 90737, 90720, 90721, or 90748) by the child's second birthday with at least one of them falling on or between the child's first and second birthdays.
- *Hepatitis B.* A member must receive at least three hepatitis B vaccinations (*CPT-4* code 90731, 90744, 90747, or 90748) with different dates of service by the child's second birthday (with at least one of them falling on or between the child's six month and second birthday); and
- *Chicken pox.* A member must receive at least one chicken pox vaccination (*CPT-4* code 90710 or 90716) with a date of service falling on or between the child's first and second birthday. In lieu of a vaccination, acceptable evidence is a documented history of the chicken pox (*ICD-9* 052) by the child's second birthday or a seropositive test result for the chicken pox rendered on or before the child's second birthday.

These administrative data specifications for vaccinations for children are indicative of a typical accountability measure and how managed-care conducts quality surveillance using administrative data. In general, the process is based on the identification of a target population and the assessment of some event, process or outcome of interest. The results may be reported as a rate, a population mean or average, or in some categorical fashion dependent on the psychometric properties of the relevant data and the measurement specifications. With this type of information, decisions on quality of care can be made and subsequent actions taken to make improvements, if necessary.

Comparison of HEDIS and the Behavioral Risk Factor Surveillance System

In addition to being an accountability system, HEDIS is a prime example of how managed-care data can be used for public health surveillance within a managed-care plan. The substantial overlap between the HEDIS and common public health measures allows managed-care plans to compare their HEDIS specifications with other public health surveillance efforts. In performing such comparisons there are methodology concerns that must be considered. In one published report, the HEDIS results on the "Advice to Quit Smoking" measure were compared with the same question from the Behavioral Risk Factor Surveillance System (BRFSS). When this report was published there were four methodological concerns with making such a comparison. Some of these concerns have been addressed in recent versions of the HEDIS. First, there was a concern on the representativeness and validity of the HEDIS results since they are not randomly collected and are not audited. This has been partially addressed with the implementation of HEDIS audit standards (*61*). Second, it was impossible to make an apples-to-apples comparison between the two results since the HEDIS results could not be standardized to the BRFSS population because the HEDIS does not include information on age and sex. The HEDIS reporting now provides more detailed information by age and sex categories. Third, there were differences in mode of administration and the wording of questions between the HEDIS and the BRFSS. This remains an area of potential concern that depends on the specific comparison being made. Fourth, the low response rate for the HEDIS survey may create non-response bias. The HEDIS now requires commercial (i.e., non-Medicaid) health plans to achieve at least a 60% response rate in their survey administration process (62). However, despite these concerns, the results from 12 states represented by the HEDIS compared to data on insured respondents from the corresponding 12 states surveyed by the BRFSS showed good agreement. The HEDIS reported that a median percentage of 63.2% of respondents received advice to quit smoking compared to the median BRFSS results of 62.4%. While the methodological issues discussed must be carefully considered, the concurrent comparability is quite good (63).

QUALITY SURVEILLANCE: WHO NEEDS THIS INFORMATION? WHAT DO THEY DO WITH IT?

The final step in surveillance is taking action on the acquired information. We will examine the uses of the quality surveillance results by the different consumers of the information—employers, managed-care organizations, and consumers.

Employers

Because of their fiduciary responsibility for the selection and management of health-care benefits for their employees and retirees, employers have been a major catalyst and supporter of the recent emphasis on quality improvement (64–66). This trend continues. A growing number of large companies are developing health benefit management strategies based on value (i.e., the combination of quality and cost). Many large employers require NCQA accreditation, an onsite review of a health plan's infrastructure and operating procedures, and the HEDIS report information as prerequisites for offering a managed-care plan to employees (67–68). In addition, these employers provide "health-care report cards" to help their employees select a health plan (69). Report cards will be discussed below in the section or on consumers' use of quality information.

In addition to the efforts of employers, there has been a dramatic increase in purchasing coalitions (i.e., individual employers that have combined forces to increase their buying power). Coalitions use their size and leverage not only to secure favorable premiums but also to integrate requirements for demonstrated quality into their contracts (70–72). A notable example is the Pacific Business Group on Health (PBGH), an alliance of seventeen large employers on the West Coast. In 1996 PBGH instituted required performance targets on quality measures as an integral part of its contracting strategy. The group established a risk pool of over $8 million that would be distributed dependent on how the HMOs performed on the quality measures. The quality measures included member satisfaction, cesarean section rates, immunization, mammography and Pap smear screening rates, and delivery of prenatal care. In general, the HMOs performed quite well. However, they did refund almost $2 million, or 23% of the premium at risk, to the

PBGH because of missed performance targets. Performance on the immunization measure was particularly poor; eight of the 13 HMOs missed their performance targets and refunded 86% of the premiums at risk. (73).

Managed-Care Organizations

The prime use of quality surveillance data by an MCO is for quality improvement purposes. In line with Deming's adage, "That which gets measured gets done," the HEDIS and other quality measurements are often the catalysts for programs to improve performance on quality measures.

Such quality improvement programs are illustrated by two examples based on the HEDIS immunization measure. The first example comes from a southern California health plan that used the HEDIS childhood immunization measure to assess its overall compliance with rates for vaccination of children for DTP, OPV, MMR, and HiB (74). The overall rate of compliance was assessed at 44%. The performance on the overall vaccination rate for other California health plans ranged from 39% to 85% and the plan felt that their performance was unacceptably low. Medical record reviews and a physician survey were initiated to determine causes for and barriers to achieving a higher rate. On the basis of this inventory of barriers and gaps in physicians' knowledge, interventions were initiated to improve the overall rate.

In a second example, a health plan in the eastern United States undertook a quality improvement program to improve a subset of the HEDIS preventive health measures. Outcome measures consisted of rates of MMR vaccination and screening for cholesterol levels. The study design used a pre–post assessment of performance. Physicians included in the study received comparative reports based on peer review in conjunction with financial incentives for improved performance on the measures. Offices that met the MMR vaccination standards improved over the three-year period from 78% to 96% (p < 0.05); screening for cholesterol improved from 92% to 95%. Noncompliance on a measure was defined as performance less than 90%. The percentage of practices not in compliance for MMR immunizations decreased from 57% to 12%; for the cholesterol screening measure non-compliant offices decreased from 21% to 11%.

The catalyst of quality measures has been a powerful incentive for performance improvement. Investment and improvements in information systems and the continued development of quality measures will continue this trend.

Consumers

Quality report cards, mentioned above, are intended to help the consumer choose a health plan. The introduction of the consumer as a market force in health care is part of a growing movement to make health care more market driven. Consumers use the following criteria when selecting a health plan (75–77).

- quality
- cost to the consumer

- benefit packages (i.e., covered services) offered to the member
- availability of preferred physicians
- administrative requirement of the health plan (i.e., the health plan's policies and procedures on what you have to do to get the care you need)

This shift to make consumers an active part of the health-care decision-making process is a recent development and complex learning process for all involved. The current report cards used by consumers are at a very preliminary and rudimentary phase; they will require both continual evaluation and evolution to adequately fulfill their intended purpose (78).

CONCLUSION

The concepts, development, and implementation of quality surveillance standards and methods are still evolving. There are clear incentives that will continue to foster development and growth of quality surveillance efforts. Concerns over health-care costs continue to be an important issue and high priorities for consumers, payers and providers. Despite the previous success of managed care at controlling costs there is increasing evidence that health-care costs are on the rise (79). Whether the trend will approach the double-digit rates of inflation seen in late 1980 is uncertain. With the cost pressures remaining and quality measures still evolving, concerns about managed care continue. Some argue that the use of techniques such as utilization management and capitation with their perverse incentives to withhold care is evidence that managed care has subverted quality in an attempt to cut costs. Others argue that managed care's emphasis on preventive services and their burgeoning efforts in quality surveillance is evidence that they have enhanced quality compared to the traditional fee-for-service system. While the debate rages, the consistent thread is that everyone wants evidence that quality is not being sacrificed to achieve lower costs. This question can only be answered as the quality surveillance systems are enhanced and used more broadly.

This chapter has focused on managed-care quality surveillance as if it were the only area of activity and concern in our health-care system. This, of course, is not true. Although managed care has grown significantly, it is not the only form of health insurance. Many people continue to be uninsured. The emphasis of this chapter on managed care is one of convenience because of a) the feasibility of quality surveillance in managed care, which has led to b) the relatively advanced development of quality surveillance systems with clear units of accountability under managed care. However, the need for quality surveillance obviously extends beyond managed care. There is no reason to believe that the same quality concerns about the adequate and appropriate provision of comprehensive health-care services do not exist under other forms of health insurance. Fee-for-service and some permutations of managed-care arrangements still have limitations for performing comprehensive quality surveillance but are the next frontier. A notable example is the Medicare system, where the 15% of beneficiaries in managed care have access to quality information through the HEDIS and other quality surveillance efforts, whereas the remaining 85% of Medicare beneficiaries do not. This is not to say that quality efforts have been entirely missing under alternative forms of insurance; significant efforts occur within delivery sites (e.g., large group practices, hospitals), but they are not comprehensive across beneficiaries' experience. They lack comparability against other measurement efforts since different measures are implemented in different ways in different settings. These are useful for internal efforts but are not amenable to a population-based approach that allows valid comparisons across settings. Research and development efforts must tackle the problems of defining a population and relevant quality measures for which providers and insurers providing care under other insurance forms and within different settings can be held completely or partially accountable for the quality of care provided.

Though quality measurement and improvement has a history that goes back at least to Codman in the early 1900s, quality surveillance in health care is still in the early and rudimentary phases of development and implementation. Unlike in the past, however, current tensions over costs and quality are not likely to disappear soon. Efforts to make health care more market-driven will help insure that cost and quality stay at the forefront. What has been described here will lead to new advances, broader dissemination of quality measurement, and more effective improvement efforts.

REFERENCES

1. Goran MJ. The evolution of the PSRO hospital review system. *Med Care* 1979;17: 1–47.
2. Hayes RP, Lundberg MT, Ballard DJ. Peer review organizations: scientific challenges in HCFA's health care quality improvement initiative. *Med Care Rev* 1994;51:39–60.
3. McGuire TE. DRGs: the state of the art, circa 1990. *Health Policy* 1991;17:97–119.
4. Pauly MV. The changing health-care environment. *Am J Med* 1986;81:3–8.
5. Gaskin DJ, Hadley J. The impact of HMO penetration on the rate of hospital cost inflation, 1985–1993. *Inquiry* 1997;34:205–16.
6. Lazenby HC, Letsch SW. National health expenditures, 1989. *Health Care Financ Rev* 1990;12:1–26.
7. Levit KR, Lazenby HC, Braden BR *et al.* National health expenditures, 1995. *Health Care Financ Rev* 1996;18:175–214.
8. Chernew ME, Hirth RA, Sonnad SS, Ermann R, Fendrick AM. Managed care, medical technology, and health-care cost growth: a review of the evidence. *Med Care Res Rev* 1998;55:259–88; discussion 289–97.
9. Levit KR, Sensenig AL, Cowan CA *et al.* National health expenditures, 1993. *Health Care Financ Rev* 1994;16:247–94.
10. Levit KR, Lazenby HC, Braden BR *et al.* National health expenditures, 1996. *Health Care Financ Rev* 1997;19:161–200.
11. Scutchfield FD, Lee J, Patton D. Managed care in the United States. *J Public Health Med* 1997;19:251–4.
12. Zwanziger J, Melnick GA. Can managed care plans control health-care costs? *Health Aff (Millwood)* 1996;15:185–99.

13. Levit KR, Cowan CA, Lazenby HC *et al.* National health spending trends, 1960–1993. *Health Aff (Millwood)* 1994;13:14–31.
14. Levit KR, Lazenby HC, Sivarajan L. Health-care spending in 1994: slowest in decades. *Health Aff (Millwood)* 1996;15:130–44.
15. Staines VS. Potential impact of managed care on national health spending. *Health Aff (Millwood)* 1993;12(Suppl):248–57.
16. Feldstein PJ, Wickizer TM, Wheeler JR. Private cost containment. The effects of utilization review programs on health-care use and expenditures. *N Engl J Med* 1988;318:1310–4.
17. Reinhardt UE. Managed care, capitation, and managed competition: a brief primer. *Compend Contin Educ Dent* 1995;Spec No:6-10.
18. Stuart B, Yesalis C. On taking chances with the law of large numbers. *Health Serv Manage Res* 1988;1:135–44.
19. Wilensky GR, Rossiter LF. Alternative units of payment for physician services: an overview of the issues *Med Care Rev* 1986;43:133–56.
20. Donabedian A. The end results of health care: Ernest Codman's contribution to quality assessment and beyond. *Milbank Q* 1989;67:233–56; discussion 257–67.
21. Neuhauser D. Ernest Amory Codman, M.D., and end results of medical care. *Int J Technol Assess Health Care* 1990;6:307–25.
22. Donabedian A. Definition of quality and approaches to its assessment. In: Explorations in quality assessment and monitoring. Ann Arbor, Mich.: Health Administration Press, 1969:178.
23. Donabedian A. The criteria and standards of quality. In: Explorations in quality assessment and monitoring. Ann Arbor, Mich.: Health Administration Press, 1969.
24. Donabedian A. Methods and findings of quality assessment and monitoring: an illustrated analysis. In: Explorations in quality assessment and monitoring. Ann Arbor, Mich.: Health Administration Press, 1969.
25. Batalden PB, Nelson EC, Roberts JS. Linking outcomes measurement to continual improvement: the serial "V" way of thinking about improving clinical care. *J Comm J Qual Improv* 1994;20:167–80.
26. Berwick DM. The clinical process and the quality process. *Qual Manag Health Care* 1992;1:1–8.
27. Plsek PE. Quality improvement methods in clinical medicine. *Pediatrics* 1999;103:203–14.
28. Batalden PB, Mohr JJ, Nelson EC, Plume SK. Improving health care, Part 4: concepts for improving any clinical process. *J Comm J Qual Improv* 1996;22:651–9.
29. Mohr JJ, Mahoney CC, Nelson EC, Batalden PB, Plume SK. Improving health care, Part 3: clinical benchmarking for best patient care. *J Comm J Qual Improv* 1996;22:599–616.
30. Nelson EC, Batalden PB, Plume SK, Mohr JJ. Improving health care, Part 2: a clinical improvement worksheet and users' manual. *J Comm J Qual Improv* 1996;22:531–48.
31. Deming WE. Out of the crisis. Cambridge, Mass.: MIT Center for Advanced Engineering Study, 1986.
32. Selby JV. Linking automated data bases for research in managed care settings. *Ann Intern Med* 1997;127:719–24.
33. Dresser MV, Feingold L, Rosenkranz SL, Coltin KL. Clinical quality measurement. Comparing chart review and automated methodologies. *Med Care* 1997;35:539–52.
34. Kashner TM. Agreement between administrative files and written medical records. *Medical Care* 1998;36:1324–36.

35. Rubin DB. Estimating causal effects from large data sets using propensity scores. *Ann Intern Med* 1997;127:757–63.
36. Rubin DB, Thomas N. Matching using estimated propensity scores: relating theory to practice. *Biometrics* 1996;52:249–64.
37. Crown WH *et al.* The application of sample selection models to outcomes research: the case of evaluating the effects of antidepressant therapy on resource utilization. *Stat Med* 1998;17:1943–58.
38. Armstrong EP, Manuchehri F. Ambulatory care data bases for managed care organizations. *Am J Health Syst Pharm* 1997;54:1973–83; quiz 2004–5.
39. Lohr KN, Brook RH, Kamberg CJ *et al.* Use of medical care in the Rand Health Insurance Experiment. Diagnosis- and service-specific analyses in a randomized controlled trial. *Med Care* 1986;24:S1–87.
40. Wingert TD, Kralewski JE, Lindquist TJ, Knutson DJ. Constructing episodes of care from encounter and claims data: some methodological issues. *Inquiry* 1995;32: 430–43.
41. Rosen AK, Mayer-Oakes A. Episodes of care: theoretical frameworks versus current operational realities. *Jt Comm J Qual Improv* 1999;25:111–28.
42. Fink R. HMO data systems in population studies of access to care. *Health Serv Res* 1998;33:741–59; discussion 761–6.
43. Nordstrom DL, Remington PL, Layde PM. The utility of HMO data for the surveillance of chronic diseases. *Am J Public Health* 1994;84:995–7.
44. Hanchak NA, Murray JF, Hirsch A, McDermott PD, Schlackman N. USQA Health profile data base as a tool for health plan quality improvement. *Manag Care Q* 1996;4:58–69.
45. NCQA. HEDIS 2000 technical specifications. Washington, D.C.: National Committee for Quality Assurance, 1999.
46. Quam L, Ellis LB, Venus P, Clouse J, Taylor CG, Leatherman S. Using claims data for epidemiologic research. The concordance of claims-based criteria with the medical record and patient survey for identifying a hypertensive population. *Med Care* 1993;31:498–507.
47. NCQA. HEDIS 3.0 Narrative: What's in it and why it matters. Washington, D.C.: National Committee for Quality Assurance, 1997:128.
48. McGlynn EA. Choosing and evaluating clinical performance measures. *Jt Comm J Qual Improv* 1998;24:470–9.
49. McGlynn EA, Asch SM. Developing a clinical performance measure. *Am J Prev Med* 1998;14:14–21.
50. Gold M, Siegel J, Russell L, Weinstein M. Cost-effectiveness in health and medicine. New York: Oxford University Press; 1996:425.
51. Davis J, Meyer D, Murray J. Obtaining stable estimates for quality of care measures. 16th Annual Meeting of the North American Primary Care Research Group (NAPCRG), Ottawa, 1988.
52. Cohen J. Statistical power analysis for the behavioral sciences. Second edition. Hillsdale, N.J.: Lawrence Erlbaum Associates, 1988:567.
53. Siu AL, McGlynn EA, Morgenstern H *et al.* Choosing quality of care measures based on the expected impact of improved care on health. *Health Serv Res* 1992;27:619–50.
54. Salem-Schatz S, Moore G, Rucker M, Pearson SD. The case for case-mix adjustment in practice profiling. When good apples look bad [see comments]. *JAMA* 1994;272: 871–4.
55. Siu AL, McGlynn EA, Morgenstern H, Brook RH. A fair approach to comparing quality of care. *Health Aff (Millwood)* 1991;10:62–75.

56. Iezzoni L. Case mix and risk adjustment. Second edition. Hillsdale, N.J.: Lawrence Erlbaum Associates, 1998.
57. Cooper JK. Accountability for clinical preventive services. *Mil Med* 1995;160:297–9.
58. Sennett C. An introduction to HEDIS. *Hosp Pract (Off Ed)* 1996;31:147–8.
59. Grimaldi PL. New HEDIS means more information about HMOs. *J Health Care Finance* 1997;23:40–50.
60. NCQA. The health of seniors: Technical specifications and survey administration. First edition. Washington, D.C.: National Committee for Quality Assurance, 1999.
61. NCQA. HEDIS compliance audit; standards, policies and procedures. First edition. Washington, D.C.: National Committee for Quality Assurance, 1999.
62. NCQA. HEDIS protocol for administering CAHPS 2.0H survey. First edition. Washington, D.C.: National Committee for Quality Assurance, 1999.
63. Centers for Disease Control and Prevention. Use of clinical preventive services by adults aged <65 years enrolled in health-maintenance organizations—United States, 1996. *MMWR* 1998;47:613–9.
64. Lynne D. Employer initiatives to examine cost and quality in health care. *Empl Benefits J* 1993;18:11–4.
65. Rontal R. Information and decision support in managed care. *Manag Care Q* 1993;1: 3–14.
66. Harvey CS. Making employees partners in the health-care purchasing decision. *Empl Benefits J* 1993;18:25–6.
67. Keister LW. Big employers back new drive for comparable quality measures. *Manag Care* 1995;4:20–4.
68. NCQA. Quality at work: 1998 annual report. Washington, D.C.: National Committee for Quality Assurance, 1999.
69. Kenkel PJ. New England HMOs, employers proceed with 'report card.' *Mod Healthc* 1994;24:18.
70. Robinow AL. The buyers health-care action group: creating a competitive care system model. *Manag Care Q* 1997;5:61–4.
71. Carlson B. Clinical care with a retail flavor: Twin Cities employer group tries a bold new experiment. *Healthc Forum J* 1997;40:17, 26–9.
72. Schroeder J, Lamb S. Data initiatives: HEDIS and the New England business coalition. *Am J Med Qual* 1996;11:S58-62.
73. Schauffler HH, Brown C, Milstein A. Raising the bar: the use of performance guarantees by the Pacific Business Group on Health. *Health Aff (Millwood)* 1999;18: 134–42.
74. Centers for Disease Control and Prevention. Use of a data-based approach by a health maintenance organization to identify and address physician barriers to pediatric vaccination—California, 1995. *MMWR* 1996;45:188–93.
75. Edgman-Levitan S, Cleary PD. What information do consumers want and need? *Health Aff (Millwood)* 1996;15:42–56.
76. Cleary PD, Edgman-Levitan S. Health-care quality. Incorporating consumer perspectives. *JAMA* 1997;278:1608–12.
77. Sainfort F, Booske BC. Role of information in consumer selection of health plans. *Health Care Financ Rev* 1996;18:31–54.
78. Epstein AM. Rolling down the runway: the challenges ahead for quality report cards. *JAMA* 1998;279:1691–6.
79. Vincenzino JV. Trends in medical care costs—evolving market forces. *Stat Bull Metrop Insur Co* 1998;79:8–15.

15

Post-Market Safety Surveillance for Pharmaceuticals

JANET ARROWSMITH-LOWE

The significant problems we face today cannot be solved at the same level of thinking we were at when we created them.

Albert Einstein

It is generally accepted that the safety profile of any drug or pharmaceutical product is incomplete at the time of approval and initial marketing (*1*). Post-market surveillance allows providers, government, and industry to take measures to enhance the appropriate and safe use of medications. Since 1962, pharmaceutical drug products approved for U.S. marketing have been required to meet certain standards for safety and effectiveness. The pharmaceutical development process encompasses several years, during which extensive information on the chemical structure and manufacturing of a drug to be marketed in the United States and its effects in single-cell systems and animal models are collected before clinical trials involving humans are conducted. Most pharmaceutical products reach the U.S. market after a number of years of data collection, including investigational studies involving humans. These pre-market clinical trials are designed to establish the safety and effectiveness of a drug for healthy volunteers and for the target population for which marketing approval will be sought.

Pre-market clinical trials are traditionally short in duration and are randomized, controlled studies. The nature of the randomized, controlled clinical trial requires as homogenous a population as possible so that events that occur during treatment are more likely to be attributable to differences among the treatments and less likely to be attributable to differences among participants. Historically, persons with complicated medical problems that require multiple concomitant medications, children, and pregnant women are excluded from these clinical trials. The elderly are also frequently excluded from participation in clinical trials conducted to support initial approval. Typically, a drug is approved for U.S. marketing on the basis of clinical data derived for its use in 3,000–4,000 persons.

Pre-market clinical trials can usually detect adverse events that occur at a frequency in excess of one per 4,000 persons exposed and that develop within the

343

short time frame of the typical pre-market clinical trial (2). In order to detect with certainty ($p < 0.05$) an event that affects only one person per 10,000 exposed, which is comparable to the rate at which anaphylaxis occurs in association with penicillin, at least 30,000 persons must be exposed to the drug for the appropriate length of time.

Once a drug is approved for marketing in the United States, licensed healthcare professionals may recommend or prescribe the drug according to their clinical judgement. This generally means that the populations that receive an approved product are less homogeneous than the more restricted clinical trial population in which most pre-market safety and effectiveness data have been obtained. In the United States, the Food and Drug Administration (FDA) has distanced itself from regulating actual use of the drug once the product reaches the market. By the time of product approval, a label has been developed that contains information on the pharmacology, mechanisms of action, warnings and precautions, dosing, and indications, as well as other information needed for the safe use of the product. All product approvals are predicated on the premise that the benefits of the drug outweigh the known risks of the drug, when it is used in accordance with the labeled indications, dosing, precautions, etc. The actual clinical use of a drug is considered to be in the realm of the practice of medicine and is not regulated by FDA (3).

Post-market safety surveillance allows additional safety data to accrue as the drug is used in the larger, more complex patient populations comprise actual clinical practice.

ADVERSE DRUG REACTIONS

Adverse drug reactions are undesirable or toxic effects produced or contributed to by a marketed drug or other pharmaceutical product. An adverse reaction can be an event that occurs with use of the drug during normal professional practice, or it might be related to drug overdose, accidental or otherwise. It could be an adverse effect that occurs during drug withdrawal or an event that results from abuse of the drug. In the United States, adverse drug events also include situations in which there is a failure of the expected pharmacologic action. Adverse drug reactions range from the trivial to the fatal or permanently disabling. It is estimated that between 3% and 11% of all hospital admissions are attributable to adverse drug events (4). They are the fifth leading cause of mortality in the United States, according to a recent study (5). The post-market safety issues associated with the use of all medical products are major public health concerns.

The more common types of adverse drug reactions are those that occur as an extension of the pharmacologic action of the drug (6). The bradycardia and exacerbation-of-reactive-airways disease among persons exposed to non-selective beta adrenergic receptor blocking agents and the adverse effects on kidney function, platelet aggregation, and the gastrointestinal tract with use of non-steroidal anti-inflammatory drugs are examples of this first type of adverse reaction. Many of these more common types of adverse reactions are dose dependent and may

be included in the initial drug label because they may be detected in the pre-market trials. Some, such as the unusual occurrence of torsades de pointes with concomitant use of terfenadine and other drugs such as erythromycin or ketoconazole, occur only in the presence of other concomitant pharmaceutical products or in the setting of concomitant medical problems.

The less common types of adverse drug. These are the idiosyncratic reactions, reactions mediated by immunologic or allergic mechanisms and carcinogenic or teratogenic events. These idiosyncratic reactions are often the most serious and life-threatening events and are a major cause of drug-induced morbidity and mortality (6).

There are certain body systems, such as the liver, the skin, and bone marrow that are frequently affected by idiosyncratic reactions. In fact, certain types of events are frequently attributable to drug exposure. Of all reported cases of liver failure, 20% to 30% may be drug related (7); up to two-thirds of all cases of aplastic anemia are drug induced (8); and rare but serious skin diseases such as erythema multiforme, toxic epidermal necrolysis, and Stevens-Johnson syndrome are commonly drug-induced (9).

It is important to note that not all events reported in association with the use of a drug or other medical product are actual adverse reactions attributed to it. Attribution of the event to the drug or other product may require additional investigation beyond recognition of a potential relationship between exposure and event. A distinction must be made between *adverse drug events,* which occur in association with exposure to a drug, and *adverse drug reactions,* a term that implies a causal association.

POST-MARKET SAFETY SURVEILLANCE IN THE UNITED STATES

In the United States, FDA's Center for Drug Evaluation and Research (CDER) manages what may be the largest public health surveillance data base in the world. The Adverse Event Reporting System (AERS) contains over 2 million adverse drug event reports received from health-care providers, consumers, and the mandatory adverse event reporting system from pharmaceutical manufacturers in the United States. The AERS was brought on line in November 1997, replacing older technology. Managed by the Office of Post-market Drug Risk Assessment (OPDRA), in CDER, the precursor to AERS was first established in the early 1960s following a number of less successful attempts of post-market safety surveillance (10). There are approximately 30 years of accessible data in AERS on adverse events reported in association with the use of drugs marketed in the United States (11).

Adverse event reports from physicians, dentists, nurses, and pharmacists form the backbone of the reporting system in the United States. Of reports submitted directly from the reporter to FDA and included in the AERS data base, 59% were from pharmacists, 15% from physicians, 9% from nurses, and 6% from other sources. Over a quarter million adverse drug event reports were added to the

AERS in 1998. Most of the adverse event reports submitted to FDA from manufacturers originate from health-care providers, primarily pharmacists and physicians (*10*).

MANDATORY MANUFACTURER REPORTING REQUIREMENTS

Manufacturers or sponsors of drugs marketed in the United States are required to actively seek new safety information concerning their marketed products and to report that information to FDA in a timely fashion. Over 90% of all reports in the AERS data base come from drug manufacturers; most of the manufacturers' reports originate from health-care providers. Manufacturers are required to review the scientific literature, domestic and foreign marketing experience, clinical trials, or epidemiologic studies conducted after marketing approval for new, important safety information. Manufacturers are also mandated to monitor the spontaneous or voluntary reports submitted to them by health-care providers and consumers. For an overview of the manufacturer's requirements, see Table 15–1. The 1962 Kefauver-Harris Amendments to the Food, Drug and Cosmetic Act established the legal requirement for post-market safety reporting by drug manufacturers (*11*). These amendments were passed by Congress following the epidemic of phocomelia in Europe associated with the widespread use of thalidomide among pregnant women. Regulations governing post-market safety reporting were enacted in the mid-1980s and have undergone change in a number of aspects. These regulations are published in the Code of Federal Regulations (CFR), Title 21, parts 310.305, 314.80, and 314.98, and will probably be updated again in the near future. The basic requirements for active mon-

Table 15–1 Requirements for Reporting Adverse Events for Pharmaceutical Manufacturers in the United States

---

15-Day Serious and Unexpected Adverse Drug Events
Each adverse event known to the manufacturer as both serious and unexpected (in accordance with regulatory definitions) must be reported FDA within 15 calendar days.
Periodic Adverse Event Reports
Serious adverse events, which are known and in the current label, and newly identified events that do not meet the regulatory criteria for "serious" must be reported periodically. The reporting period is quarterly for the first 3 years and annually thereafter.
Other
The frequency of reports that are serious and expected, and reports of therapeutic failures must be monitored. Any significant increase is reported to FDA.
Scientific Literature Review
Serious adverse events not in the label and derived from case reports, clinical trials, epidemiological studies, or other "analyses of experience in a monitored series of patients" must be reported in accordance with the 15-day requirement.
Post-Market Studies
If the manufacturer assesses a serious, unlabeled event occurring during a trial as likely to be caused or contributed to by the drug, then it must be reported under the 15-day requirement.

---

itoring, follow up, and reporting of important new information to FDA remain, with most changes having to do with format, the addition of electronic submissions, and changes that will facilitate data compatibility with international adverse event reporting systems. One major change in mandatory reporting effected by the new regulations was eliminating the requirement for 15-day reporting of increased frequency of serious adverse events that are included in the current label. This requirement, based on manufacturer's calculations of reporting rates, was cumbersome and not found to contribute significantly to safety surveillance. The updated version of the regulations can be viewed online at the MedWatch Website: www.fda.gov/medwatch/report/regs.htm.

The regulations spell out a number of procedural and record-keeping requirements as well as defining who must report, what is reportable, and time frames for submitting reports. Mandatory manufacturer adverse-event monitoring and reporting is now in effect for all products regulated by FDA except cosmetics, nutritional and dietary supplements, and over the counter (OTC) drug products marketed prior to 1938, when the Pure Food and Drug Act was enacted. Some regulatory changes are anticipated that will require adverse-event reporting for all OTC drug products.

Currently, the reporting regulations apply to all marketed prescription drugs and all OTC drugs that originally required a prescription. These so-called OTC switch drugs include single-entity products such as ibuprofen as well as combination products like Drixoral™ and others. They establish categories of reports and specify the reporting requirements for each category.

REPORTS OF GREATEST INTEREST: SERIOUS AND UNEXPECTED

There are several categories of adverse event reporting for manufacturers. The most important is *serious and unexpected*. The regulatory definitions for *serious* are contained in Table 15–2.

Table 15–2 Regulatory Definitions of *Serious* as It Applies to Adverse Drug Event Reporting (21 CFR 314.80, effective April 6, 1998)

A serious adverse drug event is defined as any event that occurs at any dose and results in one or more of the following:
- death
- a life-threatening event
- an event resulting in inpatient hospitalization
- an event which prolongs a current hospitalization
- a persistent or significant disability or incapacity
- a congenital anomaly or birth defect
- any event that, based on appropriate medical judgement, may jeopardize the patient and for which medical or surgical intervention may be required to prevent one of the outcomes listed above

Unexpected means that it is an event or effect not in the current product label. The category also includes events or effects that may be related to a labeled event but differ from the label because of greater severity or greater specificity. The examples provided in the regulations are of hepatic necrosis being called "unexpected" because it is more severe than expected, even though elevated liver enzymes or hepatitis are listed on the label. In terms of greater specificity, a report of cerebral thromboembolism or cerebral vasculitis would be considered unexpected for a drug whose label mentions cerebrovascular accidents. *Unexpected* really means that the event or effect has not been observed in connection with use of the particular drug and relates more to the product label than to the pharmacologic actions of the drug.

A spontaneously reported, serious, unexpected adverse event must be reported to FDA by the manufacturer within 15 days from the time the manufacturer becomes aware of the event and can classify it appropriately. Submission of a report does not constitute attribution of the event to the drug. However, a newly identified, serious, unexpected adverse event is considered a signal of a potential safety problem with the drug and is treated as a real event until additional information is available to confirm or refute the association.

PRODUCTS OF GREATEST INTEREST

Newly approved products (usually defined as those within 3 years of initial market entry, new molecular entities [NMEs], and products with known bioavailability or pharmacokinetic problems) receive the greatest attention for postmarket safety issues (*12*). As a general rule, the highest rate of adverse event reporting for a pharmaceutical product occurs in the first 3 years of marketing. The peak of adverse event reporting occurs at the end of the second year of marketing. From that point on, reporting declines even though use of the product may increase or remain stable, and even though reports of adverse events continue as expected (*13*). It is for this reason that manufacturers' periodic safety updates are required more frequently during the first three years of marketing (see Table 15–1).

The first approvals within a new class of drugs are also monitored closely for unexpected and serious adverse events associated with their initial use. These are referred to as *new molecular entities,* or NMEs. An NME constitutes a new development in pharmaceutical products. Recent examples of NMEs are the so-called COX-2 inhibitors for the treatment of rheumatoid and osteoarthritis. The products are relative unknowns as their use moves from the controlled clinical trials into the arena of the unselected general population.

In addition to drugs in the first 3 years of marketing and to NMEs, products with known or suspected bioavailability or bioequivalence problems are also under greater scrutiny, particularly for failure of expected effect. A product whose bioavailability is low would undoubtedly undergo close post-market scrutiny for effectiveness.

The issue of lack of effect is also of particular interest among drugs that could cause serious medical outcomes if they fail to produce their expected pharma-

cologic actions. Drugs such as antibiotics and antiviral agents, cancer chemotherapeutic agents, and other products approved for the treatment of serious illnesses may be monitored carefully for lack of effect.

For drugs with known or suspected safety problems, special postmarket studies may be requested or the manufacturer may be asked to provide more frequent updates on adverse event reports submitted directly to them. The antiviral drug acyclovir was monitored for congenital defects in the early post-market period using a data-collection system managed collaboratively with the Centers for Disease Control and Prevention (CDC) (12).

Another separate category of drug-related (and other medical product-related) safety issues are those situations in which drugs are given by the wrong route of administration, at the wrong dose, or the wrong drug is administered due to name confusion. Confusion about names of drugs can occur as a result of similarities in names of two or more drugs. The Medication Errors Committee tracks these events in CDER. This issue was part of "Minimizing Medical Product Errors: A Systems Approach," a workshop sponsored by FDA January 8, 1998. A summary of that workshop is available on the MedWatch Web site: http:/www.fda.gov/medwatch.

REPORTING RESPONSIBILITIES OF HEALTH-CARE PROFESSIONALS

Health-care professionals in the United States are not required by law to report adverse drug reactions. However, professional organizations such as the American Medical Association and the American Dental Association encourage reporting of adverse medical product events (14,15). The Joint Commission on Accreditation of Health-Care Organizations includes post-market problem monitoring for drugs, biologics, and medical devices as a requirement for institutional accreditation (16). The International Committee of Medical Journal Editors revised their "Uniform Requirements for Manuscripts Submitted to Biomedical Journals" to encourage authors to provide any information concerning adverse medical product events to FDA or other appropriate regulatory authority (10). However, there is no legal mandate for U.S. health-care professionals to report suspected adverse reactions. It is considered an ethical obligation, but not one enforced by law.

The one exception is adverse event reporting for certain vaccines used among children. Event reporting is a legal obligation for health-care professionals, mandated by the National Childhood Vaccine Injury Act of 1986. The Vaccine Adverse Event Reporting System (VAERS) is a program administered jointly by FDA and CDC (17).

Adverse drug event reports submitted by health-care professionals and consumers are usually referred to as "spontaneous" reports and are recorded in the terminology of the reporter. This simply means that these reports are derived from clinical observations and not from study or literature reports. These are also referred to as "voluntary" reports. Most spontaneous reports are initially sub-

mitted to the manufacturer, who then reviews the data to determine how and when the report is to be transmitted to FDA.

Adverse event reports from health-care professionals are critical to the success of the post-market surveillance programs. Adverse event reports submitted directly to FDA from health-care professionals are triaged for immediate review, along with 15-day, serious, and unexpected event reports submitted by manufacturers.

In 1993, the FDA launched the MedWatch program to enhance the effectiveness of post-market safety surveillance for all medical products that it regulates (*18*). The goals of the program included increasing health-care providers' awareness of adverse medical product events, providing guidance on what should be reported to FDA, establishing a single contact point for reporting medical prod-

ADVICE ABOUT VOLUNTARY REPORTING

Report experiences with:
- medications (drugs or biologics)
- medical devices (including in-vitro diagnostics)
- special nutritional products (dietary supplements, medical foods, infant formulas)
- other products regulated by FDA

Report SERIOUS adverse events. An event is serious when the patient outcome is:
- death
- life-threatening (real risk of dying)
- hospitalization (initial or prolonged)
- disability (significant, persistent or permanent)
- congenital anomaly
- required intervention to prevent permanent impairment or damage

Report even if:
- you're not certain the product caused the event
- you don't have all the details

Report product problems – quality, performance or safety concerns such as:
- suspected contamination
- questionable stability
- defective components
- poor packaging or labeling

How to report:
- just fill in the sections that apply to your report
- use section C for all products except medical devices
- attach additional blank pages if needed
- use a separate form for each patient
- report either to FDA or the manufacturer (or both)

Important numbers:
- 1-800-FDA-0178   to FAX report
- 1-800-FDA-7737   to report by modem
- 1-800-FDA-1088   for more information or to report quality problems
- 1-800-822-7967   for a VAERS form for vaccines

If your report involves a serious adverse event with a device and it occurred in a facility outside a doctor's office, that facility may be legally required to report to FDA and/or the manufacturer. Please notify the person in that facility who would handle such reporting.

Confidentiality: The patient's identity is held in strict confidence by FDA and protected to the fullest extent of the law. The reporter's identity may be shared with the manufacturer unless requested otherwise. However, FDA will not disclose the reporter's identity in response to a request from the public, pursuant to the Freedom of Information Act.

The public reporting burden for this collection of information has been estimated to average 30 minutes per response, including the time for reviewing instructions, searching existing data sources, gathering and maintaining the data needed, and completing and reviewing the collection of information. Send your comments regarding this burden estimate or any other aspect of this collection of information, including suggestions for reducing this burden to:

Reports Clearance Officer, PHS
Hubert H. Humphrey Building,
Room 721-B
200 Independence Avenue, S.W.
Washington, DC 20201
ATTN: PRA

and to:
Office of Management and Budget
Paperwork Reduction Project
(0910-0230)
Washington, DC 20503

Please do NOT return this form to either of these addresses.

FDA Form 3500-back   **Please Use Address Provided Below – Just Fold In Thirds, Tape and Mail**

**Department of
Health and Human Services**
Public Health Service
Food and Drug Administration
Rockville, MD 20857

Official Business
Penalty for Private Use $300

NO POSTAGE
NECESSARY
IF MAILED
IN THE
UNITED STATES
OR APO/FPO

BUSINESS REPLY MAIL
FIRST CLASS MAIL   PERMIT NO. 946   ROCKVILLE, MD

POSTAGE WILL BE PAID BY FOOD AND DRUG ADMINISTRATION

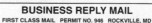

MEDWATCH
The FDA Medical Products Reporting Program
Food and Drug Administration
5600 Fishers Lane
Rockville, MD 20852-9787

Figure 15–1 Form 3500.

uct problems, and providing information for the public on medical-product safety issues.

MedWatch has been very successful and has markedly improved the methodologies for reporting adverse product events and the accessibility of safety-related product information. The program has established Form 3500 (Figure 15–1) to be used for all voluntary product-problem reports, and Form 3500A (Figure 15–2) to be used for mandatory product-problem reporting. The data may be submitted by voice using a prompted voice-mail recording, by FAX, over the Internet using on-line data entry, or by prepaid mail using a form found in the back

MEDWATCH
THE FDA MEDICAL PRODUCTS REPORTING PROGRAM

For VOLUNTARY reporting by health professionals of adverse events and product problems

Page ___ of ___

Form Approved: OMB No. 0910-0291 Expires:12/31/94
See OMB statement on reverse

FDA Use Only
Triage unit sequence #

A. Patient information
1. Patient identifier — In confidence
2. Age at time of event: ___ or Date of birth:
3. Sex ☐ female ☐ male
4. Weight ___ lbs or ___ kgs

B. Adverse event or product problem
1. ☐ Adverse event and/or ☐ Product problem (e.g., defects/malfunctions)
2. Outcomes attributed to adverse event (check all that apply)
☐ death ___ (mo/day/yr)
☐ life-threatening
☐ hospitalization – initial or prolonged
☐ disability
☐ congenital anomaly
☐ required intervention to prevent permanent impairment/damage
☐ other: ___
3. Date of event (mo/day/yr)
4. Date of this report (mo/day/yr)
5. Describe event or problem
6. Relevant tests/laboratory data, including dates
7. Other relevant history, including preexisting medical conditions (e.g., allergies, race, pregnancy, smoking and alcohol use, hepatic/renal dysfunction, etc.)

PLEASE TYPE OR USE BLACK INK

C. Suspect medication(s)
1. Name (give labeled strength & mfr/labeler, if known) #1 #2
2. Dose, frequency & route used #1 #2
3. Therapy dates (if unknown, give duration) from/to (or best estimate) #1 #2
4. Diagnosis for use (indication) #1 #2
5. Event abated after use stopped or dose reduced #1 ☐ yes ☐ no ☐ doesn't apply #2 ☐ yes ☐ no ☐ doesn't apply
6. Lot # (if known) #1 #2
7. Exp. date (if known) #1 #2
8. Event reappeared after reintroduction #1 ☐ yes ☐ no ☐ doesn't apply #2 ☐ yes ☐ no ☐ doesn't apply
9. NDC # (for product problems only) – –
10. Concomitant medical products and therapy dates (exclude treatment of event)

D. Suspect medical device
1. Brand name
2. Type of device
3. Manufacturer name & address
4. Operator of device ☐ health professional ☐ lay user/patient ☐ other: ___
5. Expiration date (mo/day/yr)
6. model # ___ catalog # ___ serial # ___ lot # ___ other # ___
7. If implanted, give date (mo/day/yr)
8. If explanted, give date (mo/day/yr)
9. Device available for evaluation? (Do not send to FDA) ☐ yes ☐ no ☐ returned to manufacturer on ___ (mo/day/yr)
10. Concomitant medical products and therapy dates (exclude treatment of event)

E. Reporter (see confidentiality section on back)
1. Name, address & phone #
2. Health professional? ☐ yes ☐ no
3. Occupation
4. Also reported to ☐ manufacturer ☐ user facility ☐ distributor
5. If you do NOT want your identity disclosed to the manufacturer, place an " X " in this box. ☐

FDA
Mail to: MEDWATCH 5600 Fishers Lane Rockville, MD 20852-9787 *or* FAX to: 1-800-FDA-0178

FDA Form 3500 (6/93) Submission of a report does not constitute an admission that medical personnel or the product caused or contributed to the event.

Figure 15–1 (Continued)

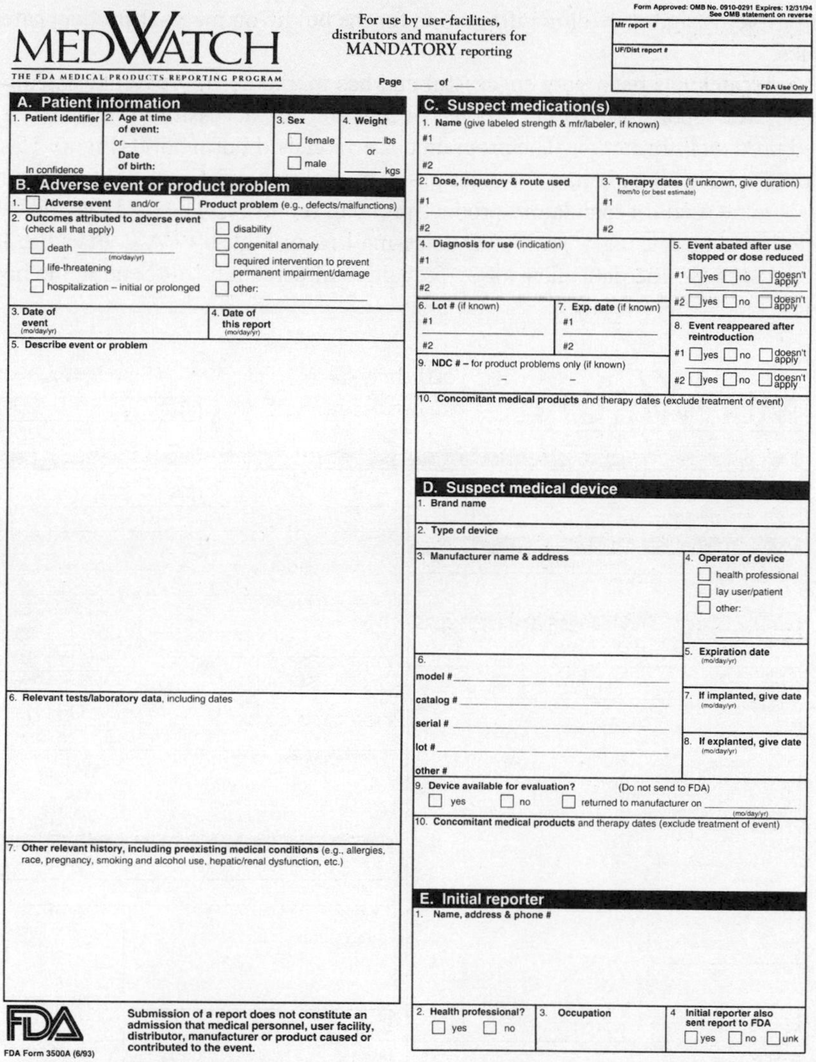

MEDWATCH
THE FDA MEDICAL PRODUCTS REPORTING PROGRAM

For use by user-facilities, distributors and manufacturers for MANDATORY reporting

Page ___ of ___

Form Approved: OMB No. 0910-0291 Expires: 12/31/94
See OMB statement on reverse

Mfr report #

UF/Dist report #

FDA Use Only

A. Patient information

1. Patient identifier — In confidence
2. Age at time of event: or — Date of birth:
3. Sex — female / male
4. Weight — ___ lbs or ___ kgs

B. Adverse event or product problem

1. Adverse event and/or Product problem (e.g., defects/malfunctions)
2. Outcomes attributed to adverse event (check all that apply)
   - death ___ (mo/day/yr)
   - life-threatening
   - hospitalization – initial or prolonged
   - disability
   - congenital anomaly
   - required intervention to prevent permanent impairment/damage
   - other:
3. Date of event (mo/day/yr)
4. Date of this report (mo/day/yr)
5. Describe event or problem
6. Relevant tests/laboratory data, including dates
7. Other relevant history, including preexisting medical conditions (e.g., allergies, race, pregnancy, smoking and alcohol use, hepatic/renal dysfunction, etc.)

C. Suspect medication(s)

1. Name (give labeled strength & mfr/labeler, if known) #1 #2
2. Dose, frequency & route used #1 #2
3. Therapy dates (if unknown, give duration) from/to (or best estimate) #1 #2
4. Diagnosis for use (indication) #1 #2
5. Event abated after use stopped or dose reduced — #1 yes no doesn't apply — #2 yes no doesn't apply
6. Lot # (if known) #1 #2
7. Exp. date (if known) #1 #2
8. Event reappeared after reintroduction — #1 yes no doesn't apply — #2 yes no doesn't apply
9. NDC # – for product problems only (if known) – –
10. Concomitant medical products and therapy dates (exclude treatment of event)

D. Suspect medical device

1. Brand name
2. Type of device
3. Manufacturer name & address
4. Operator of device — health professional / lay user/patient / other:
5. Expiration date (mo/day/yr)
6. model # / catalog # / serial # / lot # / other #
7. If implanted, give date (mo/day/yr)
8. If explanted, give date (mo/day/yr)
9. Device available for evaluation? (Do not send to FDA) — yes / no / returned to manufacturer on ___ (mo/day/yr)
10. Concomitant medical products and therapy dates (exclude treatment of event)

E. Initial reporter

1. Name, address & phone #
2. Health professional? yes / no
3. Occupation
4. Initial reporter also sent report to FDA — yes / no / unk

FDA

FDA Form 3500A (6/93)

Submission of a report does not constitute an admission that medical personnel, user facility, distributor, manufacturer or product caused or contributed to the event.

Figure 15–2 Form 3500A.

page of the *Physicians' Desk Reference,* or using a form requested from MedWatch by telephone (800-332-1088).

MedWatch also provides a free continuing education program available in the MedWatch newsletter or on the MedWatch Web site. Changes in the product labels due to safety concerns, the text of "Dear Health Professional" letters, and other safety notifications can be reviewed online or downloaded for more detailed review from the Web site. In addition, the 140 organizations that are part of the MedWatch partners use their journals and newsletters to provide safety information to health-care providers and industry. Interested individuals can sub-

Medication and Device Experience Report
(continued)

Submission of a report does not constitute an admission that medical personnel, user facility, distributor, manufacturer or product caused or contributed to the event.

U.S. DEPARTMENT OF HEALTH AND HUMAN SERVICES
Public Health Service • Food and Drug Administration

Refer to guidelines for specific instructions

Page _____ of _____

FDA Use Only

F. For use by user facility/distributor–devices only

1. Check one
   - [ ] user facility
   - [ ] distributor

2. UF/Dist report number

3. User facility or distributor name/address

4. Contact person

5. Phone Number

6. Date user facility or distributor became aware of event
   (mo/day/yr)

7. Type of report
   - [ ] initial
   - [ ] follow-up #

8. Date of this report
   (mo/day/yr)

9. Approximate age of device

10. Event problem codes (refer to coding manual)
    - patient code ___ – ___ – ___
    - device code ___ – ___ – ___

11. Report sent to FDA?
    - [ ] yes (mo/day/yr)
    - [ ] no

12. Location where event occurred
    - [ ] hospital
    - [ ] home
    - [ ] nursing home
    - [ ] outpatient treatment facility
    - [ ] outpatient diagnostic facility
    - [ ] ambulatory surgical facility
    - [ ] other: _____ specify

13. Report sent to manufacturer?
    - [ ] yes
    - [ ] no (mo/day/yr)

14. Manufacturer name/address

G. All manufacturers

1. Contact office – name/address (& mfring site for devices)

2. Phone number

3. Report source (check all that apply)
   - [ ] foreign
   - [ ] study
   - [ ] literature
   - [ ] consumer
   - [ ] health professional
   - [ ] user facility
   - [ ] company representative
   - [ ] distributor
   - [ ] other:

4. Date received by manufacturer
   (mo/day/yr)

5. (A)NDA # _____
   IND # _____
   PLA # _____
   pre-1938 [ ] yes
   OTC product [ ] yes

6. If IND, protocol #

7. Type of report (check all that apply)
   - [ ] 5-day
   - [ ] 15-day
   - [ ] 10-day
   - [ ] periodic
   - [ ] Initial
   - [ ] follow-up # _____

8. Adverse event term(s)

9. Mfr. report number

H. Device manufacturers only

1. Type of reportable event
   - [ ] death
   - [ ] serious injury
   - [ ] malfunction (see guidelines)
   - [ ] other: _____

2. If follow-up, what type?
   - [ ] correction
   - [ ] additional information
   - [ ] response to FDA request
   - [ ] device evaluation

3. Device evaluated by mfr?
   - [ ] not returned to mfr.
   - [ ] yes [ ] evaluation summary attached
   - [ ] no (attach page to explain why not) or provide code:

4. Device manufacture date
   (mo/yr)

5. Labeled for single use?
   - [ ] yes [ ] no

6. Evaluation codes (refer to coding manual)
   - method ___ – ___ – ___ – ___
   - results ___ – ___ – ___ – ___
   - conclusions ___ – ___ – ___ – ___

7. If remedial action initiated, check type
   - [ ] recall
   - [ ] repair
   - [ ] replace
   - [ ] relabeling
   - [ ] other: _____
   - [ ] notification
   - [ ] inspection
   - [ ] patient monitoring
   - [ ] modification/ adjustment

8. Usage of device
   - [ ] initial use of device
   - [ ] reuse
   - [ ] unknown

9. If action reported to FDA under 21 USC 360i(f), list correction/removal reporting number:

10. [ ] Additional manufacturer narrative and/or 11. [ ] Corrected data

The public reporting burden for this collection of information has been estimated to average one-hour per response, including the time for reviewing instructions, searching existing data sources, gathering and maintaining the data needed, and completing and reviewing the collection of information. Send your comments regarding this burden estimate or any other aspect of this collection of information, including suggestions for reducing this burden to:

Reports Clearance Officer, PHS
Hubert H. Humphrey Building, Room 721-B
200 Independence Avenue, S.W.
Washington, DC 20201
ATTN: PRA

and to:
Office of Management and Budget
Paperwork Reduction Project (0910-0291)
Washington, DC 20503

Please do NOT return this form to either of these addresses.

FDA Form 3500A - back

Figure 15–2 (Continued)

scribe to MedWatch free of charge from the FDA, by sending a message to www.fdalists@archie.fda.gov. For the message body, enter "subscribe medwatch" followed by a space and your complete e-mail address.

PROCESSING OF REPORTS

The FDA receives adverse drug reports on Form 3500A from manufacturers or on Form 3500 from health-care providers and consumers. The Form 3500 comes to the FDA either from the manufacturer or via MedWatch. Each report is assigned a unique and permanent report number, is imaged and stored in a searchable imaging system for later review, as needed. The report of the clinical event is coded by using standardized terms and entered verbatim into the AERS data base. In the AERS data base, each report represents one person and the same report may be received from more than one source, e.g., from the manufacturer and directly from the reporter. Duplicate reports can be eliminated from specific data sets by matching on dates, drugs, description of the event, and other data elements, rather than at the time of data entry.

The event coding is done manually, assigning a maximum of five standardized terms to the descriptive narrative on the report. The terminology is from *The Medical Dictionary for Drug Regulatory Affairs (MEDDRA)* and has replaced the FDA's COSTART (Coded Symbols for Thesaurus of Adverse Reaction Terms) dictionary in coding the adverse event descriptions. MEDDRA has been developed through the International Conference on Harmonization of Technical Requirements for Registration of Pharmaceuticals for Human Use, conveniently abbreviated as ICH (*10*). These coding languages are useful for the purpose of automated searches; MEDDRA will allow reports to be shared with other regulatory bodies worldwide.

Automated quality assurance is performed to evaluate reports for timeliness, completeness, and accuracy of coding. In addition, there are a number of canned and ad hoc queries that can be performed on the AERS database to enhance the value of the system in detecting new safety signals.

Adverse events reported to the AERS data base are available to the public through the Freedom of Information Office of the FDA. Confidential information such as patient identifiers, the name of the reporter, and the facility in which the event occurred are redacted. The Freedom of Information Office can be contacted via the FDA Web site or toll-free by telephone (888-463-6332).

DETECTING SIGNALS OF NEW SAFETY INFORMATION

All 15-day reports of serious, unexpected events and reports from health-care providers are triaged for immediate review by one of the safety evaluators in OPDRA. These safety evaluators are physicians or pharmacists who have a clinical perspective and who are familiar with the use, limits, and effectiveness of pharmaceutical safety surveillance data.

If the report or group of reports is believed to provide new safety information, it is considered a "signal" and may trigger a number of responses. Additional information may be sought from the reporter or from the manufacturer. The AERS database or the World Health Organization (WHO) data base of adverse drug events may be queried for similar reports associated with the same or similar products. If the signal is of sufficient strength and importance, it is termed a *monitored adverse reaction* (MAR) and is usually discussed with the pre-market review division responsible for premarket evaluation and approval of the suspect drug.

Table 15–3 Factors Important in Causality Assessment for Adverse Events Reported in Association with Marketed Pharmaceutical Drug Products

- timing of drug administration such that exposure precedes onset of the event
- abatement or resolution of the event with discontinuation of the suspect drug (de-challenge)
- recurrence or recrudescence of the event with re-exposure to the suspect drug (re-challenge)
- biologic plausibility of the event in association with the drug
- confirmatory or supporting laboratory or other objective evidence
- previous known toxicity of the suspect drug

A MAR of sufficient concern may trigger further epidemiologic investigation using one or more databases managed by outside organizations. The MAR serves to generate a hypothesis, which can be tested using other methodologies, either sponsored by the manufacturer or instigated by FDA (*11*).

ASSESSING CAUSALITY

The factors most useful in assessing causality are listed in Table 15–3. Absolute proof is rarely provided in a single report. However, there are some factors whose presence helps strengthen the signal for a possible causal relationship. First, for rare or unique clinical events, the association between drug exposure and occurrence of the event may be so striking that a very clear signal may be perceived with as few as four high-quality reports (*6*). In the event that the timing of the drug exposure clearly precedes the onset of the event, and the event resolves or abates with withdrawal of the suspected drug (de-challenge) and then is found to recur or intensify with re-exposure to the suspect drug, an isolated report can produce a signal of sufficient strength and clarity that causality is essentially proven (*14*). In general, adverse event reports generate signals of greater or lesser strength and are pursued on the basis on the factors listed in Table 15–3.

Some adverse events are recognized with comparative ease, such as potentially drug-related skin reactions, nausea or diarrhea with oral medications, abnormal liver function tests or hepatitis, or aplastic anemia. Less classical abnormalities—such as torsades de pointes with terfenadine, or clear-cell vaginal carcinoma in the female children of women who used diethylstilbesterol (DES) during pregnancy—even when observed, might not be attributed initially to a drug exposure. There often are unique circumstances that permit the most unusual adverse drug reactions to be correctly attributed to an exposure. Practitioners' lethargy and the absence of a readily available reporting form do not account for the totality of under-reporting biases.

ADDITIONAL METHODOLOGIES FOR INVESTIGATING SIGNALS OF ADVERSE DRUG EVENTS

FDA and drug manufacturers have supported, in whole or in part, a number of epidemiologic studies for testing specific drug-reaction hypotheses. The study

Table 15–4 Epidemiologic Study Designs Used in Estimating Risks in Adverse Drug Event Assessments

Research Question	Study Design
For rare events	Case-control design
Hypothesis testing	Cohort, case-control designs
Meta-analysis of existing data from clinical trials or epidemiologic data	
Obtaining numerator and denominator data	Descriptive studies using commercial marketing data bases
Outbreak investigations	Case-control studies

designs employed by the U.S. agency and manufacturers represent the types of studies used worldwide (*13,19*). Table 15–4 lists the general types of study designs used in investigating the strength of a drug-event relationship. Investigations designed to investigate drug-event hypotheses fall under the rubric of pharmacoepidemiology, coined to acknowledge the contributions of both clinical pharmacology and epidemiology.

Sample size considerations have directed many pharmacoepidemiologic investigations to the use of large, computerized patient-prescription data bases. Data bases employing Medicare or Medicaid patient profiles as well as computer-linked drug-diagnosis data from large health-maintenance organizations—like Kaiser-Permanente and Group Health of Puget Sound—have proven their usefulness in cohort and case-control study designs. Databases targeting special populations such as pregnant women, children, and the elderly have been specifically developed for use in generating hypotheses and in assessing associations between drugs and adverse outcomes. Other data bases to assess short- or long-term drug effects have been developed to meet the needs of clinical investigators and regulatory agencies in the United States. In addition, the classical outbreak investigation has proven useful in assessing reported clusters of adverse drug events. As with all epidemiologic investigations, methodology must be chosen based on the question that has been raised.

MANDATORY POST-MARKET SAFETY INVESTIGATIONS

At the time of approval, if a safety question is unresolved but does not appear to adversely affect the risk–benefit ratio for drug approval, FDA or the manufacturer may request that a post-market study be initiated to quantify the magnitude of the safety concern. These types of post-market or phase-4 studies may be required when a drug has been approved for marketing under the accelerated-approval mechanism (*20*), and if there are lingering safety or effectiveness concerns (*13,21*).

REGULATORY OUTCOMES OF POST-MARKET SAFETY SURVEILLANCE

Data from adverse events are used to determine if an approved product continues to be as safe as currently labeled. That is, do the benefits continue to outweigh the risks of use when the drug is prescribed and used according to the labeled instructions? There are a number of venues used to convey important new safety information on a marketed drug or medical product. Efforts by industry and FDA are intended to alert the health professional community and the public to a possible public health problem.

The several mechanisms available to the FDA and manufacturers to provide new safety information include the use of "Dear Health-Care Professional" letters, press notifications using the FDA Talk Paper format, and other uses of mass media. The MedWatch Web site provides information on safety issues and outcomes. MedWatch also has developed a "MedWatch Partners" program with over 140 health-care professional organizations such as the AMA and the ADA. Safety information may also be provided to health-care professionals by industry and through participating organizations' newsletters, journals, etc. Obtained from the MedWatch Web site is a sample of recent "Dear Health Professional" and labeling changes effected during the first half of 1999 (Table 15–5). Approximately 25 to 35 drug products undergo safety-related labeling changes each month. Subscribers to MedWatch are automatically notified about new safety information on a monthly basis.

Post-market safety data are used to determine if modifications to the label are necessary to help assure safe use. New information may be added to the product label to help prescibers use the drug safely. Label changes are effected by agreement between manufacturers and FDA; FDA usually reviews and responds to these changes before inclusion in the product packaging. Content, placement

Table 15–5 A Sample of "Dear Health-Care Professional" Letters and Associated Regulatory Outcomes in 1999, MedWatch Web Site

Regulatory Outcomes	Product	Indication- Drug Class	Safety Issue
Patient information and consent form	Cylert™	Attention deficit disorder	Liver Toxicity
Labeling changes	Rezulin™	Diabetes	Liver Toxicity
Restricted use, labeling	Trovan™	Antibiotic	Liver Toxicity
Labeling changes, contraindications	Propulsid™	Gastrointestinal agent	Drug Interactions Adverse cardiac events
Label change	Cerebyx™	Seizures	Overdose, Death
Label change	Mirapex™	Parkinson's disease	Unexpected sleep

of information, and use of bold lettering and black boxes to present safety information are important tools in conveying information. The regulations governing product labeling can be found in 21 CFR, sections 201.56 and 201.57.

Decisions on wording, placement, and typeface have implications for drug advertising. For instance, if a drug has a serious, life-threatening adverse event associated with its use, the FDA or the manufacturer might request that information be presented in a black-box warning such as the warning against use of angiotensin converting enzyme (ACE) inhibitors during the second and third trimesters of pregnancy. Other specific examples of black-box warnings can be found in a number of references (6,10,14). To the practitioner, the black-box warning implies a very serious health risk. To the manufacturer, the black-box warning must accompany all promotional materials, even the ubiquitous pens, penlights, and paperweights, as well as all print advertising in journals or other venues.

Other outcomes that can result from new safety information include restricting the use of the drug by label changes or, in rare instances, withdrawing the drug from the U.S. market. From 1980 through 1998, there were a total of 13 drugs removed from the U.S. market due to safety concerns (22). Far more common than market withdrawal are changes in the warning, precautions, or other label information and modifications in use or indication.

STRENGTHS OF DRUG SAFETY SURVEILLANCE DATA

The major strengths of the current system for U.S. post-market safety surveillance derive from the size and heterogeneity of the population from which the data are obtained, and from the relatively low cost of obtaining the data. With the initiation of the MedWatch program, among other factors, post-market adverse event reporting in the United States has increased dramatically. In 1970 and 1980, 14,000 and 18,000 reports, respectively, were added to the AERS database. In 1998, over 230,000 new reports were included into the AERS (10). Increased feedback to reporters, the ease with which reports can be submitted, and the increasing emphasis on adverse event reporting effected by MedWatch and its partner professional organizations has undoubtedly contributed to the increase in adverse drug event reporting. Even though the major emphasis of adverse drug event reporting is on the early marketing of the product, the spontaneous reporting system provides continuous monitoring throughout the life of the product. It provides real-world information on the actual population exposed and provider prescribing habits. The homogeneous populations and the controlled circumstances of clinical trials are supplemented by actual clinical use.

The size of the exposed population following drug approval and marketing provides the best opportunity for detecting rare events, such as those occurring at rates of 1 in 10,000 or less. The heterogeneous population can also help define at-risk populations for specific types of adverse drug events, such as the elderly, patients with certain types of concomitant medicines, and other specific risk factors that could not be evaluated in the pre-market clinical trials.

LIMITATIONS OF SURVEILLANCE DATA

There are several important limitations in safety surveillance based on spontaneous reporting of events. Most stem from the fact that data are collected in an uncontrolled manner and reporting is affected by biases that may be suspected but which usually cannot be quantified.

Under-reporting may arise from a number of biases (2). If the health-care professional does not suspect that an event may be related to drug or other product exposure, a report will not be generated. If the event and the drug exposure are relatively common, an association may not be made. If the event occurs close in time to product exposure, suspicion of causation is more likely. Conversely, if the event occurs only after prolonged exposure to the drug, attribution is less likely. If the event is distinctive, like clear-cell carcinoma in women whose mothers used DES, then attribution is more likely, regardless of the time between exposure and outcome.

Spontaneous reporting data cannot be used to calculate rates of occurrence. Essentially, the data are case reports. A number of factors can affect reporting. Ascertainment bias can lead to under-reporting. Media attention, recently promulgated "Dear Healthcare Professional" letters, articles in the scientific literature describing adverse drug events, and other sources of information can increase reporting. As noted above, the length of time a product is on the market can affect reporting.

Likewise, denominator data are difficult to estimate. There are inpatient and outpatient databases linking prescribed drug use and diagnoses in defined patient populations, which can be used to estimate rates of occurrence. In addition, commercial data bases for marketing research can be used to estimate drug use based on wholesale purchases and drug purchases by certain types of outpatient pharmacies, as well as information on the use or recommendations for marketed prescription and OTC drug products for certain diagnoses. Actual use of the drug for the diagnosis may not be verified, but general information on the uses and volume of drug distribution for marketed drugs can be estimated using commercially available data bases. In addition, the FDA and product manufacturers may help fund data bases and research organizations for the purpose of better defining incidence rates and at-risk populations.

Another of the major limitations in the usefulness of post-market safety surveillance data is in the unpredictable quality of the reports. FDA's Forms 3500 and 3500A request the essential information to help assess causality. This information includes product name, patient identifiers and demographics, narrative description of the event, relevant laboratory and supportive data, information on confounders such as past medical history and concomitant medications, sequence of exposure/event based on dates of event onset and use of product, doses and duration of administration of the suspect and other drugs, de-challenge and re-challenge information, and outcome. A few complete, succinct reports can serve as the basis for regulatory action by the FDA or a manufacturer in the case of a serious, previously unidentified adverse event. However, an analysis of report quality conducted by the FDA shows the completion rate of selected data elements may be less than 50% for the start data and dose of drug, and date of onset of the adverse event (*11*).

Again, while the data can be used to detect signals of important new safety issues and generate hypotheses to be explored using other data sources, they rarely provide solid evidence of causality.

DRUG SAFETY SURVEILLANCE IN OTHER COUNTRIES

The basic principles of drug safety surveillance as applied to data collection and analysis are the same in other countries engaged in post-market drug safety surveillance. The drugs of greatest interest are newly marketed drugs and the events of greatest interest are serious, previously unknown events. Most countries use a central monitoring agency associated with the drug licensing body. In some countries, like France, Norway, and Sweden, physicians are required by law to report adverse drug events observed during normal clinical use. In other countries, like England, Denmark, and New Zealand, newly marketed drugs and drugs meeting certain other criteria are placed under special reporting programs to increase physician awareness of the need to monitor them for adverse events during use. Many countries with national formularies or other forms of linked prescription and diagnosis data bases, like England and Finland, are able to monitor or study the rates of certain diagnoses associated with prescription drug use, not unlike health-maintenance organizations and the federal Medicaid program in the United States (*23*).

In England, a "yellow card" system is used to stimulate reporting. Physicians are provided with yellow postcards for use in reporting adverse events (*24*). Newly marketed drugs or drugs with special safety concerns at the time of market approval are indicated with a black triangle in the national formulary. The black triangle is intended to increase the likelihood of reporting adverse events noted with their use. Even so, it has been estimated that British physicians report only about 10% of serious adverse drug events and 2% to 4% of other types of adverse drug events (*25*).

The advantages and limitations of the U.S. post-market drug safety surveillance system apply to spontaneous reporting systems in other countries. In general, these are large, cost-effective efforts that allow events to be monitored in heterogeneous populations not usually included in pre-market trials. The surveillance systems produce signals of potential problems that require further study for validation. In general, drugs recently approved or marketed and drugs that may have safety issues due to known toxicity or with safety concerns at the time of market entry are targeted for more intensive surveillance. The same biases acting in the U.S. system tend to affect data submission in other countries, even those in which adverse event reporting is required by law.

THE WORLD HEALTH ORGANIZATION DATA BASE

In 1968, WHO established an international data base for safety surveillance of drugs and other pharmaceutical products (*26*). The initial data were provided by

10 countries including the United States, Australia, Canada, Sweden, and Great Britain. The intent of the WHO data base, formally known as the WHO International Programme on Drug Monitoring, was to increase the population from which safety information on pharmaceutical products could be drawn. As of 1998 there were 49 participating countries and another 11 countries enrolled but not yet submitting reports. The WHO data base receives about 150,000 reports each year. Most countries transmit only those reports for which the outcome is clear and, in the case of some participating countries, for which causality is considered likely. The data in the WHO data base are submitted using the MEDDRA language for coding and facilitating automated searches of the data by participating regulatory agencies. Information derived from this database is used by regulatory agencies and can be reported in the scientific and medical literature (27,28). The intent of the data base is to improve communication concerning drug safety issues among participating countries and worldwide pharmacovigilance.

DRUG SAFETY SURVEILLANCE IN THE FUTURE

The future of drug safety surveillance is in increased information sharing worldwide. Large, cooperative data bases, such as WHO's, and more data sources linking prescriptions to diagnoses will allow more rapid hypothesis generation and testing. The technologic barriers to international information transfer have largely been solved through the efforts of the International Committee on Harmonization of Technical Requirements for Registration of Pharmaceuticals for Human Use (ICH). The ICH is committed to continued harmonization efforts for data standards and data transmission to improve global pharmacovigilance.

New data sources for formal evaluation of potential adverse drug events are needed. The closed formularies and computer billing and data management systems that are now commonplace in managed-care systems in the United States may lend themselves to drug safety surveillance. Improved computerized data management and analytic capabilities will enhance use of data sources. Improving access to data bases linking inpatient diagnoses to drug exposures as well as outpatient databases will increase the size of the observed populations as the analytic capabilities improve.

Even so, postmarket safety surveillance is an imperfect discipline. Recently, the FDA postmarket program has been criticized for its deficiencies, and alternatives have been proposed (29). However, the minimal cost of the program, innovations such as the MedWatch program, coordination of premarket and postmarket data in decision making, and the overall success of the AERS system, are all arguments against major institutional change (22,30).

Medical products, including pharmaceutical drug products, will always be subject to postmarket safety issues by the very nature of pre-market data collection. The costs of pre-market evaluation will deter increasing pre-market, controlled, clinical trial data collection strategies. If the FDA is representative of regulatory agencies worldwide, the pressure to speed up approval of products is increasing, allowing pharmaceutical products to enter the market with fewer clinical studies. Therefore, it is clear that the need for post-market safety surveillance will increase. It is likely that the methodologies for evaluating signals will improve. However, signal detection will likely remain the province of the large observational data systems.

The author of this chapter wishes to thank Diane L. Kennedy, RPh., M.P.H., founding director of the FDA MedWatch program, for her thoughtful review of this manuscript.

REFERENCES

1. Faich GA. Adverse drug-reaction monitoring. *N Engl J Med* 1986;279:678–79.
2. Strom BL, Tugwell P. Pharmacoepidemiology: current status, prospects, and problems. *Ann Intern Med* 1990;113(3):179–81.
3. Nies AS, Spielberg SP. Principles of therapeutics. In: Hardman JG, Limbird LE, Molinoff PB, Ruddon RW, Gilman AG (eds.). The pharmacologic basis of therapeutics. New York: McGraw-Hill, 1996:43–62.
4. Beard K. Adverse reactions as a cause of hospital admissions in the aged. *Drugs Aging* 1992;2:356–67.
5. Lazarou J, Pomeranz BH, Corey PN. Incidence of adverse drug reactions in hospitalized patients: a meta-analysis of prospective studies. *JAMA* 1998;279:2005.
6. MedWatch Continuing Education Article. Clinical therapeutics and recognition of drug-induced disease. Goldman SA, Kennedy DL, Graham DJ, Gross TP, Kapit RM, Love LA, White GG (eds.). Rockville Md.: Food and Drug Administration, 1996.
7. Zimmerman HJ. Hepatotoxicity: the adverse effects of drugs and other chemicals on the liver. New York: Appleton-Century-Crofts, 1978.
8. Vincent PC. Drug-induced aplastic anemia and agranulocytosis: incidence and mechanisms. *Drugs* 1986;31:52–63.
9. Chan H-L, Stern RS, Arndt KA, Langlois J, Jick SS, Jick H *et al.* The incidence of erythema multiforme, Stevens-Johnson Syndrome, and toxic epidermal necrolysis: a population-based study with particular reference to reactions caused by drugs among outpatients. *Arch Dermatol* 1990;126:43–47.
10. Kennedy DL, Goldman SA, Lillie RB. Spontaneous reporting in the United States. In: Strom BL (ed.). Pharmacoepidemiology. New York: John Wiley & Sons, 2000.
11. Baum C, Kweder SA, Anello C. The spontaneous reporting system in the United States. In: Strom BL (ed.). Pharmacoepidemiology. New York: John Wiley & Sons, 1994:125–37.
12. Enforcement of the post-marketing adverse experience reporting regulations. Website: http://www.fda.gov/cder/regguide.htm.
13. Arrowsmith-Lowe JB, Anello CA. View from a regulatory agency. In: Strom BL (ed.). Pharmacoepidemiology. New York: John Wiley & Sons, 1994:87–97.
14. MedWatch. Continuing Education Article. Clinical impact of adverse event reporting. Goldman SA, Kennedy DL, Graham DJ, Gross TP, Kapit RM, Love LA, White GG (eds.). Rockville, Md.: Food and Drug Administration, 1996.
15. Devices and therapeutic methods of the American Dental Association principles of ethics and code of conduct. Advisory Opinion No. 1 to section 4-A.
16. Accreditation manual, 1993. Oakbrook Terrace, Ill.: Joint Commission on Accreditation of Health Care Organizations, 1993.
17. Chen RT, Rastogi SC, Mullen JR, Hayes SW, Cochi SL, Donlon JA *et al.* The vaccine adverse event reporting system (VAERS). *Vaccine* 1994;12:542–50.

18. Kessler DA. Introducing MedWatch: a new approach to reporting medication and device adverse effects and product problems. *JAMA* 1993;269:2765–68.
19. Carson JL, Strom BL, Maislin G. Screening for unknown effects of newly marketed drugs. In: Strom BL (ed.). Pharmacoepidemiology. New York: John Wiley & Sons, 1994:431–47.
20. 21 CFR 314.500.
21. Psaty BM, Weiss NS, Furberg TD, Koepsell TD, Siscovick DS, Rosendaal FR *et al.* Surrogate end points, health outcomes, and the drug approval process for the treatment of risk factors for cardiovascular disease. *JAMA* 1999;282:786–90.
22. Friedman MJ, Woodcock J, Lumpkin MM, Shuren JE, Hass A, Thompson LJ. The safety of newly approved medicines: do recent market removals mean there is a problem? *JAMA* 1999; 281:1728–34.
23. Wiholm BE, Olsson S, Moore N, Wood S. Spontaneous reporting systems outside the United States. In: Strom BL (ed.). Pharmacoepidemiology. New York: John Wiley & Sons, 1994:139–55.
24. Finney DJ. The detection of adverse reactions to therapeutic drugs. *Statistics in Medicine* 1982;1:153–61.
25. Rawlins MD. Pharmacovigilance: paradise lost or regained? The William Withering Lecture 1994. *J R Coll Physicians Lond* 1995;29:41–49.
26. Olsson S. The role of the WHO programme on international drug monitoring in coordinating worldwide drug safety efforts. *Drug Saf* 1998 July:19(1):1–10.
27. Stahl MM, Lindquist M, Pettersson M, Edwards IR, Sanderson JH, Taylor NF *et al.* Withdrawal reactions with selective serotonin re-uptake inhibitors as reported to the WHO system. *Eur J Clin Pharmacol* 1997;53(3–4):163–69.
28. Routledge PA, Lindquist M, Edwards IR. Spontaneous reporting of suspected reactions to antihistamines: a national and international perspective. *Clin Exp Allergy* 1999;29 (suppl 3):240–46.
29. Wood AJJ, Stein CM, Woosley R. Making medicines safer: the need for an independent drug safety board. *New Engl J Med* 1998;330:1851–53.
30. Rossi AC, Knapp DE. Discovery of new adverse drug reactions: a review of the Food and Drug Administration's spontaneous reporting system. *JAMA* 1984;252:1030–33.

16

Using Surveillance Information in Communications, Marketing, and Advocacy

R. ELLIOTT CHURCHILL

The difference between the right word and the almost-right word is the same as the difference between lightning and the lightning bug.

Mark Twain

Information is the primary tool of public health practice.* Surveillance is the primary means of obtaining the data that are analyzed and translated into information. In moving one step further into the realm of influencing policy and decisions made by governments or by individuals, information is translated into messages—units of communications science that tell their audiences how to respond to particular pieces of information. This process sounds deceptively simple. Unfortunately, it is so difficult that wars, failed personal relationships, broken businesses, and other disastrous or painful consequences have been associated with inadequate or inappropriate communications, marketing, and advocacy throughout human history. With increasing urgency, public health professionals have begun to understand their need to become adept in the art and science of using surveillance information in communications, marketing, and advocacy. In the world of the 21st century, these areas are not reserved for the commercial sector alone. Scientists must understand the principles of the two-way passage of information. Time-honored practice in public health has involved a great deal of *dissemination of information* (a one-way process) but very little *communication* (a two-way process) involving disseminated information, followed by feedback.

As is the case with much of public health practice, the principles and practice of communications science, marketing, and advocacy are similar in domestic and international settings. However, public health practitioners everywhere should be aware that though the concept of the "global village" may be trite, it is also ac-

---

*A great deal has been written about dissemination of information in government settings—both in domestic and international contexts. Unfortunately, to date, very little is available in the peer-reviewed literature on the art and science of communications in the public health arena. The author has included a number of guidelines, checklists, models, and other resource materials that she has developed over the past 30 years for classroom use at several academic institutions.

curate. Things that happen in health in one country are likely to have an effect on at least the adjoining countries and may have an effect half-way around the world. Airplanes are efficient "hosts" for the transmission of infection and other problems of public health consequence.

In the sections that follow, communications, marketing, and advocacy strategies that are based on surveillance information and will be applied in numerous public health settings will be discussed in the context of data, information, and messages (see also Chapter 7 for a discussion of communications efforts within the public health system).

SOME PITFALLS IN COMMUNICATIONS

Communications can be helped or hindered by relations between the public health system and the mass media. It is wise for public health staff to remember at all times that they do not have in common all the goals and objectives aspired to by representatives of the mass media. The latter view themselves as watchdogs for the public and are also in a competitive, entrepreneurial system. The public health system is certainly vitally concerned about the welfare of the public, but, whereas the approach of the mass media tends to be "the news regardless," the approach of the public health system is often constrained by the dictate of "do no harm" (from the Hippocratic oath). This lack of intersection of goals and objectives on the part of the two groups, a different approach to deadlines (the journalist *must* meet deadlines; the health scientist will work as long as necessary to try to find top-quality results), and a different set of terminology (Madison Avenue jargon versus scientific jargon—each a language within itself) make collaboration between public health scientist and professional journalist a massive challenge. Fortunately, the tension created by these points of non-correspondence between public health and mass media can be used to good effect—and with the public as the ultimate beneficiary of the efforts of people in both categories. However, the interrelationships must be carefully cultivated, gently managed, and constantly reviewed and revised as needed.

Another important issue is the level of security (and secrecy) assigned to health-related information. In the political system of the former Soviet Union, for example, all surveillance data were considered classified information and were controlled by the military authorities. Reports from surveillance systems throughout 11 time zones were collected, compiled, shipped to Moscow, and stored in locked rooms for security purposes. The concept of putting the information to use in order to improve the system never occurred to the managers of the public health system and certainly never occurred to the military (personal communication, Deputy Minister of Health, Russian Federation, 1995).

A third problem occurs when a public health system includes a punitive aspect. If data collectors (or data analysts) know that the reaction to their sending in reports of unusually high numbers of cases of rabies among humans this year will lead to jail time or a reduced paycheck, the chances are that the number of reported cases of rabies will closely resemble last year's reported number. This manipulation of numbers leads very quickly to a general distrust for any conclusions or recommendations derived from the surveillance system in question. An example of this type of distortion in a surveillance system is provided by the results of a recent epidemiologic study conducted in the Central Asian Republic of Kazakhstan. Results from this study showed that the infant mortality rates reported by the system, over time, were approximately one-half the rates that would be calculated if World Health Organization parameters were applied. This optional use of definitions made the level of the problem represented by infant mortality appear to be relatively small when, in fact, in WHO terms, it would represent a serious problem (personal communication, USAID liaison officer, Almaty, Kazakhstan).

THE ROLE OF COMMUNICATIONS IN PUBLIC HEALTH SURVEILLANCE IN DEVELOPING COUNTRIES

Problems of Perception

One reason a surveillance system may not function at its optimal level is that the people who manage it are trained that it is enough to provide information to health officials without translating, communicating, explicating, and advocating for the results obtained through their data. In many countries, problems associated with this orientation are often compounded by problems created by firmly established patterns for the flow of information (e.g., orders flow down from the top of a strongly centralized system, while data and information flow upward). Nothing flows across (e.g., between regional health centers, between village data registrars, and the like). No information or messages are returned from the central depository to the source of the data (at the bottom of the system), and the people at the base level of the system have no idea that the information they send to the top could have useful applications for their own programs. Furthermore, the idea of sharing information with peers in neighboring villages (states, provinces) is not likely to occur because there is no tradition for such openness. Instead, they wait for a directive to be sent from the central office, for a shipment of drugs and other standard supplies, and continue to do business as usual. They count the number of condoms distributed, the number of oral-rehydration kits given out, and the number of vaccinations administered. This is passive public health.

An effective communications program, applied in the context of an at least partially devolved public health system, can go a long way toward creating an environment in which data and information are translated into messages that are used throughout the public health system and beyond—to attain the goal of improving the public's health.

Three serious problems that are present in many public health systems in the developing world are not problems of science, not problems of fact. Instead, they are problems of perception, of attitude. First, many people do not want to change—they are, if not comfortable with the way they do their work, at least accustomed to it.

Second, if one asks who the decision makers are in a public health system, many staff members will identify people above themselves in the system. They use the pronoun *we* to describe the people who do the work, but they use the pronoun *they* to describe the people who make decisions. In fact, in a devolved, de-centralized system, this perception can be not only dangerous but destructive. It is important to make a commitment to accuracy, to precision, to dissemination of information and the conveying of messages in a timely fashion and to the appropriate audiences. But public health staff must also make a commitment to make decisions and to provide resources in the form of reports and recommendations to the managers of the health system who are above them. The attitude of health staff must not be "That's not my job" but "How can I help?"

The third problem relates to the belief on the part of many people that technology is magic. "If only I had enough computers" is a common statement in many public health systems. Computers *are* useful tools—but it is a big mistake to assume that they do things *better*. They make it possible for people to do *more* things and to do *more things faster*, but they do not do anything *better* than can one human being equipped with the appropriate knowledge and a piece of paper and a pencil.

Problems of Management

Communicating with others about important health messages, and seeing those messages acted upon through changes in policy, allocation of resources, or changes in behavior, is the culmination of a long process of collection, analysis, communication, and follow-up. Successful communications requires that someone apply marketing, human psychology, interpersonal relations, persuasion, and other subjective strategies, in addition to all of the tools and techniques of science.

Problems of Definition

Public health surveillance has often been interpreted to mean dissemination of information within the public health system. Since the advent of HIV/AIDS, however, CDC has aimed at addressing a far more wide-reaching target audience than its original one of "state and local health departments." (CDC Mission Statement, 1985). Traditionally, public health surveillance managers have focused on the dissemination of information within the public health system. The distinction between *communications* and *dissemination* is critical to understanding what actually happens with public health information versus what public health workers *think* happens with it. The distinction is also key in planning, implementing, and evaluating programs that involve communications in public health practice.

The paragraphs below *a*) define communications in the context of public health practice, *b*) discuss how communications can be integrated into the infrastructure and the operational structure of public health information systems, and *c*) provide some guidelines for evaluating and modifying communications strategies as needed.

Defining Communications

Communications is a process that involves at least two people in an effort to convey, receive, interpret, and agree upon the meaning of *data, information,* or *messages.* The purpose of this process from the point of view of the person or agency that disseminates data, information, or message may be to inform, to influence, to motivate, to persuade, or some combination of these or other activities. The purpose of this process from the point of view of the person or agency that receives data, information, or messages may be to learn, to use as the basis for decision making, to reject, to discredit, to reinterpret and use for other purposes, to sell, or some combination of these or other activities. In other words, we use the term *communications* to mean *the process in which we use language or images (symbols) to share meaning with other people.*

The basic reporting unit of science is the *fact* (a piece of information), whereas the basic reporting unit of communications is the *message.* This is one reason that scientists and communicators must struggle in their efforts to collaborate— or even to understand each other. Scientists are trained to discover, to record, and to convey facts—not messages. And how do facts and messages differ?

Communications takes facts and packages them to convey meaning. When everyone agrees on that meaning, there should be no problem. However, recipients often receive different messages from a single communications effort. Communications may be unsuccessful because information is not sent at the proper time or not made available to the appropriate audience. Communications is a strong and powerful tool. In looking at communications, we also need to be aware that there is a difference between the medium and the message, and that technology does not necessarily bring correct answers to our problems.

How Data, Information, and Messages from Surveillance Systems Fit into the Communications Construct

Communications involves *data, information,* and *messages* (Table 16–1). *Data* are the smallest units of description; they may be presented as words, numbers, or other symbols. *Information* is made up of data that have been interpreted to provide meaning and context. Finally, information is aimed at a particular audience and given a particular slant in order to elicit a desired result. This product is a *message.*

These examples show the progression from data to message. The data are simply values. There is not enough context provided to evaluate the import of the data. What is the time period? Who is the population affected? How does the number compare with reports for previous years? When we move on to information, we are given the data but are also provided with enough context (time, place, person) to be able to do at least *some* assessment of the meaning of the data. We know, for example, that if 1,000 cases of measles represents 50% more than were reported last year, there is some sort of a problem of public health relevance. The message is based on the information provided, but the message goes a step further than information does and tells people what they are supposed to think about the information or why they are supposed to care about it. Why is it

Table 16–1 The Communications Process, Data through Information
to Message

Data	→	Information	→	Message
(the smallest units of measurement; numbers, symbols, words—no context provided)		(data with enough context provided to allow people to analyze and determine meaning)		(information with the addition of interpretation. Answers such questions as "What does this mean to me?" "Why should I care?" "What am I supposed to do about it?")

An example of this data–information–message series from public health.

| 1,000 cases of measles | | "This is a 50% increase from last year" | | "Have all infants vaccinated for measles before their first birthday." |

Or

| 1,000 cases of measles | | "This is a 50% increase from last year. Five cases have been fatal" | | "Every infant in this country can be vaccinated for measles for less money than it takes to care for five cases that lead to complications and death" |

important to me? What am I supposed to do with this? Why should I care? One set of data and file of information can be used to craft many different messages. The points that are emphasized depend on many factors including interest, resources, and audience.

The statement "Let the data speak for themselves" is insufficient. Surveillance provides information for action. We therefore need to supply the content and message to provide the basis for appropriate and conclusive actions. Often the critical step of translating the data through information into a clear message is omitted, which leads to frustration on the part of the transmitter ("Why don't people use my information?") and the recipient ("What should I do with this information?").

Officials who convey their data (or even *information*) to media representatives, elected officials, or the general public often cannot understand why these groups do not immediately comprehend the meaning, value, and relevance of the data or information they have provided. Their target audience (the sub-group of the population that they most want to reach and convert to their point of view), in the meantime, may not understand the meaning of information conveyed in terms of risks, rates, or other biostatistically derived relationships, or they may not appreciate the relevance of things reported in terms of "...per 100,000 population" or "...per 1,000 live births." They may not appreciate the value of the information they receive because they do not know whether or how this information relates to them in particular—either as individuals or as members of a group. Finally, elected officials or other persons who set policy and allocate resources usually have limited knowledge of the subject matter. Thus, it is difficult for them to compare the gravity, relevance, and value added by recommendations based on public health information and messages with the gravity, relevance, and value added by material that relates to competing priorities. These competing priorities often include

- a water supply that is adequate for personal, commercial, and industrial needs
- pollutants in the environment
- adequate road, rail, and water shipping
- expansion of industrial zones
- shifting populations and displaced populations
- quality and capacity of schools

With these things in mind, it becomes easier to see why policy setters and legislators want to know costs, the true value of the benefits of those costs, and how reliable the information is.

THE MECHANICS OF COMMUNICATIONS

Communications is a process—not a product (Figure 16–1). Because the process of communications is a loop, it requires not only the effort of the communicator to convey the desired information, it also requires the attention, the cooperation, and the understanding of the recipient before communication can actually occur.

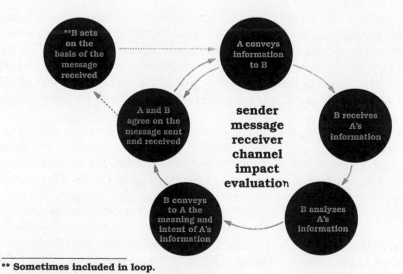

** Sometimes included in loop.

Figure 16–1 The communications loop.

In the model of communications that follows, there are at least six components: the sender, the message, the receiver, the channel, the impact, and the evaluation. In order to succeed at communications, all of these factors must be taken into consideration and decisions made about each.

SENDER	Who is the most appropriate person (organization) to convey this message?
MESSAGE	Exactly what message is it you want to convey? "It is 10 o'clock" is a fact, or a piece of information—not a message. "It is 10 o'clock; do you know where your children are?" is a message.
RECEIVER	How can you describe the targeted audience or audiences? Is it one population (e.g., teenagers), or is it components of several different populations (e.g., all people who smoke cigarettes)? What are these people like? Is it, in fact, an audience that represents part of the public? Or is the targeted audience part of the "establishment" (for example, politicians or public health officials)?
CHANNEL	How best can you reach your intended audience? Can you reach them through any mass communications medium? What do they read? Do they watch television more than they read?
IMPACT	What do you want to happen as a result of your message being sent and received? What action do you wish to be taken?
EVALUATION	What will you change before trying to share this message with this audience again?

PUBLIC HEALTH STRATEGIES AND PROGRAMS IN THE OPEN MARKETPLACE

One of public health's most important messages is this: "By modifying behavior and changing life style, the public can make substantial gains in their overall health and live longer, more active lives." Public health would like for this message to be applicable to every man, woman, and child in the world. The question is how to *reach* people with the message, how to *persuade* them that the message is true and that it applies to them, and how to *convince* them to take the required actions to reach the health objective carried in the message. The research component of this process is called *marketing* and the application component is called *advocacy*.

The Marketing Component

Countries throughout the world have a successful communications model for marketing in the form of advertising for commercial goods. Advertising campaigns are carefully researched, attractively packaged, directed very carefully at a well-defined audience, and evaluated painstakingly and extensively. Why? Money, of course. If you don't do these things, your competition will, and his or her product will capture the imagination of the public, and your product will likely fail. Marketing, whether it is applied to commercial products or to life-style choices for healthful living, is the process of researching what approaches will work most effectively with which targeted audiences in order to achieve the originator's desired result (i.e., the purchase of a product or the "purchase" of an idea that leads a person away from a behavior that puts him or her at risk of having a health problem).

How does this relate to public health communications based on surveillance information? Public health planners can learn what advertising technology and psychology do and how the process works. Public health is competing with messages from the mass communications industry, which tries to persuade people to buy a product. Very often, public health messages ask people to change often pleasurable types of behavior (e.g., eating fatty foods, smoking, or consuming alcoholic beverages).

So how can public health ever hope to succeed with messages that people would prefer not to hear? Several factors are important.

- Public health workers must develop a rapport with our public that is based on reliability and truthfulness. The public must believe that public health messages tell the truth and do so because the public health system wants what is best for its clients.
- Public health workers must be patient and persistent. A public health information campaign usually requires several years to become successful; people generally will not pay attention to or believe messages that advocate changes in behavior right away. (An exception to this pattern is represented by bulletins or public service announcements provided to the public during or immediately following an emergency situation. People generally do respond quickly to such messages—if they can understand what it is they are supposed to do.)
- Public health workers must repeat, modify, and update. The main points of the message must be presented repeatedly, but in novel and different ways over time. The messages must be couched in current idiom and presented through up-to-date technology.
- Public health workers must use all appropriate avenues. A multimedia approach is more likely to capture the attention of the audience and to reach all components of a diverse audience.
- Public health workers must ultimately speak person-to-person. The mass media effort must be augmented by more personal interventions and the organization of community resources at the local level. Public health must recruit persons in every community it seeks to serve who can serve as spokespersons for the messages the community needs to hear.

For example, in 1993, one of America's professional basketball superstars announced that he was HIV positive. He denied being a homosexual or injecting

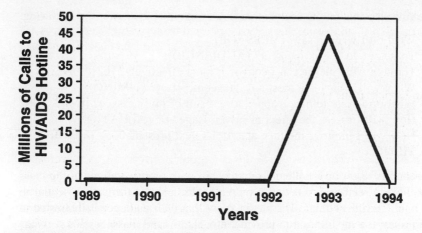

Figure 16–2 Pattern of use of CDC's HIV/AIDS telephone hotline.

drugs, and the public was left to assume that he was infected through a hetero-
sexual contact. A national AIDS hotline had been established a few years earlier by CDC so that persons could use a telephone and receive information and
be directed for counseling about HIV/AIDS. Figure 16–2 shows what happened
to the pattern of the use of this hotline after Ervin "Magic" Johnson held his
press conference. After many months of fairly consistent call-in rates of 2,000
attempted calls per day, in the 24-hour period following Magic's press conference there were 151,000 attempts to use the HIV/AIDS hotline. This level
of use continued to rise throughout 1992. Public health officials had been warning for several years that HIV/AIDS was not just a problem for homosexual
males and users of intravenously injected drugs, and had insisted that it was a
threat to the entire country. Now, suddenly, people believed. If this could happen to Magic Johnson, it could happen to them. Figure 16–2 also demonstrates
that this initial level of concern does not usually continue without reinforce-
ment. The pattern of use of the hotline returned to pre-Magic levels by the end
of 1994.

The Advocacy Component

Communications campaigns should be attractive, appealing, and persuasive. They
must overcome the public's suspicion about the motives of the public health system (learned partly from experience with the commercial world and, unfortunately, learned partly from negative experiences with public officials). *Why* does
the public health system care what happens to them? *What* does the public health
system (or the politicians) expect to get out of this? More important, *what* will
the public (target audience) get out of this that they actually want?

The first step in a public health advocacy program is to answer the following.

- What do I want to say? (MESSAGE)
- To whom do I want to say it? (AUDIENCE)
- Through what means can I convey it most effectively? (CHANNEL)
- When will it have the most advantageous effect? (TIMING)
- What do I want to have happen as a result of my message? (IMPACT)
- How will I assess the effect of my message? (EVALUATION)
- How will I improve the message for its next presentation? (MODIFICA-TION)

The second is to set up a collegial relationship with representatives of the mass media. Such a relationship between public health and the media is essential in many public health settings. The media know that their audience is interested in health issues; the media want to provide information and messages about things of interest to their public; the media (at least in most countries) are supported by advertising or foundation funding and can conduct more expensive and extensive campaigns than most ministries of health or local health agencies. The key in this setting is to establish the common campaign goal that suits the interests of both the media (owners, investors, audiences) and public health.

EFFECTIVE MEDIA RELATIONS IN PUBLIC HEALTH MARKETING AND ADVOCACY PROGRAMS

When people speak of "the media," they generally mean the channels through which people convey information and attempt to communicate with individuals or groups of people. The office telephone, for example, is a simple communications medium or channel, and it is primarily designed to allow one person to make voice contact with one other person. It has little amplification capability over a face-to-face discussion between two people. Commercial television, on the other hand, is a medium or channel through which a person has the potential of reaching millions of other people—verbally and visually and in a current time frame. Television is an excellent example of a "mass communications" medium. Other mass media currently in widespread use include radio, print, and computer-based telecommunications. All of these media represent potential tools for public health communications, marketing, and advocacy strategies. The key is in finding out how to access, recruit, and use them.

Science and the Media

Public health officials—indeed, scientists in general—are often reluctant to deal with representatives of the mass media. There are many reasons for this. First, scientists as a group prefer controlled, measured settings and processes. The more people are involved in a process, the less predictable that process becomes. For more-or-less complete predictability, a scientist is safest in the controlled confines of the research laboratory.

Second, scientists spend a great deal of time and effort learning their science. With their understanding comes an entire system of jargon—terms, expressions, and descriptions that they and other scientists in their field understand readily. It is not necessarily easy to translate the language of science into everyday language. Most scientists prefer to "talk science" to other scientists because the effort they must expend in conveying their messages is considerably less than that required to make their information understandable to people outside their particular field of science.

Third, many scientists have had disappointments in their dealings with the media—because of misquotations, distortion, broken promises to publish or broadcast a message, and the like. At least some of these disappointments result from the media's need to convey information in a novel way, which enables them to make a financial profit in an extremely competitive business. Many such disappointments thus reflect the unfortunate consequences of the conflicting priorities of the scientist and the reporter.

While admitting the validity of these concerns, and the many others that may apply in the scientist's dealing with media representatives, the fact remains that we live in an era of mass communications, and a great many people receive their health messages through these media. People around the world view CNN. Electronic mail and other telecommunications devices connect even very remote areas with the mainstream of information with which the world's people are being bombarded.

Public Health Science and the Media

Perhaps more than scientists in general, public health scientists in particular must get their messages—their advocacy—about control and prevention of illness, disability, and death to the people who need to hear them. Typically, this means working with media representatives—producers, editors, and reporters.

At the receiving end of the information are the target audiences—those of public health and those of the media. A *target audience* is that sub-group of a population for which a particular message is believed to have the most relevance. A message may also be directed at secondary (less accessible, less well-defined, less important) or even tertiary target audiences, but it is of extreme importance to determine the primary target audience for every public health message and to ensure that the message is appropriately crafted, timed for greatest impact, and conveyed through the medium most likely to reach that audience.

An extremely important concept in managing the creation and dissemination of public health messages is the *single overriding communications objective*, or "SOCO," developed at CDC several years ago by staff in the Office of Health Communications. The SOCO is the essence of the message that needs to be conveyed. The SOCO needs to be simply and clearly stated—so that the media and the target audience reached through the media have no problem in understanding the meaning of the SOCO, as well as which attitudes or actions of the target audience represent the focus of the message.

Public health scientists should not only learn to be responsive to media representatives, but to *seek out* and cultivate positive relationships with the media. They should become proactive rather than remaining reactive, and they should learn to operate on a positive and straightforward basis in order to retain control of the agenda and the content and tone of the messages they want conveyed.

Just as many scientists are reluctant to deal with media representatives because of past negative experiences, media representatives also often justifiably complain that scientists are not receptive to the constraints and demands under which the mass media operate: extremely short turnaround times, changing priorities, and pressure to compete for media market share with radio or television stations or other media units.

Most members of the news media are ethical, conscientious, hard-working people who serve as representatives for the public in its ongoing quest for an improved quality of life. The mistakes they make—the misquotations, the incorrect interpretations—often result from the fact that, despite their best efforts, they do not really understand what the scientists are saying. Scientists often speak in technical, perhaps jargonistic language. They may also overwhelm media representatives with too much information or present information in vague, general terms and couched in risks and probabilities that do not make clearly convey the intended message (the SOCO).

All of these problems can be minimized if participants hold to the following principles.

- Truth and honesty, on the part of all participants in the process.
- Trust, developed among scientists and media representatives, that all are out to achieve the same objective: good information provided in a responsible manner to the targeted audience in an appropriate time frame. The motivations may differ (e.g., profit for the media and public health for the scientist), but that is not a problem if the mutual trust is established, earned, and maintained.
- Sensitivity to time; enough to allow the scientist to be comfortable with the quality of the information provided but not so much that the media's deadlines are missed. Compromises are required on all sides.

COMMUNICATIONS PROGRAMS BASED ON SURVEILLANCE INFORMATION

Effective use of existing health-related information, including that from surveillance systems, requires that communication occur among health-care professionals, health-related organizations, government agencies, the private sector, the media, and the individual citizen. Leaders in health, education, government, industry, labor, and the community must all be involved if a comprehensive and effective health communications strategy is to be implemented.

Health communications strategies can be designed to inform, influence, and motivate target audiences in setting policy or making other decisions that have a positive impact on public health.

Health communications CAN

- remind audiences of knowledge, attitudes, or behavior that have an impact on health
- create attitudes to support change for a particular policy or action
- increase awareness of a health problem, concern, or solution
- demonstrate skills or technology
- increase demand for health services and for health-affirming policies

Health communications CANNOT

- take the place of adequate or appropriate health services
- produce changes in attitudes and behavior unless other program elements support and sustain the changes
- be equally effective in addressing all health problems for all people

Therefore, health communications (marketing and advocacy components) should be included as only one key element in an integrated program designed to address a health problem or to convert health policy to action.

Public health communications has much in common with commercial communications—that is, to shopping, to buying (or spending), and to selling. What is being shopped for is health—by the individual and his or her public health program. What is being sold are ways to obtain that health. And the buying (or spending) involves public health providers (who "spend" their efforts and their resources to provide health) and all of the recipients of public health programs (the people who "buy" health—including government, the private sector, and the individual).

Crafting a Public Health Communications Plan

Effective health communications strategies must be based on a clear understanding of the needs and perceptions (attitudes) of the target audience(s). This means that considerations about the audience must be built into the communications strategy from the beginning, and it means that evaluation and revision, as needed, are critical components of the successful communications program. (See Appendix 16A for material on the creation and use of a health communications plan and Appendix 16B for guidelines and checklists for communications programs and strategies.)

Evaluating Public Health Marketing and Advocacy Programs and Projects

Integral to health communications marketing and advocacy programs is an assessment of its impact. Evaluation should be incorporated early into the overall communications plan and not left as an afterthought. Evaluation may continue for

Appendix 16A
The Health Communications Planning Process

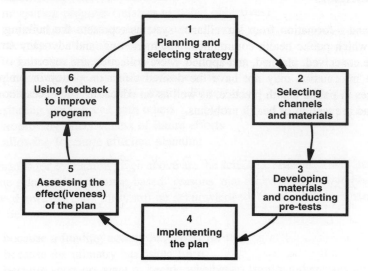

Figure 16–A The Health Communications Planning Process

Step 1. Planning and Selecting Strategy

1. What is the status of the health problem of concern? What is known about it (including scientific data and public perceptions)?
2. What additional (or new) information is needed before the program can be planned?
3. Who is (are) the targeted audience(s)? What is known about these people? How reliable is the information? How stable (likely to change) is the information?
4. What is the proposed change in (policy, treatment, legislation, service, or other activity that is proposed to solve or decrease the problem)?
5. What measurable objectives can be used to define and then to assess the level of success of the program?
6. How can progress be measured—i.e., what evaluation tools will be used?
7. What should the target audience be told?

Step 2. Selecting Channels and Materials

Note: If step 1 is not done carefully and accurately, step 2 becomes more difficult. This magnification of error, omission, or flawed logic continues and amplifies throughout the communication process. It is clearly to the advantage of program managers to plan and implement each step carefully and deliberately. In this setting, surprises are likely always to be unpleasant.

1. What existing materials can be adapted for use for the program?
2. What channels (e.g., mass media, worksite, face-to-face) are most appropriate for reaching the targeted audience(s) with this information?
3. What formats are most appropriate for the messages and the selected channels (e.g., booklets, videotapes, town meetings, telephone interviews)?

Step 3. Developing Materials and Conducting Pre-Tests

Steps 1 and 2 represent most of the planning. At step 3 program messages begin to craft the actual program.

1. What are the different ways in which the message can be presented (e.g., primarily visual, primarily language, encouragement, warnings)? Medium, level, tone, frequency of message, context of message (What other messages appear near this message?), and many other factors affect this subtype.
2. How does the target audience react to the message concept(s)?
3. Does the audience
   - understand the message?
   - remember the message? for how long?
   - accept the importance of the message?
   - agree to the proposed solution to the problem described in the message?
4. How does the audience respond to the format of the message?
5. Does feedback from the audience indicate that message or format needs to be modified?
6. How can the message be promoted, the materials be distributed, and progress of the strategy be tracked?

Step 4. Implementing the Plan and Preparing for Evaluation

1. Does the message move appropriately and effectively through the intended communications channels?
2. Does the target audience react as it is intended to (i.e., by paying attention, by being interested, by understanding the message, by being convinced of the importance of the message)?
3. Do any existing channels need to be replaced or new channels added?
4. What aspects of the program seem to be having the strongest effect?
5. Do changes need to be made to enhance the effect of the program?

Step 5. Assessing the Effect(iveness) of the Plan

1. Are the program's objectives being met?
2. Can the results that are being measured be attributed completely to the program, or are other factors playing a role? If the latter, take time to assess these contributing factors insofar as possible.
3. How effectively and efficiently has each step of the program of planning, implementation, and assessment been handled so far?

Step 6. Using Feedback To Improve the Program

Using all of the information gathered during steps 1 through 5, answer the following questions:

1. Why did the program work or not work as it was intended to?
2. What changes in the program are needed to improve the likelihood (or level) of success?
3. What lessons have been learned about the public health network, the target audience, the media, or the message that can be usefully applied to a revised version of this program or to another public health communications program?

Appendix 16B
Guidelines and Checklists for Public Health
Communications Programs and Strategies

Checklist for Public Health Practitioners To Use in Dealing with Media Representatives

1. Prepare fact sheets (statements about problem to be discussed) for reporters about all problems to be covered. Keep them updated.
2. Avoid jargon.
3. Respect reporters' deadlines.
4. Always be polite and straightforward.
5. Always tell the truth. If information is not available or unreliable, say so.
6. Always set the SOCO (or message you need to convey) according to your own agenda, and stick to it. Answer the reporter's questions insofar as possible, but return to your own agenda.
7. If you are not sure about a question (the meaning of the question, or you simply do not hear it), ask the reporter to repeat it.
8. If you do not know an answer, but it is within your area of responsibility, try to find it. If it is outside your area, do not try to answer it. Admit that you do not know.
9. Stick to facts; do not offer your own opinions.
10. Explain the context and relevance of your message (e.g., public health significance).
11. Make notes (or a tape) of the meeting (interview).
12. Provide feedback to the reporter and his or her editor on the results of your interaction.

A Proactive Approach to Media Relations for the Public Health Practitioner

1. Study the patterns and type of reporting in the area, and determine which media representatives appear to be most knowledgeable, most responsible, and most effective. Then contact them.
2. Write and state clearly and concisely the facts and the desired messages.
3. Explain the relative importance of the issues discussed and how they fit into the overall context of public health practice.
4. Maintain an image (and the integrity to back it up) of truthfulness, expertise, and candor.
5. Respond to media representatives when contacted.

Guidelines for News Releases

News releases are intended to take the place of a person-to-person interview. The subject must be of sufficient interest and very current.

1. Make sure the item is of sufficient interest and scope to make it worthwhile for media representatives to use it.
2. Distribute only to a list of media representatives pre-selected on the basis of a) their documented interest in public health issues, b) the appropriateness of their target audiences for your purposes, and c) their past responsiveness and responsibility.
3. Use the inverted pyramid style of writing: Most important items first, tapering down to detail.
4. Open the press release with a summary lead: a paragraph in which you answer Who? What? When? Where? Who cares? and How? Depending on the subject matter, there may not be a need to answer Why?
5. Make the news release no longer than two pages.
6. Use short, straightforward sentences. Define any necessary specialized terms, but generally avoid using jargon or specialized vocabulary.
7. Provide direct quotations, with the source and credentials of that source provided.
8. Consider providing audio or video segments to accompany the news release, if appropriate. If not feasible, supply appropriate still photographs and useful graphic material to illustrate or dramatize the message in the press release.

Guidelines for Fact Sheets

The public health fact sheet is a brief (no more than two pages) report that describes background and context for a particular health problem. For example, a fact sheet on hurricanes, intended for general audiences in the United States, would

- describe the mechanisms that cause hurricanes,
- tell when and where hurricanes usually occur,
- give some examples of detailed (unusual, particularly hazardous, etc.) problems associated with hurricanes, and
- provide recommendations for actions to be taken by target audiences if a hurricane occurs.

Fact sheets (sometimes called "back-grounders") are often used by journalists and other media representatives as reference material when they prepare their reports. They may be kept and used several times before they need to be replaced with more current information. They are also useful to the public health staff who prepare them, because fact sheets in reporters' files can obviate the need for public health staff to answer the same questions over and over again as different reporters (and members of target audiences) call with inquiries.

Guidelines for Dealing with a Health Crisis

A health crisis is an unplanned event that triggers a real, perceived, or possible threat to the well-being of the public (or some segment of it), the environment, or the affected health agency.

Many times, organizations do not handle crisis situations as effectively as they might. Two major problems related to such failures can be solved by foresight and planning.

1. *Failure to react quickly enough.* In a crisis, the first 24 hours are critical. If you do not provide the facts and the implications of those facts, the media and the public will speculate and form opinions on their own.
2. *Failure to name a primary person* (and one who is experienced in media matters) to be "the voice" for your organization. Multiple voices, even when delivering the same information, may be perceived as conveying different messages. If a reporter states that "Dr. Jones *said* everything was fine—but he *looked* worried and seemed to be in a big hurry," Dr. Jones may have done more harm than good by serving as agency spokesperson. Of course, in this case one might also accuse the reporter of being irresponsible for speculating on the mood behind the scientist's words.

To define the problem accurately, organizations must remember

- If there are delays in response on the part of the appropriate agency, the media and the public will define the problem for themselves—perhaps inaccurately.
- On the premise that bad news is *always* news, it is important to remember that a shift from "safety violation" to "a history of cover-ups" can occur easily and rapidly.
- It is important to anticipate or determine how (and when) the media will report the problem so your agency can react calmly or responsibly *or* make an appropriate announcement before the story appears in the popular media.

Enlisting the aid of the media

Since the media *will* be involved, regardless of whether you want them to be, acknowledge the role they can play in assisting you to deal with the problem.

Some of the ways to channel the media's interest and efforts include

- assisting in pre-crisis education
- conveying warnings
- conveying instructions or other information to target audiences
- reassuring the public
- defusing inaccurate rumors
- assisting in the response effort
- providing health officials with updated information on conditions beyond the health agency
- soliciting and obtaining help from the outside as needed

The most frequently asked questions by media and public include

- What happened?
- When and where?
- Who was involved?
- What caused the situation?
- How was this allowed to happen?
- What are you doing (going to do) about it?
- How much (what kind) of damage is there?
- What safety measures are being (will be) taken?
- Who (what) is to blame?
- Do you (your agency) accept responsibility?
- Has this ever happened before? With what result?
- What do you have to say to those who were injured (endangered, inconvenienced, etc.)?
- How does (will) this problem affect your operations?

Guidelines for the agency spokesperson:

- Do not give names of injured or dead until next-of-kin have been officially notified.
- Acknowledge responsibility, but avoid prematurely assigning blame. Assure the media that results of the investigation will be given to them.
- Avoid conjecture, speculation, and your own personal opinions.
- Always tell the truth. Admit it if you do not know the answer to a question.
- Prepare a brief written statement, and make it available to the media representatives (include background information and accompanying photos, audio and video tapes, as appropriate).
- Do not give exclusive interviews. Schedule a press conference for all media representatives, and give them all the same information at the same time. If a prepared statement will be read (and no questions will be answered until later), say so at the beginning.
- Be as accessible as possible to take follow-up inquiries from the media so that it does not appear that you are hiding from them.
- Stay calm.

Naming the Agency Spokesperson

Many people cannot be effective representatives of their agencies to the media. The primary spokesperson should have the following attributes:

- key position (administration or public affairs)
- experience in dealing with media
- responsible, calm, and confident manner
- ability to speak clearly (accent, quality of voice) and convincingly

Summary

- Silence kills. It is equated by the media and the public alike with guilt.
- Do not delay. The first 24 hours are critical.

- Permit controlled access to the site (or the agency premises) as soon as possible.
- Only speak the facts and messages that apply.
- If a question cannot be answered because the spokesperson does not know the answer or because the answer is confidential information, say so. Follow up on promises to get answers to questions.
- Monitor media reports. Correct any erroneous information and clarify points of confusion as needed.

Sample News Release with Simulated Information

Called *Dateline*	May 20, 1994 Centers for Disease Control and Prevention
Source *Organization*	Contact: Dr. S. A. Smith Investigative Epidemiologist National Center for Infectious Disease Telephone: (404) 933-2121
Summary *Lead*	Infectious disease investigators at CDC announced today that an outbreak of meningitis at the U. of Ga. Athens Campus is now under control.
Text	More than 100 students and staff at the University have had a laboratory-confirmed diagnosis of meningitis in the past week. Meningitis, a potentially serious infection, is caused by a bacterium. More than 50% of all known cases of this disease have led to complications, and 10% of patients have died.
Text	"This outbreak at (U of) Georgia is certainly serious," acknowledges investigative epidemiologist, Dr. S. A. Jones, "but we are now confident that it is under control." Ill students and staff have been hospitalized and placed in strict isolation for their protection and the protection of other patients and hospital staff. In addition, all known contacts of students and staff with meningitis have been given chemoprophylaxis against meningitis. This means that even if they do become infected and have the illness, they should have only mild cases. "Each year," says Dr. Jones, "we see outbreaks of meningitis on college campuses. Groups settings and the age of the university population make the risk of this infection higher for these people than it is for the population in general." CDC does not recommend that all school- and college-age young people be vaccinated at this time.
Attachments	Attachments—[List]
Close	30

RECOMMENDED READING

Ambron A, Hooper K (eds.). Interactive multimedia. Redmond, Wash.: Microsoft Press, 1988.

Bourque LB, Russell LA, Goltz JD. Human behavior during and immediately after the Loma Prieta earthquake. In: Bolton P (ed.). The Loma Prieta, California, earthquake of October 17, 1989: Public response. USGS Professional paper 1553-B. Washington, D.C.: U.S. Government Printing Office, 1993:B3–B322.

Burkett W. News reporting: science, medicine, and high technology. Ames: University of Iowa Press, 1986.

Churchill RE. MOD:Comm—a communications module. Atlanta: Centers for Disease Control and Prevention, 1995.

Committee on Disasters and the Mass Media. Disasters and the media. Proceedings of the Committee on Disasters and the Mass Media Workshop, February 1979. Washington, D.C.: National Academy of Sciences, 1980.

Imperato PJ. Dealing with the press and the media. In: The administration of a public health agency: a case study of the New York City Department of Health. New York: Human Sciences Press, 1983.

Kotler P, Roberto EL. Social marketing. New York: Free Press, 1989.

Lipson GL, Kroloff GK. Understanding the news media and public relations in Washington (a reference manual). Washington, DC: Washington Monitor, 1977.

Wurman RS. Information anxiety. New York: Bantam Books, 1990.

Index